Cultural Psychology and Psychoanalysis: Pathways to Synthesis

A volume in:
Advances in Cultural Psychology
Jaan Valsiner, *Series Editor*

Advances in Cultural Psychology

Jaan Valsiner, Editor

Becoming Other: From Social Interaction to Self-Reflection (2006)
edited by Alex Gillespie

Transitions: Symbolic Resources in Development (2006)
edited by Tania Zittoun

Discovering Cultural Psychology: A Profile and Selected Readings of Ernest E. Boesch (2007)
edited by Walter J. Lonner and Susanna A. Hayes

Otherness in Question: Development of the Self (2007)
edited by Livia Mathias Simão and Jaan Valsiner

Semiotic Rotations: Modes of Meanings in Cultural Worlds (2007)
edited by SunHee Kim Gertz, Jaan Valsiner, and Jean-Paul Breaux

Trust and Distrust: Sociocultural perspectives (2007)
edited by Ivana Markova and Alex Gillespie

Innovating Genesis: Microgenesis and the Constructive Mind in Action (2008)
edited by Emily Abbey and Rainer Diriwächter

Challenges and Strategies for Studying Human Development in Cultural Contexts (2009)
edited by Cynthia Lightfoot, Maria Lyra, and Jaan Valsiner

Rethinking Language, Mind, and World Dialogically (2009)
edited by Per Linell

cultural-psychodynamic theorisation of mental processes, the theory and the analysis of psychological intervention in clinical, scholastic, organisational and social fields, psychotherapy research and the methodology of empirical analysis of sociosymbolic dynamics. Associate Editor of *Integrative Psychological and Behavioral Science,Rivista Psicologia Clinica/Journal of Clinic Psychology and Psicologia Scolastica*. Address: Department of Educational, Psychological and Teaching Science, Via Stampacchia, 45, 73100 Lecce. Email: sergio.salvatore@unisalento.it.

Pietro Stampa. Clinical psychologist and psychotherapist in private practice, Rome. Professor of Psychology of educational organisations and institutions, University of Chieti; Professor of Ethics and psychological issues, SPS School of psychoanalitic psychotherapy, Rome. Co-editor of *Rivista di Psicologia Clinica/Journal of Clinical* Psychology (On Line Journal). Email: p.stampa@freudian.com.

Jaan Valsiner. Cultural psychologist with a consistently developmental axiomatic base that is brought to analyses of any psychological or social phenomena. He is the founding editor (1995) of the Sage journal, *Culture & Psychology*. He is currently professor of psychology at the Department of Psychology, Clark University, USA, He has published many books, among which *The guided mind* (Cambridge, MA: Harvard University Press, 1998) and *Culture in minds and societies* (New Delhi: Sage, 2007). He has edited (with Kevin Connolly) the *Handbook of Developmental Psychology* (London: Sage, 2003) as well as the *Cambridge Handbook of Socio-Cultural Psychology* (2007, with Alberto Rosa). He is the Editor-in-Chief of *Integrative Psychological and Behavioural Sciences* (Springer, from 2007) and *History and Theory of Psychology* (from 2008, with Transaction Publishers). In 1995, he was awarded the *Alexander von Humboldt Prize* in Germany for his interdisciplinary work on human development, and Senior Fulbright Lecturing Award in Brazil 1995–1997. He has been a visiting professor in Brazil, Japan, Australia, Estonia. Germany, Italy, United Kingdom, and the Netherlands. Email: jvalsiner@clarku.edu.

René van der Veer. Professor of the history of education at Leiden University in the Netherlands. He has written a dozen books and hundreds of papers on the history, theory and methodology of child psychology. Several of these books address the history of Russian and Soviet psychology and, more specifically, Vygotsky's thinking. More recently, he also published on the history of attachment theory and on the advice presented in baby care manuals. Email: veer@fsw.leidenuniv.nl.

Tania Zittoun. Professor of education at the University of Neuchâtel, Switzerland. She is a developmental psychologist with a focus on the role of cultural mediation in the life course. Her interest for semiotic processes has brought her to explore people's uses of novels, music and films as symbolic resources. At a theoretical level, it has brought her articulate sociocultural and psychoanalytical models. This has led her to explore various empirical issues—people naming their children, youth transitions, personal relationship to philosophy and religion, etc. She is Associate Editor of the Sage journal *Culture & Psychology*, and the author of *Donner la vie, choisir un nom* (L'Harmattan, 2005), *Insertions* (Peter Lang, 2006), *Transitions* (InfoAge, 2006). Email: tania.zittoun@unine.ch.

CULTURAL PSYCHOLOGY AND PSYCHOANALYSIS: PATHWAYS TO SYNTHESIS

edited by

Sergio Salvatore
University of Salento

and

Tania Zittoun
University of Neuchâtel, Switzerland

IAP

Information Age Publishing, Inc.
Charlotte, North Carolina • www.infoagepub.com

Library of Congress Cataloging-in-Publication Data

Cultural psychology and psychoanalysis : pathways to synthesis / editors,
Sergio Salvatore and Tania Zittoun.
p. cm.
Includes bibliographical references.
ISBN 978-1-61735-514-1 (pbk.) -- ISBN 978-1-61735-515-8 (hbk.) --
ISBN 978-1-61735-516-5 (e-book)
1. Psychoanalysis--Social aspects. 2. Psychoanalysis and culture.
3. Social psychology. 4. Social psychiatry. 5. Cultural psychiatry.
6. Psychotherapy--Social aspects. I. Salvatore, Sergio. II. Zittoun, Tania.
BF175.C86 2011
150.19'5--dc23 2011028003

Printed and bound by CPI Group (UK) Ltd, Croydon, CR0 4YY

CONTENTS

PREFACE BY SERIES EDITOR

Uneasiness of Culture: The Discontent with Quantifying Civilization in Cultural Psychology

Jaan Valsiner

Cultural psychology has much to discover in the vast desert of psychoanalysis where the sandstorms of the unconscious are interspersed with the oases of deep insights into the human *psyche*. Yet, psychology—as a self-proclaimed science—has been ill at ease in its relations with psychoanalysis. Psychology over the last century has shown great ambivalence in its relation to psychoanalysis—borrowing unashamedly from it, while denigrating it so as it cannot enter psychological science as an equal partner. Cultural psychology—in its quest for new solutions—is courageous enough to recognize the relevance of psychodynamic perspectives for understanding how cultural phenomena organize our psychological functions. There are numerous examples of how psychoanalytic perspectives have played a major role in cultural psychology (Kakar, 1989, Obeyesekere, 1990, Roland, 1988). In this volume, we can observe how our scientific thinking can be based on psychoanalysis without being reduced to it—or to any other orthodoxy that plagues contemporary psychology.

Among the latter, it is the pervasive imperative—introduced by "the empire of chance" (see Gigerenzer et al., 1989, also Lamiell, 2009—to obligatory quantification of qualitative and unique phenomena. What the reader can find in this volume is the consistent line of proving the inadequacy of making "*the statistical* method" into "*the scientific* method" in psychology (in this volume—see Chapter 9 by Massimo Grasso and Pietro Stampa). This continues the line of argumentation that was most prominent in our somewhat rhetorical question—*have the last 60 years of psychology gone astray* (Toomela and Valsiner, 2010)? Unfortunately, the answer to this question continues to be affirmative. However, as we look at the work published in the present volume, we can observe new efforts to break down the existing civil order of seemingly "scientific" psychology.

Civilization often leads to rigid thinking. It has become a social habit—of that part of psychology that attempts to become "scientific" by wearing the "civil" uniforms of statistical inference—to dismiss all other directions of knowledge making. The result is a powerful—yet sterile—machinery of producing ever-increasing numbers of quantified data that have lost touch with the phenomena from which they were derived. Yet, the rewards for *appearing* "scientific" are well set in the social practices of the discipline. Such civilization of keeping up apperances raises serious sentiments of discontent in new emerging fields—such as cultural psycholology—since it is attempting to make sense of the intricate qualitative phenomena that cultural processes abundantly produce (Valsiner, 2011). From that perspective, the attempts to "measure" quantitatively the phenomena that break down in their qualities when arbitrary numbers are attached to them is similar to letting an elephant loose in a porcelain cabinet.

The present unification of psychodynamic and cultural perspectives in psychology take an alternative path. The psychodynamic perspectives in this volume reflect the focus on uniqueness amplification of all developmental processes that was explicated within the tradition of "second cybernetics" half a century ago (Maruyama, 1963). The basic idea of generating uniqueness as the universal principle of psychological, social, and biological systems has been conveniently overlooked in what has become established as "science of psychology" over the twentieth century. As Maruyama has clearly explained—psychology's axioms need a radical change:

> The uncritical use of the assumption of normal distribution—the bell-shaped curve—dominated psychology and social sciences. But, in this assumption, something important was overlooked. Researchers tended to forget or never learned how the bell-shaped curve had been mathematically derived and defined. The normal distribution occurs when both the following conditions are satisfied: (1) The fluctuations are *random*; (2) they are *independent* of one another. But psychological and social events are neither random nor independent. Therefore, it is *illogical* to assume a normal distribution. (Maruyama, 1999, p. 53)

The axiomatic notion that all phenomena strive towards being distributed around the mean value is also challenged in contemporary physical chemistry of Ilya Prigogine (1973). A return to the psychodynamic perspectives in this volume is a step in the direction of re-vamping psychology's underlying assumptions. Cultural psychology here leads the way.

And changes are already on their way. Restoration of the focus on uniqueness as a systematic pattern is in the making in the 21st century (Lamiell, 2009, Molenaar, 2004). It takes the form of creating a seeming contradiction in terms by formulating the notion of idiographic science (Salvatore, Valsiner, Strout-Yagodzinsky, & Clegg, 2009). Our new series within the Information Age books program—*Yearbook of Idiographic Science* (Salvatore, Gennaro, & Valsiner, 2011) is an indicator of how such efforts to break through antiquated methodological traditions in psychology are gaining momentum. Looking into individual cases in depth—and with the focus on generalization—brings psychology back to the realm of real sciences where the single object is sufficient for generalization. There is no reason to find more than one Mars in order to send a Mars Lander to that planet for purposes of basic science.

The present volume also continues the coverage of qualitative breakthroughs in the human psyche (Zittoun, 2006) and the exploration of otherness (Simão and Valsiner, 2007) in our book series. It constitutes a step forward into the realm of the dynamic and deep processes of the human experiences in their living realities. The uneasiness of culture is turning out to be fruitful in this new look at psychoanalysis.

Worcester, November, 2010
Jaan Valsiner

REFERENCES

Gigerenzer, G., Swijtink, Z., Porter, T., Daston, L., Beatty, J. & Krüger, L. (1989). *The empire of chance*. Cambridge: Cambridge University Press.

Kakar, S. (1989). *Intimate relations: Exploring Indian sexuality.* New Delhi: Penguin.

Lamiell, J. T. (2009). Reviving person-centered inquiry in psychology: why its erstwhile dormancy? In J. Valsiner, P. Molenaar, M. Lyra & N. Chaudhary (Eds.), *Dynamic process methodology in the social and developmental sciences* (pp. 31–43). New York: Springer.

Maruyama, M. (1963). The second cybernetics: Deviation amplifying mutual causal processes. *American Scientist, 51*, 164–179.

Maruyama, M. (1999). Heterogram analysis: Where the assumption of normal distribution is illogical. *Human Systems Management, 18*, 53–60.

Molenaar, P. C. M. (2004). A manifesto on psychology as idiographic science: Bringing the person back into scientific psychology, this time forever, *Measurement: Interdisciplinary research and perspectives*, 2, 201–218.

Obeyesekere, G. (1990). *The work of culture*. Chicago: University of Chicago Press.
Prigogine, I. (1973). Irreversibility as a symmetry-breaking process. *Nature, 246*, 67–71.
Roland, A. (1988). *In search of self in India and Japan*. Princeton: Princeton University Press.
Salvatore, S., Valsiner, J., Strout-Yagodzinsky, S., & Clegg, J. (Eds.) (2009). *YIS: Yearbook of Idiographic Science—2008*. (Vol. 1). Rome: Fireira Publishing.
Salvatore, S., Gennaro, A, & Valsiner, J. (Eds.) (2011). *YIS: Yearbook of Idiographic Science*. (Vol. 4). Charlotte, NC: Information Age Publishers.
Simão, L. M., & Valsiner, J. (2007). *Otherness in question: Labyrinths of the self*. Greenwich, CT: InfoAge Publishing.
Toomela, A., & Valsiner, J. (Eds.). (2010). *Methodological thinking in psychology: 60 years gone astray?* Charlotte, NC: Information Age Publishing.
Valsiner, J. (Ed.) (2011). *Oxford handbook of psychology and culture*. New York: Oxford University Press.
Zittoun, T. (2006). *Transitions*. Greenwich, CT: InfoAge Publishing.

EDITORS' INTRODUCTION

Cultural Psychology and Psychoanalysis: Pathways to Synthesis

Tania Zittoun and Sergio Salvatore

The hard work of living evolves as the world changes. In all times, groups of specialists—priests, philosophers, medicine men, and more recently, social scientists and psychologists—have tried to describe, understand, and perhaps help to solve the intricacies of people's lives. Yet, theories are often too slow to adjust to realities, and researchers are often impatient with existing models—looking for new ones, they often forget what older models might bring.

Our venture clearly belongs to the currently developing field of sociocultural psychology: a psychology that tries to understand the mutual constitution of human beings and their cultural worlds, with a strong focus on how people actively make sense of these. Part of the development of that field, over the past ten years, has been made possible thanks to a careful examination of previous authors, too-soon forgotten for historical and political reasons, or because fashion led researchers elsewhere (inter alia, Diriwächter & Valsiner, 2008; Valsiner, 2005; Valsiner & Van der Veer, 2000). However, there is a field of psychology that has still not been considered crucial in relation to the core project of cultural psychology—that of psychoanalysis.

In our understanding, one of the central challenges of cultural psychology is that of describing the complexity of the way humans make sense of human experience. Humans, as we are permanently reminded by the world's present state, are far from being only rational thinkers. They decide to invest or to borrow money because they desire better lives, and they sell their houses because they are scared of losing them; they vote against the construction of minarets, when they are in fact afraid of a being invaded by massive herds of wild people; they construct walls to circumscribe a problem they cannot solve. In our daily lives, we willingly miss unpleasant dental appointments, we are aggressive with a waiter when we have been annoyed by our boss, we pretend that the pain we have in our teeth does not exist, or we might have a terrible morning just because we had a bad dream. We all have our little madnesses—yet we are not crazy. Hence, as humans, a great part of our sense-making seems to escape from our total free will. This has finally been acknowledged by psychologists; however, over the past twenty years, they have been more ready to admit that human behavior was guided by genes, synaptic connections and social class, than by emotions. Even sociocultural psychologists until recently repeatedly overlooked the few texts inviting them to pay attention to affective processes (see for instance the "rediscoveries" of Vygotksy's work on emotions, Vygotsky, 1925/1999). We believe that a psychology that wants to address sense-making has to account for this nonrational part of human thinking and activity—and to do this, we need to look closely at affective processes.

In this book, we directly address the role of affective processes in sense-making. In order to do so, we propose to explore psychoanalysis—a field of enquiry that has generally been kept at a careful distance by sociocultural psychologists. Psychoanalysis, the analysis of unconscious psychological processes, was born as a self-standing domain thanks to the systematic work of Sigmund Freud (1856–1939). Freud defined psychoanalysis as (a) a method of investigation of the psyche; (b) a theory of the psyche, and (c) a therapeutic technique (Freud, 1915–1917/1963). Freud's work has been developed along various lines, in France and in Latin countries, in the United Kingdom and in the United States. These developments have given rise to brilliant theoretical advances, enriched through fertile interdisciplinary work with neighbouring scientific fields. However, the Freudian heritage has also led to sect-like phenomena, clan-like wars and fratricide conflicts; it has led to theoretical absurdities, and clinical issues that were debated with great furor in public. Like any difficult science touching upon unpleasant sides of humans, psychoanalysis has been spread in society, giving rise to numerous social representations (Moscovici, 1961/2008). Today, psychoanalysis is presented in many films and TV series as something admired and desired, mocked and feared. In sociocultural psychology as well, although it has been inspirational for some authors (see Boesch, 1991; Valsiner, 2005), it is still looked upon with some defiance—for instance because of the ethnocentric bias it might have (Rey, 2004).

However, we consider here psychoanalysis from a different standpoint: we believe that some psychoanalytical traditions share with cultural psychology a core epistemological stance: the idea of the centrality of sense-making in human activity, which demands attention to semiotic processes—the processes by which signs (or symbols) are both constructing and constituted by cultural phenomena and psychological processes.

This book thus sets out to explore how psychoanalysis can enrich and complement sociocultural psychology. It presents theoretical integrations of psychoanalytical notions in the sociocultural framework, explores the historical similarities, if not intricacies, of the two fields, and presents papers that have tried to apply an enriched theoretical framework in developmental and clinical empirical work. It is organized in three sections that can be roughly described as follows.

The first section presents our theoretical proposition for an integration of one particular stream of psychoanalysis within sociocultural psychology, which emphasizes both the dialogical and the semiotic nature of psychological dynamics. Opening the book, it has both the function of presenting current debates and issues within psychoanalysis to a readership which might not be fully familiar with it, and to present an original theorization of the role of the affective context in sense-making (Chapter 1).

The second section pursues this theoretical dialogue through a historical perspective. It might be known that Vygotsky, considered one of the fathers of contemporary cultural psychology, had some knowledge of psychoanalysis. His work on the psychology of art is informed by an understanding of the unconscious (Vygtosky, 1925/1971), and his famous paper on adolescent creativity closely follows one of Freud's papers on creativity (Vygotsky, 1931/1994). But how far does this Freudian inspiration go, and how much is it worth to pursue a dialogue that was just sketched out? This section starts with an exploration of the place of psychoanalysis in the actual genesis of the ideas that would become sociocultural psychology. René Van der Veer thus brings us back to the diffusion of psychoanalysis in Russia, and the intellectual context in which Vygotsky and Voloshinov developed their ideas (Chapter 2). Taking a reverse stance, Tania Zittoun shows how the germ of some of the key issues addressed by Vygotsky and still pursued by cultural psychologists today—the mediation of cultural tools in human activity, semiotic processes, the role of play, and the so-called "higher mental functions" —were actually present in Freud's work on dreams and on culture (Chapter 3). This grounding invites us to find further ways in which psychoanalysis might actually complement cultural psychologists' quest. In their chapter, Kenneth Cabell and Jaan Valsiner thus propose to reopen Freud's famous *Anna O.* case, and his reflection on the *Unheimlich,* to develop a reflection on the process of affective hypergeneralization (Chapter 4).

The third section pursues the implications of this parallel reasoning. It invites researchers who propose further syntheses between some strands of psychoanalysis and approaches within social and cultural psychology. The contributions collected in this section show how sociocultural psychology and psychoanalysis can complement each other, when it comes to tracing the emergence of meaning in actual interactive settings. Renzo Carli and Fiammetta Giovagnoli derive a reframing of clinical psychology from their joint psychoanalytic and cultural approach. They propose to consider the centrality of the notion of *analysis of the demand*, and on this basis, a new way of considering methods and objectives of the psychological intervention with individuals as well as groups and social structures (Chapter 5). By examining research interviews, Tania Zittoun shows how an understanding of unconscious dynamics enables the researcher to make hypothesis about dynamics of semiotic elaboration that usually escape explicitation (Chapter 6). Nicolas Favez takes a developmental stance to show how children develop narrative capacities in interactions, and how these are modulated by the modalities of the mother's emotional response (Chapter 7). Also interested in narratives, Maria Francesca Freda suggests seeing them as offering a transitional zone for the linking of conscious and unconscious dynamics; she thus proposes to reconsider the role of narrative in the clinical setting (Chapter 8). Finally, Massimo Grasso and Pietro Stampa's provocative exploration shows the dramatic consequences deriving when physicians ignore the person's perspective or when psychologists fail to consider the symbolic context of the person's experience (Chapter 9). This last paper can thus be read as a *reductio ad absurdum* showing the necessities of taking in account both the subjective, emotional experience of individuals and their material and social context when we want to understand the meaning people confer to their experience.

Hence, showing historical common roots, epistemological similarities, and theoretical complementarities, this book hopes to open the route for further investigations. We hope that this book suggests how the encounter and reciprocal contamination between cultural psychology and psychoanalysis could provide innovative theoretical and methodological syntheses. Through the various contributions three directions of development emerge as particularly promising for psychological science.

Firstly, the semiotic conceptualization of affects, emerging from several of the contributors, appears to be a significant step ahead in the understanding of the dynamics of sense-making. It enables the role played by affective semiosis within the more general processes of communication and thinking to be recognized, thus empowering the capability of cultural psychology to grasp the weft of feeling, memories, wishes and plans sustaining the semiotic constitution of (inter)subjectivity. Moreover, taking the affective dimension into account provides the way to address conceptual issues that are central to cultural psychology: the microdynamics (micro-genetic) of sense-making—that is, how the combination of signs enables meaning to emerge—and the circularity between persons and intersubjective context, as well as between the micro and macrosocial level of meaning-making.

A second promising direction of development concerns methodology. The reader will find several invitations to rethink the way of analyzing the phenomena of sense-making. The recognition of an affective (unconscious) dimension of sense-making does not only mean inserting a new object in the agenda of the analysis. Above all, it entails an innovative hermeneutical approach, consistent with the contextuality, dynamicity and fuzziness of its object.

Finally, the volume highlights how the connection between theory and practice in psychology is not a mere matter of application. Rather, the psychological intervention could be—needs to be—a theoretical object for cultural psychology, as it already is for psychoanalysis. At the same time, the intervention could be a fertile domain where a psychological practice endowed with reflexive capability generates new theoretical constructions.

August, 2010
Neuchâtel & Lecce

REFERENCES

Boesch, E. E. (1991). *Symbolic action theory and cultural psychology*. Berlin: Springer Verlag.

Diriwächter, R., & Valsiner, J. (Eds.). (2008). *Striving for the whole: Creating theoretical syntheses*. Somerset, NJ: Transaction Publishers.

Freud, S. (1963). Introductory lectures on psycho-analysis. In J. Strachey (Ed. and Trans.), *The standard edition of the complete psychological works of Sigmund Freud* (Vols. 15–16). London: The Hogarth Press and the Institute of Psycho-analysis. (Original work published 1915–1917)

Moscovici, S. (2008). *Psychoanalysis: Its image and its public* (G. Duveen, Trans.). Cambridge: Polity Press. (Original work published 1961)

Rey, F. L. G. (2004). Subjectivity in communication. Development in personality. In A. U. Branco & J. Valsiner (Eds.), *Communication and metacommunication and human development* (pp. 249–270). Charlotte, NC: Information Age Publishing.

Valsiner, J. (2005). *Heinz Werner and developmental science*. New York: Kluwer/Plenum.

Valsiner, J., & Van der Veer, R. (2000). *The social mind: Construction of the idea*. New York: Cambridge University Press.

Vygotsky, L. S. (1971). *The psychology of art* (Scripta Technica Inc., Trans.). Cambridge, MA & London: MIT press. (Original work published 1925)

Vygotsky, L. S. (1994). Imagination and creativity of the adolescent. In R. Van der Veer & J. Valsiner (Eds. and Trans.), *The Vygotsky reader* (pp. 266–288). Oxford: Blackwell. (Original work published 1931)

Vygotsky, L. S. (1999). Consciousness as a problem in the psychology of behavior. In N. Veresov (Trans.), *Undiscovered Vygotsky: Etudes on the pre-history of cultural-historical psychology* (European studies in the history of science and ideas. Vol. 8, pp. 251–281). Peter Lang Publishing. Retrieved from http://www.marxists.org/archive/vygotsky/works/1925/consciousness.htm. (Original work published 1925)

PART I

FOUNDATIONS

CHAPTER 1

OUTLINES OF A PSYCHOANALYTICALLY INFORMED CULTURAL PSYCHOLOGY

Sergio Salvatore and Tania Zittoun

Sense-making—the process by which people turn their experience into a meaningful experience, which has a value, a relationship with other events, and about which they can think or communicate—sense-making is a core psychological phenomenon, and therefore, represents an essential challenge for psychological enquiry.

In this chapter, we present the outlines of a general model of *sense-making*. One core component of sense-making, we argue, is the affective nature of our experience. However, cultural psychology has only had a limited interest in affects (with the notable exception of Valsiner, 2007). In this chapter, we intend to consider psychoanalysis as an alternative theory of sense-making, which addresses the specific issue of affects. We consequently argue that such psychoanalytical insights can usefully complement cultural psychology and thus enable the fundamental role of affects in sense-making to be accounted for.

Cultural Psychology and Psychoanalysis: Pathways to Synthesis, pp. 3–46

This chapter is divided into four parts. Firstly, we clarify our general assumptions on sense-making, and in particular, briefly introduce the semiotic and dialogical approach to cultural psychology that we adopt as a theoretical frame. Secondly, we address the notion of *affects* as it has been elaborated within the psychoanalytic domain. After briefly reviewing the various definitions of this concept, we discuss in greater detail the definition provided by intersubjective psychoanalysis, which models affects in a processual and semiotic way—as *affective semiosis*. We ground our reflection in this model because it is "naturally" consistent and integrable within the framework of a semiotic and dialogical cultural psychology. As we will show, the semiotic interpretation of psychoanalysis considers the notion of affects as the basic concept in any attempt to model psychological processes. In so doing, it offers a powerful bridge to link cultural psychology and psychoanalysis. Thirdly, we discuss the phenomenology and dynamics of affective semiosis in the model we define. For this purpose, we refer to Matte Blanco's formal model of unconscious processes that provides conceptual devices to rethink the mind in a comprehensive way, integrating notions such as affects, emotion, and thinking. Fourthly, we make our fundamental claim concerning the role of affective semiosis in human experience—that is, that affective semiosis plays a constructive orienting function in sense-making.

THE SEMIOTIC VIEW IN CULTURAL PSYCHOLOGY

Cultural psychology can be broadly defined as an approach within psychology that examines the activities and processes of meaning making by which humans and their social and cultural environment mutually constitute each other. It is a fluid theoretical field encompassing many perspectives, with their variety of epistemological, theoretical, and methodological choices (Valsiner & Rosa, 2007). In particular, not all of them place the same importance on the processes of sense-making. Without aiming at mapping the whole field (for this the reader can refer to, *inter alia*, Heine, 2008; Ratner 1994; Valsiner & Rosa, 2007), our intention is here to make our dialogical and semiotic perspective explicit.

Semiotic Dynamics

We see the psyche as an ongoing process of shaping human experience through the mediation of semiotic devices (Zittoun, 2006). We consider these devices semiotic because whatever their source and support might be—words, images, ideas, objects, actions—they work as signs, that is, as something standing for something else, or as signifiers for some signified. Semiotic devices enable human beings to go beyond the immediacy of the experience—to live immersed in the here and now and at the same time to treat it as something else that transcends the present moment and has form, consistence, and persistence (Rosa, 2007). These semiotic devices can also be seen as traces of other people's experiences in time and space, and in that sense, are largely what culture is made of.

The meditational role of the signs consists, first of all, in orienting the person's interpretation of reality. But also, more deeply, signs shape the objects or states of experience sustaining a person's encounter with the world. This implies that sense-making is not just one of the various operations the mind performs; rather, it *is* the psychological life, the way the mind works. To use a Freudian expression: it is *the actual psychic reality*.[1]

Signs are not fixed entities with a stable content (Salvatore, Forges Davanzati, Potì & Ruggeri, 2009), their meaning is not something already given, stored in a imagined Platonic world and from there applied to human affairs. Signs are inherently polysemic—they are potentialities of signification (Linell, 2009) that are actualized according to contextual boundaries created by their use. Hence, their meaning depends on the way in which they are used (Wittgenstein, 1953/1958). Consequently, sense-making is a dynamic process.

Dialogicality

Signs have no autonomous life. They are mobilized by people as they are engaged in activities that imply inter-subjective engagement. Sense-making is thus also intrinsically intertwined with action (Harrè & Gillet, 1994) and semiotic devices. Hence, sense-making is intrinsically dialogical. The idea of dialogicality can be understood in two complementary ways. First, it implies that any utterance or use of a sign is taking place in a flow of sign exchanges and other utterances. Integrating the propositions made by Bakhtin (1975/1981), current authors consider any use of a semiotic device as an answer to an earlier utterance, or as anticipation to a future one, this utterance being made by a present interlocutor, or by an imagined or imaginary other. In addition, any utterance is charged with the "echoes" of previous uses, effects of contexts, etc. (Bakhtin, 1986). In that sense, thinking is itself always and already a dialogical activity, inherently social (Linell, 2009; Marková, 2005). Second, the idea of dialogicality invites us to consider seriously the actual, socially situated conditions of the production of signs and discourse (Marková, Linell, Grossen & Salazar Orvig, 2007). From that perspective, utterances appear to be shaped by the intersubjective circumstances motivating their activation. To use Wittgenstein's terminology, the sign's psychological value is its function of regulating the forms of life carried on by linguistic games. And it is evident that this regulative function is not inherent to the sign, but depends on the virtually infinite circumstances of the social exchange serving as setting of the speech acts (Nightingale & Cromby, 1999).[2] Of course, broader contextual dimensions (cultural models, ideologies, or structures of power; Ratner, 2008) are just as constitutive of the dialogical nature of thinking and communicating, as the here and now circumstances of these activities. However, these dimensions have to be activated within the contingence of the life of people influenced by them—and it is at this level that we examine them here.

The dialogically based social-cognitive approach of Rommetveit (1992) is a representative example of an analysis of sense-making focusing on the intersubjective level, but by no means minimizing the role played by the socially shared ecological structure of meaning. According to this author, the world as a "*not-yet-verbally described* state of affairs" (1992, p. 22, italics in the original) is subjected to socially shared categorization, generating objects of experience. This process of socially shared categorization is carried out by means of intersubjective communication. Each actor carries with him/herself his/her own perspective reflecting specific interests and commitments and leading him/her to see some aspects of the world and not others, in one out of many possible ways. Within such constraints, actors engage in a dialogical process of reciprocal syntonization: an "attunement to the attunement of the other" consisting of the creation of a joint focus of attention upon selected objects of experience. Such reciprocal adjustment of perspectives is oriented by the cultural structure of meaning ("drafts of contracts for categorization" according to Rommetveit's terminology[3]). Once and insofar as actors achieve their reciprocal syntonization, the resulting shared representation is instituted as a taken-for-granted reality and as such acquires a regulative function, allowing the actors to reduce the polysemy in which the meaning of every sign consists.

It is worth referring to the sketch Rommetveit (1992) offers as an example. He imagines a Saturday morning in Mr and Mrs Smith's house. Mr Smith is pushing a lawn-mower around their lawn. Mrs Smith is sitting in the kitchen; she is sad and angry because she feels that her husband is avoiding being with her. The telephone rings and Mrs Smith answers. It is Betty, a friend of hers, who starts the conversation by asking: " *Is that lazy husband of yours still in bed?*". Mrs Smith answers: "*No, he is working this morning, he is mowing the lawn*". After a short while, the telephone rings for a second time. It is Mr Jones. As Mrs Smith assumes he is calling as usual to ask Mr Smith to go fishing with him, when he starts: "*Is your husband working this morning?*", she answers: "*No, he is not working this morning, he is mowing the lawn*". As we can see, Mrs Smith produces two opposing utterances ("he is working" vs. "he is not working"), to depict the same state of experience.

Yet, it is not hard for us to recognize that she is telling the truth in both cases. This is because Mr Smith's action of pushing a lawn-mower in the garden can be brought into language and made meaningful by means of a variety of fashions of categorization. Mr Smith can be seen as engaged in mowing the lawn, in enjoying a leisure-time activity, in avoiding the company of his wife, as well as in disturbing the neighbours with the noise of the machine.... Each of these ways of categorizing mirrors a cultural model of activity and offers a way of shaping the field of experience, by means of which a legitimate version of the reality is created. Mrs Smith selects one way among all the possible ones, in order to try to syntonize her perspective with the perspective of the other person. She does so according to her representation of the other's dialogical intentions, then according to the sense that she attributes to the other's speech act. Thus, as for instance we can infer, she interprets the question asked by her friend Betty as a kindly way of asking about her state (e.g., something like "why are you alone, where is your husband?"); therefore, she answers by selecting a fashion of categorization that enables her to be attuned to what she feels is Betty's perspective and at the same time to perform her own communicational act (i.e., "he is working, putting constraints on his time and in doing so he is avoiding spending the weekend with me"). In the second call, Mrs Smith selects a perspective that highlights a different possible meaning of Mr Smith's action: the area of sense concerning |leisure activity|, as opposed to |constrained activity|—signifying it by means of the expression "not working." Also in this case, this selection is carried out as the way and at the same time the result of Mrs Smith's attempt to attune her perspective to Mr Jones's act, as she understands it according to the representation of his communicational intention (she takes it for granted that he usually calls in order to arrange to go fishing with Mr Smith). To conclude on this example, three points are worth underlining. Firstly, the meaning is not "held" within the sign (in this case: the word "work"). Rather, the sign is a potentiality of meaning, a bundle of possible signifiers yet to be stabilized (Visetti & Cadiot, 2002). Secondly, it is the interplay between the participants of the communication that transforms the potentiality into an actualized meaning. In this interplay, each participant responds to the communicative initiative of the other and, at the same time, she/he contributes to shaping the sense of such an initiative with feedforward and feedback projections (Linell, 2009), prompting one or the other area of the potentiality of signification—Mrs Smith's use of the sign "work" is the way of attuning to the other; on the other hand, the sense of Betty and Mr Jones' communicative initiatives is not in the words they implement; it emerges from the combination of their utterance with Mrs's Smith's answer. Thirdly, one can observe that even if the meaning emerges locally, within and through the communicative interplay, it cannot come out from nothing. Signs are potentiality, but not absolutely open—the word "work" is polysemic yet it cannot mean everything. It is a *constrained* potentiality, which can be actualized through its use. In the final analysis, this means recognizing the role of the cultural dynamics—transcending the communicative situation (Linell, 2009) —shaping the sign as constrained potentiality prompting situated sense-making.

THE ROLE OF AFFECTS: PSYCHOANALYSIS AS A SEMIOTIC THEORY

Psychoanalysis as a field is even more fragmented than cultural psychology: according to Wallerstein (2000; see also Pine, 1998) there is not one, but many forms of psychoanalysis. Therefore, we have to specify which area of the psychoanalytic discourse we are referring to. Given our interest in a cultural psychology focused on sense-making as semiotic and dialogical dynamics, our focus cannot but be on the part of psychoanalysis that can be conceived as a semiotic theory, that is, that which sees the mind as a process of unconscious/affective signification of the experience. This vision is typically espoused by a segment of contemporary psychoanalysis. Yet, a more careful look makes one realize that it is actually found throughout the whole history of the discipline, already being salient in some of Freud's seminal elaborations. In this paragraph, we will briefly outline these roots; then we will highlight how an important domain of contemporary psychoanalysis can be fully considered a semiotic theory.

Freud's Semiotic Unconscious

Psychoanalysis is usually considered as an individualistic and at the same time a biological theory. It may therefore seem very far from the semiotic and dialogical approach we are trying to develop here. One of the basic constituents of the classic psychoanalytic architecture is the intrapsychic and quasi-biological notion of drive (*inter alia:* Brenner, 1973; Ellenberger, 1970; Modell, 1984; Rapaport, 1960). Freud conceptualized drive as an element standing on the boundary between the somatic and the psychic (Freud, 1915/1957): a source of stimulation coming from the body and working on, or through, the mind. According to Freud, the drive is a demand of work addressed to the mind. The modelling of the psychic processes in terms of dynamics of drives entails an energetic conception of the mind based on the concept of *cathexis* (*Besetzung*), which constituted a constant through the various formulations and revisions to which Freud subjected his thought. Freud depicted the drive forces as distributions of libidic (or aggressive, after having introduced the death drive) charges creating conditions of disequilibrium perceived by the psychic system in terms of excitement. The activity of the psychic system is nourished by the need to restore the condition of equilibrium in the distribution of the charges, by means of motor and/or mental operations aimed at their discharge. This is what the Freudian principle of constants states: the psychic system tends to keep the stimulation as close as possible to the zero point; the satisfaction consists in the reduction, rather than the increase, of the stimulation (Freud, 1915–1917/1963).

In addition to the notion of drive, Freud also developed a semiotic conception of the mind. In *The Interpretation of Dreams*, Freud (1900/1953) conceptualized the unconscious as a *form of expression*: a language having its own syntax (characterized by the rules of condensation, displacement, plastic representation, symbolic transformation, absence of negation and absence of time) and creating a specific form of meaning. As one can see, this formulation implies a model of the unconscious which differs from Freud's topographical model (a spatial model, in which the unconscious is a place-container of the repressed thoughts) and his structural model (in which the unconscious-Id is an entity of the mind). In Freud's theorization of dream work, unconscious processes are depicted in a semiotic way: the notion of the unconscious designates a mode of combining signs, generative of images and texts.

Freud's main contribution is hence not the discovery of unconscious processes as such (Freud, 1933/1964—the concept of unconscious was already present in the scientific knowledge of his time; Bucci, 1997; Ellenberger, 1970), but rather, his description of the modes whereby the semiotic processes of the unconscious are organized. The notion of *secondary process* describes the logic of our diurnal mode of linking ideas, admitting succession, causality, no double contradiction, etc. The notion of *primary process* designates the privileged mode of working of the unconscious. This mode is not simply the weakening of the secondary process, a reduction of the constraints provided by the reality test. Rather, it is a specific, autonomous and totally different way of functioning of the mind (Freud, 1900; Matte Blanco, 1975; see below). *Primary process* is a magic and hallucinatory way the mind works, typical—yet not exclusive—of dreams. It is grounded on the possibility of freely combining (condensing, moving) representations, without the constraints imposed by the reality test and by the distinction between inner and outside world. The notion of primary process has allowed psychoanalysis to read the idiosyncratic expression of humanity not as a mere absence of thought, lacking in rationality, but as reflecting a specific modality of the mind, radically different from rationality, yet endowed with its own inner systematic logic. For us, one of the main contributions of psychoanalysis to psychology is the acknowledgement of this unconscious thinking process, and its attempt to account for its logic, different from that of rationality, however describable in semiotic terms.

The shift in the theory of anxiety is the other point in Freudian works where a semiotic standpoint is clearly evident. Initially, Freud (1895/1950) proposed the so-called "toxic" model of anxiety. According to this model, anxiety is the effect of the accumulation of instinctual energy that the mental apparatus has been unable to discharge. Yet, 30 years later (Freud, 1926) he radically changed his views, proposing that anxiety should be considered as a signal produced by the Ego in order to warn that an unconscious source of undesirable conflict is going to arise, thereby making the Ego itself ready to cope with it. This is quite a radical theoretical change, made possible and motivated by the elaboration of the second topography,[4] and the consequent centrality gained by the notion of Ego within Freudian thought.

This change has had highly relevant implications for the further development of psychoanalytic theory—and more specifically for the psychoanalytical theory of the affects. According to the toxic model, anxiety is a subjective reflex of the energetic flow—the psychological precipitate of a somatic state. The idea of anxiety as a signal entails a semiotic conception of this kind of affect: a given state of the body (i.e., the anxiety) is not treated in itself, but in its standing for something else (the emergence of an undesirable conflict).

As concerns the focus of our discussion, two aspects of the signal theory are worth underlining. First of all, this theory has opened the way to theoretical elaborations that have led the notion of affect to gain a central place within contemporary psychoanalysis. This is because with the signal theory the affects has been endowed with a specific, important role within the psychoanalytic architecture of the mind. According to the signal theory, the affects perform the function of connoting the state of the inter-systemic relationship (i.e., something like the following warning: "the relationship between the Ego and the Id is going to enter a critical condition") and consequently of triggering the response of the Ego in coherence with this connotation (i.e., in terms of activation of defense mechanism for coping with the danger coming from the Id). In the final analysis, with the signal theory the idea of the affects as an epiphenomenal correlate of the dynamic of drives is abandoned and replaced with a vision of them as a fundamental source of regulation of the psychic apparatus. Secondly, the theory of anxiety as a signal provides a semiotic perspective encompassing biological and psychological domains, making them strictly intertwined. The theory asserts that a state of the body (anxiety) works as the signifier of the psychological condition (the undesirable conflict to be coped with), the latter being its signified. In sum, with the signal theory Freud allows affects to enter within the domain of symbolic phenomena, qualifying them in terms of the signifier/signified duality.

Affects in Object Relation Theory

Melanie Klein and her followers have developed the seminal Freudian idea of the symbolic nature of affects. According to Klein (1967), from the very beginning of their life, people are engaged with an activity of affective connotation of the world leading them to feel every experience in terms of a relation with a positive (loved) or negative (hated) object (i.e., inner representation of relational experiences).[5] Indeed, Klein conceives the affects as the process of attributing basic meanings to experiences—love and hate, which she conceives as the psychological precipitates of the drive of life and the drive of death. Thus, Klein keeps the Freudian concept of drive, but uses it in a very innovative way, making it part of a semiotic dynamics where it assumes the theoretical status of a basic, bodily rooted meaning according to which the state of the self-object is shaped. This is very clear in the way Klein models the relationship between mother and infant. From the beginning of its life, the infant has to deal with the alternation of presence and absence of the mother, she/he experiences this in terms of global and intense bodily states—for example, presence as a condition of satisfaction and warmth, associated with the mother's care; absence as a state of suffering, associated with the sense of hunger. The infant has not the cognitive competences to modulate these bodily states, therefore, she/he experiences them as very intense, extreme affects—of total pleasure or of total catastrophic displeasure. As Klein maintains, these two affective conditions are not associated with the representation of the same external object—the actual mother—as she is alternately present with or absent from the child. Rather, the two affects are felt to be due to two different objects, according to the instinctual duality (life and death drives): the good object providing love and warmth, and the bad object attacking and seeking to destroy the infant. Given the centrality of the object, this model is commonly called "object-relations theory."

Hence, in object relation theory, affects do not merely connote the experience—for example, in terms of positive, joyful, unpleasant reactions to the circumstances; rather they psychologically *generate* the object (Stein, 1991). This means that the affect associated with a certain circumstance (e.g., the pleasure associated with seeing a nice landscape, or of talking with a loved friend) is experienced (at the unconscious level) *ipso facto* as relating with the object qualified by that affect. For instance, the sense of pleasantness that a person may feel is experienced by her/him as the presence of a loved, pleasant object.[6]

Unconscious Process as Symbolization

The semiotic perspective has been developed by other authors after Klein (Klein, Heimann & Money-Kyrle, 1955). The leading Italian psychoanalyst Franco Fornari (1979, 1981, 1983; for a presentation of the work of Fornari in English: Giannakoulas, 1984) proposed a model of the unconscious defined as a process of symbolization. Fornari (1981) described the unconscious as a semiotic device feeding the strive of the subject to signify itself and the world in terms of very basic affects (or "coinems" in the terminology of the author), considered as fundamental emotional, preconceptual meanings attached to fundamental vital dimensions (life, death, parental relationship, parts of the body) connoting the experience.

> "Psychoanalytic philosophy radically changes, if exploring the unconscious, we assume a subject wanting to signify her/himself, marked by a primal *facultas signatrix*, or we assume a subject that always has to hide behind the modes it manifests itself." (Fornari, 1981, p. 13, italics in the text, our translation from Italian original)

According to this author, individuals reveal two coextensive ways of signifying: one working under the socially shared rules of formal thinking—the "diurnal" side of operative categorization—and one working according to the primary process—the "onirical" side of affective symbolization, which works as the mobilization of *coinems*. In brief, affective symbolization is the process of projecting every object of experience onto *coinems*. In so doing, the individual makes every element of the experience full of affective meaning (e.g., the student projects the teacher onto the affective category of "mother," consequently feeling and interacting with him/her as if he/she were the student's mother, that is someone having a function of holding, feeding and taking care of him/her). In this model, there are only a few *coinems*—Fornari speaks of the *coinems* as "the few things oniric symbolism speaks of" (p. 73, our translation from the Italian original); they thus work as generalized classes, homogenizing the experience: patterns of experience that have no semantic linkage can be made identical by being projected onto the same coinemic category.

Fornari's model is relevant to our discussion for three reasons. Firstly, it offers a processual notion of the unconscious that leads to it being seen no longer as an entity but as a mental activity of semiosis characterized by a specific modality. Secondly, Fornari puts the notion of affects at the centre of his semiotic model of the unconscious. According to him, and thanks to him, a semiotic standpoint in psychoanalytic theory equates to a theory of the affects—better, a theory of affective semiosis.[7] Thirdly, Fornari's way of modelling affective semiosis preserves the nature of primary process.[8]

However, the model also has a fundamental limit from a dialogical standpoint: it shares with the Kleinian object relations theory a Kantian vision of the mind. In both approaches, the basic meanings sustaining the affective semiosis of experience—drives and *coinems,* respectively—are conceived as universal *a priori,* inherent properties of the individual mind. Although the content of these universal *a priori* clearly connote and therefore regulate relational contexts, nevertheless, they do not depend on the intersubjective experience provided by such a context.

From Object Relation to Triangulation

Once the centrality of affects was recognized, authors after Klein have however tried to expand the model. One of the criticisms addressed to object relations theory is the very immediate nature of the self-object relation, and the simplicity of its semiotic model: basically, any relation is reducible to a child/good-mother or child/bad-mother relationship (or the slightly more complex model of *coinems*). However, clinical work with children and adults has led authors to propose a more complex view of the semiotic processes involved. Indeed, in many cases, the problem for a child or patient is his or her inability to transform an affective experience into something "thinkable"—that is, into a sign-like experience. To account for this, Bion—another British author—has come to see the role of the mother in early interaction (the "object") as active in the relationship: her work is to contain the strong love or hate of the child, and to reflect it to the child in an already symbolized way, by a vocal or bodily expression. The mother thus "transforms" brutal affects (what Bion calls *beta-elements*) into signs (or *alpha-elements*) (Bion, 1962). In that sense, the mother is for the child like an "external" system for "digesting" experience; eventually, the child will internalize this "alpha-function"—the ability to turn affects into signs. These basic signs are a means of distancing oneself from the affect and bringing them to mind, within a relationship. They triangulate the self-object relationship.

Similarly, the model developed by Winnicott —a third British psychoanalyst—is a critique of the binary nature of the Kleinian model. For Winnicott (1971/2001), the very fact that the child can stand being separated from the mother is due to the fact that he/she can use things or movements as signifying the permanence of the relation to the mother (the object). These basic signs triangulate and mediate the self-other relationship. They become progressively more and more complex, and can stand for affects and experiences which can be semiotically externalized within a relationship: the child who plays with a toy, or who draws with his therapist, is thus using basic semiotic modes to take his distance from, and represent relationships to present and absent objects.

Some of this work pursues the vein opened by Freud, seeing the discourse on dreams as the royal road to the unconscious, and Anna Freud, seeing children's play as such a royal road. In any case, externalizations are seen as signs which, within a specific interpersonal relationship, offer a window on the semiotic dynamics of unconscious processes, a flow that can be guided through further uses of signs in the here and now of the interaction. Studies emphasizing the ternary nature of symbolization have developed in two directions. On the one hand, they have given rise to current studies on the limits of thinking in terms of various modes of symbolization (Alvarez, 1992; Segal, 1991). On the other hand, they have led to give more attention to the intersubjective nature of the relationship in which symbolization might, or might not happen (Green, 2002/2005; Tisseron, 2006). Of course, these two strands have also been combined (Fonagy, Gergely, Jurist & Target, 2005). For us, an important point to retain is the fact that humans progressively, in interactions, come to use signs, which emerge out of, designate, and control fields of intense affective experience.

Interpersonal Psychoanalysis

In parallel to these British and European developments of psychoanalysis, another development gives a more radical alternative to the over-monistic Kleinian model of mind and affect. A primarily American, postwar tradition has proposed a rereading of psychoanalysis with a strong focus on interpersonal relations (Gill, 1994; Greenberg & Mitchell, 1983; Hoffman, 1998; Mitchell & Aron, 1999; Modell, 1984). As its proponents emphasized the dialogical nature of the mind and the role of relational experiences in the organization of the psyche (Sullivan, 1953), they came to radically criticize the original Freudian theory of drives. One of the most representative authors of this approach, Mitchell (1988) thus stated that mind does not preexist relationships, but emerges within and by means of intersubjective communication. Consistently with this idea, interpersonal psychoanalysis underlines that affective meanings and the relational field are recursively linked, each being the source and the product of the other. Being part of an intersubjective field elicits patterns of experiences of self and the other made of sensations, fantasies, ideas, feelings, acts and so forth. These patterns acquire subjective meaning according to the constellation of generalized emotional and relational experiences associated with positive or negative affective value (e.g., pleasant, unpleasant; dreadful, disgusting and the like). Thus, the previous experience provides a context for giving sense to the present moment in terms of an affective meaning onto which the here and now is projected. At the same time this affective meaning works as the *interpretans* of the ongoing intersubjective field eliciting its emergence.

> In place of Freud's topographical and structural theories of mind we envision an organized totality of lived personal experience, more or less conscious and more or less contoured according to those emotional and relational experiences. Instead of a container we picture an experiential system of expectations, interpretative patterns and meanings (...). Within such a system or world, one can feel and know certain things often repetitively and with unshakable certainty. (Stolorow, Orange, & Atwood, 2001/2006, p. 675)

Within this approach, Gill (1994) provides a hermeneutic and situated view of the psychotherapeutic process for which the clinical relationship is a co-construction of meaning, performed jointly by analyst and analysant. The co-construction of meaning is carried out through communicational processes working both at the level of intentional negotiation and unconscious semiosis. This vision radically questions the classical image of the "mirror analyst," according to which the therapist would work aseptically, as if she/he were outside the relationship. On the other hand, Gill highlights how the analyst participates in the clinical exchange through her/his subjectivity which interacts with the patient's. Everything that happens within the clinical exchange has to be considered the expression of an intersubjective field (see also Odgen, 2004; see also Grossen & Perret-Clermont, 1992, for an analysis of the therapeutic encounter).

And What About the Logic of Primary Processes?

Contemporary psychoanalysis has developed a semiotic approach to the mind, giving room to the notion of affective semiosis and at the same time overcoming the hypostatization of the affective meaning entailed in the implicit reference to a transcendental subject. Nevertheless, in mainly Northern American streams of psychoanalysis, this has not been achieved without costs: a loss of the specificities of the notion of unconscious dynamics as primary process.

First, the quote by Stolorow and his colleagues above highlights that this interpersonal psychoanalysis tends to overlap the notions of *unconscious* and *unawareness*, and to conceive affective semiosis as a kind of sense-making that works according to the rules of rational thought (secondary process, in psychoanalytic terms) which keeps in touch with the reality, even if in a somehow fuzzier and less constrained way. In such terms, interpersonal psychoanalysis misses out the specificity of affective semiosis. What remains is a form of subjective reaction to the environment, and emotions commonly called happiness, sadness, or loneliness. The "experiential system of expectations, interpretative patterns and meanings" to which Stolorow, Orange, & Atwood (2001/2006, p. 675) refer to is a constellation entailing an idea of the psychological reality as strongly shaped and regulated by idiosyncratic passions and emotions, desires and relational memories. Nevertheless, this kind of constellation has nothing to do with primary process, that is, the specificity of unconscious processes as pointed out by Freud (1933/1964). Hence, this stream of contemporary psychoanalysis seems to have given up the specificity provided by the nuclear and foundational notion of primary process (Eagle, 1987).

Secondly, such developments of psychoanalysis have assumed a descriptive, nondynamic idea of the unconscious, defined in negative terms as what is *not-conscious*. Cues of this trend can be found in the work of authors revising psychoanalytic theory in the light of cognitive science (Epstein, 1998; Erderlyi, 1985; Singer, 1998). One way of losing the specificity of the notion of the unconscious is provided by models proposing a functional definition of this concept. According to this kind of definition, the unconscious is endowed with plans and goals, even though not under the control of conscious thought. A well known example of this approach is provided by Weiss, Sampson and the Mount Zion Psychotherapy Research Group (1986) with their clinical theory centered on the idea of "unconscious plans". According to this approach, the patient engages with the therapist with the unconscious aim of being confirmed in his/her own pathogenic beliefs concerning her/himself and the other. For example, a patient asks the therapist to be held and understood; yet at the same time he behaves toward the therapist in a provocative way, so as to trigger negative feelings in the clinician. According to this approach, the patient is guided by the unconscious plan of finding confirmation of his unconscious pathogenic belief that nobody can welcome and understand him. Clearly, concepts as plans, aims, beliefs, goal-oriented action entail the idea that the unconscious has, or is a reflex of, a computational competence, that is, that it works in terms of secondary process.[9]

We consider that psychoanalysis that gives up its specifi city—being a psychology of the depth (Salvatore & Pagano, 2005)—loses most of its heuristic power. In contrast, we believe that psychoanalysis can contribute to a dialogic and semiotic cultural psychology only if it can take into account both the horizontal dimension of intersubjective dynamics, and the vertical dimension of the intrapsychological processes unifying unconscious dynamics and conscious thinking (Green, 2002/2005).

AFFECTS

The discussion in the previous paragraph shows the complex role played by affects in psychoanalysis. A cultural psychology that wants to capture the dynamics of sense-making has to account for this essential component of human experience. As already stated, this means that the bridging between psychoanalysis and cultural psychology passes through the development of an integrative theory of affective semiosis capable of deepening the psychocultural understanding of sense-making. Unfortunately, the notion of affects is one of the most ambiguous and polysemic within the psychoanalytic tradition, and more generally, the psychological realm, where it is subject to a wide number of definitions and uses. It is therefore necessary to clarify our position.

A Notion Looking for a Definition

Freud did not use the notion "affects" in a unique way. In various parts of its writings, he implied a quantitative and somatic conception of affects, considering them as derivatives of the drive, as the amount of charge associated with the drive (i.e., as "sum of excitation") or as the somatic process of discharge (i.e., as cathexis) of pulsional energy. In other part of his works, especially in those concerning clinical topics, affects are conceived as feelings working as *regulators*, rather than as a mere derivative of pulsional dynamics. This is already evident in *Studies on Hysteria* (Breuer & Freud 1893/1955) as well as, even more clearly, in Freud's later work (Freud, 1926) on the signal theory, which depicts anxiety as an affective state associated with bodily sensations feeding a feeling of displeasure that pushes the subject to react.

The *reference* of these affects is another source of variability in Freud's conception. Two general ideas are traceable. On one side, affects are seen as representations and inner reproductions of experiences of the external world. Typically, in Freud's theory of trauma the affect is a quasi-hypnotic state of the mind resulting from traumatic experiences. It works to keep such experiences continuously active—somehow moving the mind outside of time, in the suspended present of the trauma. When the affect cannot be metabolized and remains, as it were, "undigested," then the traumatic experience preserves its power of colonizing the mind, and therefore of sustaining the person's psychic realty. On the other hand, Freud provided an idea of affects as inner perceptions, that is, as representations of the body's state of activation.[10]

Contemporary Evolutions of the Notion

Contemporary psychoanalysis has updated the original Freudian thesis on affects, yet the fundamental conceptual articulation found in Freud's writings is still considered valid. Thus, the initial physiological modeling of the affects in terms of drive derivatives has been updated as a result of the reelaboration of the concept of drive in accordance with advances in biology, ethology and neuroscience. For instance, Noy (1982, quoted in Stein, 1991), conceives affects as an inner program of action associated with fixed patterns of physiological activation. According to the evolutionary approach of this author, the fundamental function of affects is to regulate and coordinate the various bodily reactions to the stimuli and to activate the motivational systems, therefore to trigger behavior. The same relevance to the bodily state is entailed in the concept of *arousal* that plays a very central role in the psychological theory of affects. According to the classical theory of emotions of Schachter and Singer (1962), arousal is a state of generalized and undifferentiated neuro-vegetative activation elicited by the environment. This state is then subjected to interpretation (*appraisal*), and so doing it is differentiated in terms of a given emotion, consistently with the contextual circumstances. What is interesting to notice here is that in the final analysis the concept of arousal is germane to the notion of drive, a sort of translation of the latter into psychological language (Stein, 1991). On the other hand, the notion of appraisal paves the way to the recognition of the connections between affects and meaning. In the psychological field this connection has been highlighted in terms of the close recursive linkage between emotion and cognition. According to this view, emotions are conceptualized as innate schematic values connoting the environmental objects and events in an unreflexive and unmediated way (Lazarus, 1991). Appraisal is thus inherent to the emotion: the individual enters in touch with the world primarily and very quickly in terms of generalized judgments (pleasant, unpleasant, dangerous, awful, etc.) selecting and orienting the further analysis of the experience.

This kind of approach is consistent with neuroscientific modeling of emotions. Le Doux (1996) distinguishes two circuits through which the brain processes the information concerning a dreadful stimulus. One path (that gets to the amygdala via the thalamus) is very fast, entailing only a rough computation of the sensorial information. The other path involves the cortical structure, and a more sophisticated, slower analysis of the stimulus. Moreover, the idea of the emotion as attribution of subjective value is close to the psychoanalytic theorizations that have tried to conceptualize the notion of affects in psychological terms, that is, in terms of feelings. For instance, consistently with the Kleinian view, Sandler and Sandler (1978) pointed out that affects are the way of representing and connoting the state of the object bond, thereby performing a fundamental function of regulation of the Self (and the relationship with the Object).

Unconscious Affects and Subjective Feelings

The conceptualization of affects in terms of subjective value has constituted a major advance within psychoanalytic theory as well as a bridge between psychoanalysis and psychology for two main reasons. Firstly, this idea has allowed the recognition of the motivational and communicational valence of affects, evident for psychologists (Ekman & Rosenberg, 2005; Tomkins, 1970) and clinicians (Klein, 1976; Lichtenberg, 1989), as well as for the layperson. Emotions are subjectively felt as an impulse to act and are associated with reactions that work as very immediate signals for others, thereby working as powerful regulators of both the subject and the other. Insofar as affects are conceived as the attribution of subjective value to experiences and objects, then it is easy to understand that affects are a way of mapping the world in terms of how to engage with it. In the final analysis, the notion of value leads to recognize that affects and action are strictly intertwined: affectively feeling an object means to be ready and inclined to move towards (against, far from, on, etc.) it, and at the same time, to express such an inclination to the object. Secondly, the interpretation of affects in terms of value connotation allows us to address a basic paradox that accompanies the psychoanalytic discourse on the affects: the issue of their unconscious nature. Briefly, the point at stake is the following. As far as one conceives the affects in terms of somatic activation, their unconscious nature is preserved. Or rather, the somatic conceptualization of the affects entails the notion of a dynamic (not repressed) unconscious, that is an unconscious that is so, not because is the container of ideational content kept out of consciousness, but because its way of functioning (primary process) makes it inherently ungraspable for thought (i.e., for secondary process). Hence, the somatic conception of the affects allows affect to be considered in psychodynamic terms, that is, consistently with the "true psychic reality" of primary process. On the other hand, insofar as one conceives affects as feelings, that is, as subjective representations associated with and connoting experience, this means that one is led to a secondarization of the unconscious, which means giving up the dynamic nature of the affects and conceiving the mental process in terms of representational contents that can be computed by the subject, as the subject computes the contents of rational thinking.

Some psychoanalysts tried to address this issue, proposing the idea that affects - intended as feelings—could be unconscious. Nevertheless, insofar as affects are considered mere feelings, alongside the path paved by Freud with his definition of the affects in terms of inner perception, this solution raises more problems than it solves, because it leads to the paradox of feelings that are unfelt. The definition of feeling in semiotic terms - that is, as a process of connotation of the object, of attributing value to it—seems to enable psychoanalysis to avoid this paradox. As a matter of fact, the meaning connoting the object can be conceived as an embodied significance, which is a meaning without a discrete representational content, which however motivates a specific disposition to act. In this way, affects can be conceptualized as part of the psychological realm, as a subjective process, and at the same time in dynamic terms, as an unconscious process working according to the primary process.[11]

In sum, the psychoanalytic discourse on affects, intertwining with the psychological and neuroscientific theorization, leads to this notion being conceived in accordance with the following basic processes:

1. *Somatic activation as embodied appraisal*. Affects are dynamics of generalized bodily activation, that is, the basic way of prereflexively experiencing the world in terms of embodied meanings, in terms of

hedonic basic values (positive vs. negative, exciting vs. relaxing) qualifying and construing the experience.

2. *Self-other regulation*. The immediate appraisal of the experience has an inherent motivational and communicational valence, thereby making the affects a powerful situated, preconventional semiotic regulator of the social bond.
3. *Symbolization as subjectivization*. The patterns of sense-motor activation sustaining arousal are subjected to a continuous and recursive process of symbolization (also sometimes called mentalization). One can conceive of this process of symbolization as a process of incorporating the embodied meanings within an associative chain of signs (Green, 1973), thereby transforming raw experience (Bion, 1962) into representations, that is, the subsymbolic into the symbolic (Bucci, 1997; Damasio, 1999).
4. *Feelings* are the self-reflective output of this process, resulting from the introduction of the body into the realm of the secondary process, mainly through language. These feelings can then in turn enter the whole dynamics again, for instance as triggers for further affective activation.

This proposition results from a generic synthesis and is therefore very general. Different theories of affects could then be elaborated depending on how each of these dimensions is conceptualized and connected to the others. We will devote the next section to presenting our specific way of putting these building blocks together.

A PSYCHOANALYTICAL, SEMIOTIC VIEW OF AFFECTS

In this section, we will propose a model of affects based on the idea that affective semiosis works according to primary process. Our presentation is divided into two steps. Firstly, we present a model of the unconscious in terms of which affective semiosis works. We do this by referring to the seminal contribution of the Chilean psychoanalyst Matte Blanco (1975) who conceptualized primary process in logical terms. Secondly, we describe some characteristics of the functioning of affective semiosis in the light of Matte Blanco's model.

Matte Blanco's Bi-Logic Theory of the Unconscious

Matte Blanco (1975) proposed a theory of the unconscious to which we can refer, as we want to define a semiotic understanding of the dynamics of primary processes and their interactions with secondary processes. As far as we know, no other model addresses this central issue in such a systematic way, a circumstance that makes Matte Blanco's "bi-logic" theory a cornerstone for those interested in modeling the processes of affective semiosis.

Following the Freud of the *Interpretation of Dreams,* Matte Blanco's bi-logic theory assumes the unconscious as a specific modality of the mind's functioning. His logical formal analysis, based on the principles of the unconscious that Freud had recognized as the basis of dreams (condensation, displacement, plastic representation, symbolic transformation, absence of negation and time), shows that the unconscious logic is different from the rational mode grounded in the principle of noncontradiction, but none the less systematic.

Matte Blanco suggested that the logic and semantic relations sustaining rational thought should be called *asymmetrical,* in the sense that the positions of the terms of any relation are not changeable and cannot be inverted without affecting the truth value of the proposition. For instance, if the proposition "$A > B$" is true, then "$B > A$" cannot be true at the same time, or if "Marco is the father of Bruno," then "Bruno is the father of Marco" is not the case.

In contrast, unconscious processes are free of these constraints, and Matte Blanco called the *symmetry principle* what he saw as their fundamental rule. Unconscious thought, that is, the mental activity working mainly according to the rule of the unconscious, *does not set limits to the exchangeability between the terms of a relation*. This means that from the point of view of the unconscious all propositions generated by all possible permutations of their terms are treated as the same. Therefore, for instance, from the point of view of the unconscious, if Marco is the father of Bruno, then Bruno is also the father of Marco. Hence, the principle of symmetry highlights exchangeability as the specificity of the logic of the unconscious: the logic of the unconscious openly and radically violates the noncontradiction principle. The full application of this logic cancels any differences and produces homogeneity among the signs that are part of any relation—insofar as Marco and Bruno are at the same time father and son of each other, they are not distinguishable from one another. In the final analysis, this means *that the logic of the unconscious transforms any relation of contiguity between two signs, that is, any association between these, into a relation of identity*.

Matte Blanco does not consider these two logics—that of conscious thought and of unconscious thought—as juxtaposed, but as complementary. Conscious (asymmetrical) thought works in terms of setting categorical distinctions-relations within the homogenizing (symmetrical) way of functioning of the unconscious. Thus, conscious and unconscious processes are two *coextensive* ways of mental functioning that are antagonistic and complementary: every psychological process is the output emerging from their interaction, and therefore, thinking is always a mixture of both. One can differentiate various forms of thinking according to the proportion of the conscious and the unconscious, that is, of symmetric and asymmetric logic characterizing the mixture. In the case of formal thought asymmetric logic is strongly prevalent. However, even this mode of thinking retains a degree of symmetry, in terms of nonreflexive assumptions, analogical thinking, metaphoric linkages, unconstrained pertinentization, etc. (Matte Bon, 1999; Valsiner, 2009). Conversely, even a psychotic's thinking is never the implementation of the symmetric principle alone. This is because working in terms of pure symmetry would mean a condition where no relation, therefore no thought, would be possible. One can imagine the pure unconscious as an absolutely undifferentiated, presymbolic field of activation, produced by the encounter between the mind and the world, where no distinction has yet been made (Bucci, 1997; Valsiner, 2007).

In sum, unconscious thought is the mental activity characterized by the strong predominance of the symmetrical logic associated with a quantum of asymmetrical logic, which is however present. The asymmetrical logic introduces elements of differentiation within the unconscious totality (that is what we have mentioned above as the presymbolic field of activation), in so doing allowing the production of first basic relations, that is, the first proto-categories—in the final analysis, the first forms of experience.

Affects as Symmetrical Sets

Matte Blanco depicted this function of differentiation performed according to asymmetric logic as the creation of bags of symmetry within the unconscious totality's indistinctness.[12] They are separate (therefore asymmetrical) from each other (one bag is different from another), but each of them conserves symmetrical homogeneity inside itself. This means that relations are possible among the bags, while within any bag only symmetry works (everything is everything else). The very basic differentiation of the unconscious totality is the one producing the opposition between the class of *goodness* as opposed to the class of *badness* (Klein, 1967; see also Carli & Giovagnoli, 2011; Carli & Paniccia, 2003). In this way, a basic distinction is made in the undifferentiated field of activation, and at the same time, the foundations are laid for a hypergeneralized assimilation of experience, that is, the experience-as-a-whole understood as goodness (or badness).

The idea of "bag of symmetry" is a way of modeling the emerging of the basic significance in the mind: symmetrical classes can be seen as the first classes of meaning emerging from unconscious processes. Inspired by mathematics, Matte Blanco called these as bags or classes, "sets." Matte Blanco's idea of basic meanings as emerging from the encounter between conscious and unconscious dynamics provides a meaningful way of modelling affects. On this basis, we propose to define *affects* as *symmetrical sets*, that is, as hypergeneralized, homogenized meanings produced by asymmetrization within the undifferentiated unconscious totality. Human experience takes its basic and primary shape in terms of these affective meanings (Salvatore & Venuleo, 2008).

The conceptualization in terms of symmetrical sets offers an innovative way of looking at affects. As we have said above, psychology and psychoanalysis tend to conceive the affects as bodily states of activation endowed with hedonic basic values (positive vs. negative, exciting vs. relaxing) nourishing and shaping the subjective experience of the world as well as regulating the relational engagement with it. Matte Blanco's theory does not contradict this general vision. Rather, it can be seen as a mode of interpreting it in a way that enables us to better understand the generative function of the affects for thought. In accordance with Matte Blanco, one can see the hedonic value sustaining the affects as the basic form of asymmetrization—that is of creation of symmetrical sets of meaning. In other words, the hedonic values can be conceived as the "antagonist" of the unconscious, introducing a quantum of differentiation within the symmetrical totality.

From this point of view, affective semiosis is a way of functioning of the mind characterized by the predominance of the unconscious, with the complementary action of the asymmetrization function that creates hypergeneralized and homogeneous symmetrical classes of embodied meaning.

Phenomenology of Affective Semiosis

The reading of affects in terms of symmetrical sets enables us to conceptualize some aspects of the way they work.

Randomization of the signifier-signified linkage

Conscious thought consists of the mobilization of signs. A "sign (...) is something that stands to somebody for something, in some respect or capacity" (Peirce, 1897/1932). In the case of languages, it is generally accepted that a sign designates a link between a signifier and a signified (de Saussure, 1916/1977). Semiotics has highlighted that, for certain classes of signs, such links are conventional and stable within a given cultural system (Eco, 1975). They are conventional since nothing forces a certain signifier to be used in order to convey a certain signified: if an agreement is established, the signifier "ababa," or the signifier "vvvv" can be used for denoting the concept |dog|. The extreme variability of languages is an argument supporting the idea of the conventional nature of signs, given that each of them has its own system of sounds to label concepts. However, once defined, the conventional link between signifier and signified acquires stability and univocity for the linguistic group within which the convention keeps the value of stipulation, and for this reason works as a code grounding the interpretation of the sign.[13]

The symmetric principle is inconsistent with this property of linguistic signs. It works in terms of a *random linkage* between signifier and signified: any signifier can stand for a potentially infinite number of signifieds, and any signified can be expressed by an infinite number of signifiers.[14] Obviously, the randomness does not remain infinite. As we have already observed, the asymmetrization function tends to reduce—but not to eliminate—it. In the final analysis, this means that affective semiosis treats the signs as constrained-but-yet-infinite potentiality of combination. From the standpoint of affective semiosis no sign has an already defined content. Rather, it acquires its signified only within and through the web of connections that reduces its randomness (Carli & Paniccia, 2002, 2003; Salvatore, Tebaldi, & Potì, 2006/2009).

This statement is very clear for any psychoanalyst. Contrarily to the naïve idea of psychoanalysis, the psychoanalytic method takes as its target the contingent pattern of combination among signs as the vector of affective semiosis (Ferro, 2003; Fornari 1983; Odgen, 2004). Within the analytic situation, every sign acquires its significance in a situated and contingent way, according to the other signs it is connected to. Thus, for instance, if the patient evokes the image of an object with a cylindrical shape, this does not necessarily mean a penis. Suppose that, in his free associative flow, the patient speaks of how he is used to write with his fountain pen, even if this makes his handwriting hard to understand. Then, after a moment of silence, he goes on, telling the therapist that the day before he tried to phone his son and that the latter did not answer—and even though he thought that his son may not have heard the ring, he felt sad, as if he were purposely refusing to answer. Well, what could be the interpretation of this associative flow? A possibility is to interpret it as indicative of the patient's phantasy of having only bad things (his incomprehensible handwriting produced by the fountain pen) to offer to the loved objects (the readers of his writing; the son) and for this reason to be condemned to being rejected (readers that do not understand him, the son that does not answer his call). Obviously there could be other readings of this virtual sketch—and in the clinical reality many other aspects and data would be necessary in order to provide a valid interpretation. Nevertheless, the example provided is sufficient to highlight that the fountain pen does not necessarily mean penis. The word "pen" is a bundle of potentialities of signification, prompted by the infinite characteristics people can associate to it. Only one of these characteristics is the cylindrical form of the object at stake. Another characteristic is the quality of the handwriting consequent of its use, which in our example can be seen as triggering the chain of associations, and within it, can be symbolically interpreted as standing for the capacity of engagement with a loved object. In sum, affective semiosis can be conceived as a dynamic field: the meaning is produced by the emerging effect of the whole organization of the signs, rather than by the cumulative combination of discrete signifiers conveyed by single signs.

Reification

This characteristic is complementary to the previous. Conscious thought makes and keeps a distinction between the signifier and the signified, with the former standing for the latter. Thus, the signifier represents the signified, but does not substitute it. In other words, the picture of a portion of spaghetti can be used to denote the dish, but if one decided to eat it, one will not be fed.

On the level of affective semiosis things go differently. According to the symmetry principle, signifier and signifier are linked through an identity linkage. The signifier does not stand for the signified: *it is what it represents*. The process of wish-fulfilment described by Freud concerns this characteristic: unconscious representations (oniric images as well as phantasies) are not mere figurations of the wished goal, but their hallucinatory satisfaction. In the same way, the infant who sucks her/his thumb is doing more than self-stimulating: she/he is experiencing her/himself being nourished. The thumb is not something standing for the breast: it *is* the breast. The same mechanism is evident in many circumstances where the affective semiosis is salient. Take the example of a flag, which in many cases, is felt and used as something more than the conventional sign of the Nation: it renders the value of the Country present and alive.

Recognizing the reifying valence of the symmetrical principle leads to conceiving affective semiosis as a device of *mental hypostatization*. Affective semiosis does not attribute meaning to objects of experience that preexist to it. Rather, consistently with the Kleinian idea of affects creating the objects subjected to emotional connoting, affective semiosis generates objects within the mind, through the act of connoting them (Salvatore & Venuleo, 2010).

It is worth recalling here the observation made by Bowlby (1961) concerning the elaboration of mourning. In this kind of circumstances, a feeling of anger against the absent object often takes the place of the first reaction of grief. The model of affective semiosis we are proposing allows for an understanding of this mechanism. Anger can be interpreted as the way affective semiosis makes (hallucinates) the absent object present-for-the-mind through the act of connoting it, albeit in negative terms: because it is gone it is bad, but it is present as being bad.[15]

The semiotic principle of reification is well known by those who work in the field of advertising. In many circumstances the message on the product does not serve the function of informing about the object. Rather it is aimed at affectively construing (generating) it by making it present in the public's mental landscape (Klein, 1999). This circumstance is particularly clear in the case of paradoxical and negative advertising (i.e., "do not buy this product"; "it is a bad object").

The reifying valence of affective semiosis can be highlighted from a complementary standpoint, underlining that it has no intentionality, that is, no possibility of referring to hypothetical representations. This is an evident implication of reification. As a matter of fact, asserting that affective semiosis generates the object that it connotes is equivalent to saying that *affective semiosis always and only predicates presences*.

This comes back to Freud's seminal observation about the absence of negation in dream work (Freud, 1900/1953) as well as to Klein's model of the infant's affective transformation of the experience of the mother's absence into a present persecutory object.

Anthropomorphization

The objects generated by affective semiosis as mentally salient are not discrete pieces of the reality ("objects" in the ordinary sense). Rather, they are *embodied experiences of relationships*. In other words, objects are animated by a communicational and relational dynamism oriented toward the symbolizing subject. Affective semiosis is a kind of picturing the world shaping it as engaging with the subject. We do not feel an object as bad, rather as bad-with-me/us. Such an addressivity is already entailed in the Kleinian model of affective semiosis of the absent mother, who is not symbolized as a recognition of a fact, but as a (subjective) object endowed with a destructive agency against the person who is symbolizing. And it is also evident in the child's way of beating and saying "bad" to the table she has just run into. On the other hand, everyone who loves knows that this circumstance is not limited to infancy. One who loves does not feel the lack of commitment (interest, attention ...) from the loved one as just a fact. She/he feels this lack as something that the loved one performs against her/him—the loved one is accused of lack of commitment, and is guilty of not loving. This is evident in episodes of marital unfaithfulness, which are generally experienced as a form of betrayal, that is, as a presence occurring against the partner, rather than an absence in the conjugal relationship produced as a result of the presence of another relationship.

Generalization

Affective semiosis signifies anything in terms of generalized class: affective semiosis does not recognize a mother as an individual, but *tout court* as the whole class of all that is associable (then made identical) with being a mother—that is, in the final analysis, as *mother-ness* (Rayner, 1995). Examples of generalization are numerous: consider the awe we can feel in front of our superior or another figure with some authority over us (a teacher, a policemen, an elderly relative ...). Such a feeling cannot be related to the actual attitude and power of the figure; rather, it reflects a meaning that we attribute to the generalized class of the authoritative and powerful figures we identify our interlocutor with, rather than to the specific person.

Homogenizing through absolutization

This aspect is strictly interwoven with generalization. The fact that affective semiosis treats every element as identical to the class also means that all the qualities and characteristics of the class are attributed to the element, and that it will have them to the maximum degree (the unconscious cannot modulate!). As a consequence of this absolutization, every element is made identical—homogenized—to every other element that is part of the same generalized set of meaning. Stereotypic thought evidently shows hints of the affective mechanism we are discussing. All the objects that are projected in the stereotypical class are confused with each other regardless of their individual specificity, and treated according to all the properties associated with the class. Thus, to give another example, stereotypic thought tends to connote all Muslims as Arabs and all Arabs as extremist male chauvinists, terrorists ..., giving all of them the maximum extent of the qualities of "enemy-ness," dangerousness, wickedness that are associated with the stereotype. The experience of falling in love is another manifestation of the process of absolutizing. When a person is in this state, he/she views the loved subject in an idealized way—that is as having, to the highest extent, the totality of the qualities associated with goodness and fineness. Obviously, a person falling in love understands that reality is different, but he/she does so by means of a further operation of asymmetrization, placing some constraints on the absolutizing feeling.

Wholeness

The statement made above makes it clear that the reference of affective semiosis is never the discrete object (i.e., a person, an event, a thing) working as the focus of attention. This is because, given the symmetrical quality of affective semiosis, the discrete object is in any case assimilated within the hypergeneralized and homogenising assimilative set of signifieds. In other words, every discrete object is experienced as the whole field provided by all the elements with which the discrete object is connected and therefore "symmetrized" (i.e., made identical). Hence, affective semiosis is the reifying transformation of the encounter with the world (i.e., the ongoing flow of stimuli) as a unitary experience of a total object. One can pick up a hint of this level of experience when a new situation is encountered. In those circumstances, sometimes we can be aware of how, though very briefly, we emotionally[16] experience the situation as something of global value (as threatening, warm, distancing ...), before differentiating the experience through a specific attentive focus.

Inherent intersubjectivity

Intersubjectivity is more a quality already entailed in what has been said, than a further characteristic of affective semiosis. We present it on its own because of its theoretical relevance and for the sake of our later discussion. Affective semiosis is an inherently intersubjective process in accordance to three complementary points of view. First, affective semiosis is an emergent product of dialogical dynamics. Indeed, as we have previously stated (randomization), affective semiosis is the effect of the whole organization of signs—that is, of the way signs are combined within the dialogical stream. Given the fact that unconscious logic does not recognize differences between self and other, one has to conclude that the chain of signs that reduces the randomness and polysemy of the signs encompasses all the contributions to the dialogue, before and regardless of any distinction of their source. In this sense, affective semiosis is by definition the systemic effect of an intersubjective process. This point can be shown by coming back to the sketch of the patient and his fountain pen. In the example, the chain of signs is produced by only one person—the patient. Yet, given that the source of the signs is irrelevant at the level of affective semiosis, we can change the example and imagine that some of the signs have been provided by the therapist. For instance, it might have been the therapist who expressed concerns about her/his handwriting with the fountain pen used to write a note to the patient. At the level of affective semiosis, the result would have been the same[17]. (We will come back to this point – the dialogical emergence of affective semiosis – later). Secondly, as we have seen, affective semiosis concerns the whole field of experience, before and regardless of the distinction self-world. Then, as the Kleinian theory has clearly highlighted, affective semiosis is the way of emotionally connoting the relationship in itself. Thirdly, as the discussion on anthropomorphization should have shown, intersubjectivity is the content of affective semiosis—this was meant by the previous claim that affective semiosis shapes the field of experience in terms of relational engagement. In sum, one can say that the subject, the reference and the object of affective semiosis is the relationship.

To summarize, in this section we have focused on some characteristic of affects. In so doing we have pictured it as a dialogical-semiotic process, that we have called *affective semiosis*, whose product is the transformation of the flow of ever-changing contact with the world into a global, generalized and homogenized object of experience, endowed with an inherently subjective, anthropomorphic addressivity. Connecting this statement to the ones provided in the previous paragraphs, we can add that such addressivity is signified and shaped through and in the terms of embodied meaning, that is, of hedonic values that can be considered the first form of meaningfulness, therefore of subjective mental life.

THE ROLE OF AFFECTIVE SEMIOSIS IN SENSE-MAKING

Having defined our model of affective semiosis, we can now address the focal aim of our contribution: the conceptualization of the role played by affects in sense-making. In order to move in this direction, we first have to take a step back and refer to the whole, anthropomorphic object of experience generated by the affective semiotization of the ongoing encounter with the world.

Affective Context

We propose the term "affective context" to designate the immediate experience of the affective object. In so doing, we give a specifically psychological and psychodynamic coloring to the notion of context. According to our standpoint, the *affective context* is the subjective construction of the environment, where the latter is conceived as the source of the shapeless flow of energy-matter triggering, nourishing and constraining sense-making (but not defining it, Maturana & Varela 1980). Thus, affective context is the unitary global mental state associated with the continuous of the experience the subject is embedded in, before and regardless of the articulations between past and present; here and elsewhere; me, thou, it, us, you. In other words, the affective context is the first, immediate output of the semiotization of being-in-the-world. It is a hypergeneralized, embodied semiotic construction sustaining the mind and giving content to it—that is, conferring the felt sense of being in relationship with a live animate object.

This definition of the affective context provides a framework for conceptualizing the role of affective semiosis in sense-making. In general terms, we maintain that *the affective context works as a hypergeneralized, basic and prereflexive assumption orienting the way persons interpret experience, and therefore, their intersubjective fields.*

The affective context has to be seen as the basic, global mental state embedded within the encounter with the world, triggered and nourished by such an encounter. This means that any specific engagement with a discrete element of the reality (an object, an event, a practice, a person, etc.) occurs within the global semiotic field provided by the affective context, as its temporary specification or instantiation. And this leads us to say that any engagement with a discrete element of the world keeps the affective valence of the context of its instantiation. Hence, when a person has experience of the piece of the reality α in terms of the sign a, she/he is experiencing the context *A-ness*—that is, she/he is experiencing the infinite set of signs a_n in which the affective meaning consists of.

Affective Context as the Ground of Dialogue

The concept of affective context that we propose does not underestimate the role of dialogical mechanisms involved in sense-making. As we have seen above (and we will examine in more depth later), affective semiosis unfolds within and thanks to dialogue, as well as it concerns and grounds dialogue.

The following example intends to show how the affective context is the semiotic ground of the dialogical sense-making in which people engage, and how they themselves contribute to it (we devote another section to the complementary issue of how dialogue produces the affective context). Imagine a very simple social exchange: persons A and B meet by chance; they do not share any current ongoing activity, and engage in dialogue (they are able to use the same linguistic code). Consider the following discursive scene:

A: "I am going to Rome by car. I know you have to go there too. Maybe you would like a lift."

B: "Thank you, it is very kind of you."

We can ask ourselves: what assumptions do A and B require sharing as premises in order to understand each other and, more importantly, in order to find the communicative attempt plausible and meaningful? We will show the limits of a traditional semantic analysis; an analysis in terms of the affective context enables to account for the situation.

First, A and B have to share some assumptions concerning *what* world they speak of and *how* it works (the semantic models, see Jonhson-Laird, 1983; Sanford, 1987). From this standpoint, we can, for instance, deduce that B believes s/he lives in a world where saving effort, time etc. is a desirable event (if not B would not have described A's offer as a kind act); we can think that in such a world, the value of the act is not necessarily in itself, rather it can lie in the actor's intention to perform it (B denotes A as kind, even if A has just expressed a willingness); we might also consider that in such a world helping other people by doing something good for them is not an obligation, but a choice (otherwise the invitation would not be a sign of kindness); and so on. In sum, A and B share a certain knowledge about how the world functions. According to cognitive psychology, thanks to this knowledge, A and B can coordinate the reciprocal understanding of the content of their exchanged signs. However, this is not sufficient. In order for the dialogue to unfold and for its content to acquire a communicational meaningfulness, A and B need something more than shared semantic knowledge of the world: they need to share an underlying system of assumptions concerning the pragmatic value of the relationship. As contemporary linguistics and discourse psychology have highlighted (Austin, 1962), this system of assumptions concerns the interpretation of the activity people are involved in—*what* they are doing and *why*—which enable them to grasp the sense of their reciprocal communicational acts. In order to make their communication meaningful, each of the participants has to assume a vision of their contingent world, that is, of the other, and of being involved in relationship with the other. Moreover, they need their assumed visions to be at least partially consistent with each other.[18] In effect, the same semantic content can be interpreted in different ways. B could interpret A's speech act as just a sign of courtesy, or as a mode of courting, or an endeavour to be forgiven, or to obtain willingness, or to show off the new car, or to underline B's not having a car at his/her disposal, and so on. At the same time, A could interpret B's answer in different ways as well: as a ritualistic answer, as a sign of appreciation, as a way of saying "Yes", or even of saying "No", and so on.

Our fundamental thesis is that the selection of one path of interpretation from the huge amount of possibilities made available by the cultural domain[19] *depends in the final analysis on the perspective that A and B have on their situated, contingent exchange. And these perspectives directly depend on the affective context shared by the protagonists.* In this particular situation, we could thus say that if A and B were attuned to a pragmatic interpretation depicting their communication as a game of reciprocal agreement-seeking—or of declaration of willingness, or of courting—they would be implying a more general affective assumption consisting of the symbolization of their intersubjectivity as a friendly relationship, as an affective context of *goodness*. On the other hand, if as A and B were attuned to a communicational game of reciprocal control, or of avoidance, or of subtle reciprocal aggression, this would be possible because their pragmatic assumption would be grounded on a symbolization of their communication as an affective context of enmity—an affective context of *badness*.

On the basis of these affective contexts, A and B will define the sense of their dialogue and the pragmatic value to their utterances.[20] The affective context indeed excludes possible meanings. For example, if A and B attune themselves to a representation of their dialogue as a game of ritualized cooperation aimed at neutralizing the interpersonal involvement according to the accidental nature of the encounter, it is probable that B will interpret A's proposal as a sign of courtesy devoid of functional implication, and

A will interpret B's answer as a way of closing the ritual, devoid of an information charge. On the contrary, if A and B attune themselves to a representation of their communication as a game of reciprocal attempts to get agreement, then, for instance, B might interpret A's offer as A's way of showing interest in helping him/her. On the other hand, A and B could be attuned to a vision depicting their exchange as a competitive game; consequently, B would be led to interpret A's proposal as a way of underlining B's not having a car at his/her disposal or a tactic aimed at playing a nasty trick on him. And A will interpret B's answer as an ironic way of taking up the proposal.

Hence, in our view, *pragmatic assumptions are embedded within the affective context* that works as the intersubjective situated scenario, according to which the exchange can be performed and interpreted (Salvatore, Ligorio & De Franchis, 2005). Since the affective context is the shared affective symbolization that actors make of their relationship, we can say that it defines and constrains the domain of signification within which actors perform their reciprocal attempts to attune.

Finally, we can formulate our comprehensive model of sense-making as follows: *affective categorization generates the symbolization of intersubjectivity. Such symbolization, working as an affective context, limits the possibilities of reciprocal positioning and pragmatic interpretations of the dialogic exchanges. In so doing, it allows people to perform their dialogic strategies of reciprocal attunement, which in turn leads to activate and make relevant an area of meaning for the signs exchanged in the contingence of dialogue.*

The Salience of the Affective Context

According to our thesis, the affective context works as a constraint delimiting the landscape of the virtually infinite polysemy of signs and their combinations. Hence, it is nothing but a distribution of probability of combinations among the signs embedded within the intersubjective communication[21] (Salvatore, Tebaldi, & Potì, 2006/2009). The salience of a certain affective context is a structure of probability defining the opportunities of sign combination: it renders the generation of some combinations of signs more probable, others less probable, or very improbable. Thus, the affective context can be conceived as the first fundamental constraining of the signs within a finite region of the totally open infinite dimensional space describing their reciprocal combination—that is the virtually infinite trajectories of sense-making; such delimiting makes some combinations of meaning possible.

The role played by the affective context in sense-making is thus conceivable in terms of a catalytic form of causality: the affective context as a promoting sign (Valsiner, 2009) defining—in terms of constraining—the conditions thanks to which a given pattern of meaning is the most likely to emerge.[22] In other words, the affective context mainly performs its orienting function in an indirect way. It is not a normative rule prescribing the way of sense-making. Rather, it shapes the conditions according to which signs combine to each other and thus generate meaning.

The salience of the affective context is evident in the circumstances in which persons are in a state of strong emotional activation. In this kind of situations, ideas, evaluations, reasoning, every act of meaning appears to be "polarized" by the emotional state. Let us think a circumstance in which we feel very happy. Our attention is more easily focused on aspects of the situation consistent with the mood we are experiencing. The same happens to our interpretations and evaluations; even the commitment in the situation tends to be shaped by the emotion we are "caught" by—thus we can be willing to attempt an unpleasant task and be subjected to boring routines that we usually avoid. And one can compare this movement of sense-making to what happens when our emotional activation takes different directions: we become very competent in finding new reasons for remaining upset; our interpretations and judgment become sharp and ungenerous, and so forth.

Our previous example refers to situations in which intense feeling is involved. Most of these cases feature the capacity of our emotion to orient our evaluations, ideas, modes of thinking, as well as our way of selecting aspects of experience to be considered as pertinent. We are somehow adjusted and in various cases aware of the polarized valence of the emotions (e.g., take an expression like: "I'm sorry. I do not actually believe what I said to you yesterday. The fact is that I was very angry"). Nevertheless, emotional experiences are like the tip of the affective semiosis-iceberg. Indeed, affective semiosis is ubiquitous: it works even when we have no feeling of its working. No situation is affectively neutral. People cannot help affectively making sense, just as they cannot help perceiving or thinking. Every experiential encounter with the world triggers a movement of affective semiosis.[23] This means that the orienting function of the affective context is always in action, even if we are able to be aware of it only in situations where the affects are particularly intense.[24] Hence, people engage in an affective presemantic activity of interpretation of the experience which orients the subsequent process of thinking and judging the situation, and more in general, of conferring sense to it.

The Embeddedness of the Affective Context

It is worth highlighting one last point. The affective context is not a separate moment from other levels of sense-making: we represent the discrete elements of the reality accordingly to an affective context, and our representations constitute an experience of such reality as a whole. Thus, for instance, at this very moment I am typing on the keyboard striving to elaborate and express some ideas on sense-making. At the same time, I am "immersed" in an affective context. It emerged this morning, when I sat down at the computer, as the local stabilization of the infinite flow of interacting signs (my feeling on my activity, my ideas, how I slept, the sensation associated with the chair I am siting on, etc.). I can grasp this affective context only partially and vaguely, as it partly escapes to language. I would depict it as a state of pleasant tension. According to the model proposed in this chapter, this state is not only a feeling: it is the cue of a hypergeneralized homogenising meaning that is active in my mind and sustains the sense of myself in the present moment. Insofar as this affective meaning is an infinite set of signs, one can only give an impression of it, by resorting to metaphoric terms. In this case, the image I find useful is the following: "being in relation with a lovable and active object, activating me and enabling my enjoyment." This image encompasses a very large class of experiences through one's lifetime, unified by the fact that they share the same hedonic value. This basic affective tone can be said to have its origin in the experience of the infant playing within an interaction with its mother, thus producing a pleasant movement of increasing-decreasing tension—this tension being the content of a transmodal presymbolic experience of the intersubjective field (for an analysis of this kind of process, see Stern, 1985). The point at stake is the following: while I am typing and working on ideas that I am trying to make meaningful, obviously I am in a functional relationship with the concepts and the mediating devices - I am engaged with a discrete activity, dealing with specific object. *Yet, at the same time I am living the experience of mother-infant playing*.[25]

In conclusion, the affective context is embedded in the course of sense-making, conveyed and reproduced moment by moment by ongoing acts of meaning. Obviously, persons are usually somehow able to differentiate, to place constraints on generalization. In so doing, they generally succeed in focusing their attitudes and evaluation on the specific objects to a certain extent. Nevertheless, this does not mean that the affective contextual meaning disappears. Rather, the differentiation adds a further source-level to sense-making, but it does not cancel the salience of the affective context.

CONCLUSION

In the previous pages we have proposed a view of the affects grounded on psychoanalytic thought. Our model of the affects has taken various aspects into consideration, as they have been elaborated by different streams of psychodynamic and psychological theory (e.g., object relations theory, theory of coinems, interpersonal psychoanalysis, Matte Blanco's bi-logic theory). We have tried to integrate them in a concept of the affects as the basic semiotic process that constitutes the intersubjective dynamics of sense-making. For this purpose, we have taken as central the fundamental Freudian intuition, namely that the unconscious is something different from and beyond unawareness, being a specific way the mind works – what he called the primary process. The primary process (rather than the unconscious) is what Freud considered his fundamental discovery. Following Matte Blanco's logical formulation of the notion, the primary process is the homogenising and generalising activity of the mind, blind to any kind of difference among signs. Accordingly, affects can be defined as the modality of sense-making within which the primary process dominates over the complementary function of introducing differentiation—that is, of the secondary process. Reading the affects in terms of semiosis shaped by the primary process has allowed us to highlight some aspects characterizing the subjective and social phenomenology of the affects—namely their reifying, generalizing, absolutizing, anthropomorphizing, homogenizing valences (that can be partially retrieved in the emotions and in emotional acting). We have thus provided a view of affective semiosis as the dialogic-semiotic transformation of the flow of experience into a global, generalized and homogenized mental object, endowed with an inherently anthropomorphic addressivity, signified in terms of embodied meaning (e.g., pleasure–displeasure). We have called this mental object affective context, proposing that it be considered the basic, prereflexive assumption orienting people's way of giving sense to their intersubjective fields. Affective semiosis, therefore, represents a fundamental dynamics of sense-making, grounding, orienting and constraining the way people use signs in thinking and communicating.

In sum, in this chapter, we have tried to develop the psycho-cultural view of sense-making by taking into account the psychoanalytic lesson concerning the role affects play in personal and intersubjective feeling, thinking, dialoguing and acting. Nevertheless, before concluding, it is worth at least noting that the dialogue is not only unidirectional—also psychoanalytic theory has something to gain from the encounter with cultural psychology. As a matter of fact, the semiotic and dialogical view of sense-making provided by cultural psychology represents a promising source of development for psychoanalytic thought. As we have said above, psychoanalytic thought seems to be caught in a dilemma: to keep itself within a static, individualist conception of meaning, in order to preserve the specificity of the unconscious, or to renounce such specificity in order to grasp the dialogical nature of sense-making. As we hope our discussion has showed, our dynamic, contextual and dialogic approach to sense-making provides a theoretical framework that enables psychoanalytic theory to be re-thought in one of its central topics—the concept of affects. Moving ahead in this direction is one of the results we would like to achieve with this work.

NOTES

1. Valsiner (2007)'s model of the recursive differentiation of the field of experience highlights the latter point in an efficient way. In his semiotic reframing of sociocultural psychology the author underlines how objects of experience are the emerging products of a process of symbolic generalization transforming the shapeless flow of occurrences into complex signs, that is, into fields of signification by means of which people are enabled to grasp the "fuzzy, always floating personal experience—intra-psychological and inter-psychological" (Valsiner, 2007, p. 47; see also Valsiner, 2001). Symbolic generalization performs such a function by allowing the transfer of the value of a given object of the experience onto other objects, in so doing creating a symbolic equivalence between the elements thus becoming part of the field of meanings.
2. The latter consideration echoes Vygotsky (1934/1986)'s distinction between sense and meaning. The Russian author defines "sense" as the "totality of the psychological events aroused in our consciousness by the word," and "meaning" as "only one of the zones of sense that word acquires in the context of some kind of speaking" (p. 305, as translated by Valsiner, 2001, p. 89). Hence, Vygotsky thinks that sense and meaning are not immanent properties of the sign, but something that the sign gains in the interaction with the subject ("aroused in our consciousness") and—as regards the meaning—in the contingence of a circumstance of speaking ("... word acquires in the context of some kind of speaking"). This calls for the dynamic mutuality of these two processes to be addressed.
3. As Rommetveit (1992) highlights, "ordinary language provides us with culturally transmitted draft of contracts for categorization of states of affairs within a multifaceted 'Leibenswelt'..." (p. 23). These drafts offer different "options with respect to perspectives on states of affairs entering human discourse [that are regulated according] to the range of possible human interests, commitments and concerns with respect to those states of affairs" (p. 23).
4. Freud has proposed two "topographical" models of the psyche: the "first topography" (from 1900) sees the psyche as organized into unconscious, preconscious and conscious parts; the "second topography"(from 1920) identified the Ego and the Id.
5. In psychoanalytic terminology the term "object" is used as a generic term to mean the piece of the world the subject relates with. Therefore, the object can be a person as well as any other content of experience.
6. The generative capability of the affect is consistent with the fact that Melanie Klein conceives them as a very basic dimension working according

to the primary process. And the primary process is unable to make distinctions between the self and the object (see below). Consequently, every state of the self is experienced as a state of the undifferentiated self-world totality.

7. In so doing, Fornari goes beyond the Kleinian semiotic use of the notion of drive, radically freeing the psychoanalytic theory of this notion (substituted by a reference to linguistics and semiotics). Actually, this change of reference cannot be considered an absolute necessity. As a matter of fact, the concept of drive is not as surpassed, and its validity is not as dubious as it is often pictured. Various psychoanalysts have proposed a revision of it, in order to make it more consistent with the contemporary knowledge produced in biology and neuroscience. For instance, Kernberg (1990) (cf. Stein, 1991) has defined drive as a hierarchical system of affects, thus reversing the traditional Freudian idea of the affect as a derivative of the drive. Moreover, other authors have set out to reconceptualize the drive in terms of motive (Lichtenberg, 1989). In these approaches, the reference to the concept of drive generally entails a functionalist vision of the mind (i.e., the mind as a mechanism to be explained in terms of causes and/or goals). Therefore, despite the path of integration between drive and meaning proposed by Klein, contemporary psychoanalytical approaches referring to the concept of drive (inter alia, Brenner, 1973, 2002; Busch, 1993) are quite far from a semiotic vision of the psychological process.
8. This is for example evident in the way Fornari (1983) reconceptualizes the method of free association. The author highlights how, according to the traditional mode of using free association, what the patient says after having recounted a dream, in answer to the therapist's request to freely saying what is passing through his mind, is conceived of as a content of the unconscious connected to the images of the dream. On this basis, the content of the free association is very often used as the signified of the dream, the latter considered as the signifier. For example, if the patient says he has dreamt of a policeman getting angry with him, and afterwards, when asked by the therapist to freely associate, says that the day before he had been shouted at by his father, then the therapist would interpret that the policeman is the signifier of the father. Fornari highlights how this way of using the free association contradicts the primary process principle, because it assumes a structural difference between the patient's account of the dream—treated as a signifier—and the following statement produced in regime of free association—treated as signified. If one does not make such a distinction, in so doing keeping the "primariness" of the dreaming activity, then one cannot but assume everything said by the patient as signifiers, whose combination has to be interpreted.
9. Storolow and colleagues (2001/2006) define the unconscious as the affective dynamics that the subject subtracts from the intersubjective communication, because she/he feels incompatible with the regulation of the relationship. Typically, such a definition condenses the two previous criticisms: it is merely descriptive and negative (unconscious as what-is-kept-not-expressed); it entails the reference to a function of directionality—the unconscious does something in order to avoid overcoming a state of incompatibility. Note that this definition of the unconscious

is germane to the conceptualisation of the psychoanalytic notion of repression proposed by Billig (1999, 2003) within the frame of discursive psychology.

10. "In 1915 and in 1923, in the first and second topographical theories, affects were placed in a system and were seen not only as springing from the drives but also as being activated by the ego as well, being regarded as inner perceptions (...). They were seen as unmediated inner perceptions, more primordial and influential than external perceptions and more commensurate in intensity and quality to inner bodily processes (...)" (Stein, 1991, pp. 32–33).
11. The idea of the affects as embodied, unmediated and unreflexive connotation of experience forms a bridge between the psychoanalytic theory and the phenomenological vision of the situated and embodied nature of experience (De Leo, 2009; Ziemke, Zlatev & Frank, 2007). According to this standpoint, affects can be interpreted as the basic way of shaping experience, or more, of knowing the world—the individual unfolds through and in the terms of her/his body, that is in terms of hedonic basic values consciously or unconsciously experienced (positive vs. negative, exciting vs. relaxing). Being in the world is inherent to the body and is lived in/through the body. The affects are the first way the subject experiences the "lived" body embedded in and shaped by the world. Therefore, feeling the body and its movements is ipso facto the experience of the world. This idea is clearly expressed by Green (1973, p. 221) when he speaks of the affects as the glaze on the moved body.
12. "The fact that the classes are differentiated from one another means that there are asymmetrical relations which differentiate them. Viewed in this light, a class, if and when the principle of symmetry rules, can be considered a portion of "symmetrical being" surrounded by a layer or skin of asymmetry. As the mind and the unconscious deal with various classes, we can say that there are as many "bags" of symmetry surrounded by films of symmetry as there are classes in our unconscious." (Matte Blanco, 1975, p. 104)
13. This statement can be maintained even though one assumes a sociopragmatic and situated vision of sense-making, as we do. From this perspective the code is not an abstract a priori normative model. Rather it is embedded within the use of the signs itself (Wittgenstein, 1953/1958). This means that the significance of a sign ultimately consists of—and is provided by—the way of combining it with other signs. On the other hand, the possibilities of combination are constrained, and these constraints—which are what indeed defines the significance of the sign—even though they are not rigidly fixed, are however stable (at least in a given temporal range). For instance, the probability of combining the signifiers "dog" and "gallop" in an utterance as "The dog gallops" is quite low.
14. This characteristic has been highlighted by the Freudian conceptualization of over-determination of the symptom and more generally of oniric symbolism (Freud 1900/1953; see Cabell & Valsiner, 2011).

15. To use the terminology of linguistics, affective semiosis entails an inversion of the relationship between subject and predicate. It is not the subject that logically precedes the predicate (as happens on the asymmetrical level, where the predicate follows the subject, adding something not-yet-given to the latter). Rather, it is the predicate that precedes and produces the subject.
16. The feeling—what we can make correspond to the naïve term "emotion"—is not affective semiosis, which according to our thesis follows the rule of the primary process, for which it cannot be exhaustively represented by conscious thought. Nevertheless, feeling is one of the domains of human life—together with dream and delusion—where the clues of the symmetric quality of affective semiosis are clearer. For this reason here and later we sometimes refer to emotional experience in our examples.
17. This consideration means that the affective semiosis keeps its inherent dialogicity also when instead of an external dialogue performed by two or more people engaged in a communicative exchange, there is one person producing her/his idiosyncratic chain of signs sustaining an inner dialogue. This is consistent with the dialogical theory stating the intersubjectivity of thinking as well as of perception (Linell, 2009).
18. This does not mean that this vision has to have a representational format that is a declarative content that is reflexively conscious to the persons. Moreover, the sharedness of the assumption among the persons not necessarily—indeed rarely—is the result of an explicit negotiation (we address this topic in the final section)
19. "Ordinary language provides us with culturally transmitted drafts of contracts for categorization of states of affairs within a multifaceted 'Leibenswelt' (…) [Yet these drafts offer different] options with respect to perspectives on states of affairs entering human discourse [that are regulated according] to the range of possible human interests, commitments and concerns with respect to those states of affairs" (Rommetveit, 1992, p. 23).
20. In saying this we do not imply a logical and/or temporal separation between the system of assumptions sustaining the vision of the communicational exchange and the practice of this exchange—that is, the specific interpretation of the dialogical occurrences. Rather, the assumptions are activated and reflect the history of the intersubjective field, and are in circular linkage with the contingent acts of dialogue. In the final analysis, the assumptions are the products of the sedimentation of the previous acts of dialogue. At the same time, the assumptions active in a given moment regulate the acts of that moment. And through those acts and their consequences the assumptions reproduce and consolidate or change and are accommodated. In sum, the fact that the system of assumptions performs a regulative function on the participation of the people in dialogue does not necessarily mean a static idea of these assumptions, as if they came from the outside. Rather, we maintain a dynamic and situated idea of them as interwoven with the process that at the same time they regulate, emerging from them (for a similar approach, see Bickhard, 2009; Christopher &

Bickhard, 2007). The concept of symmetrical hierarchy discussed by Valsiner (2007, 2009) is consistent with the vision just proposed.

21. We are led to think that our definition of context is consistent with Bartlett's interpretation of the notion of "schema," stressing the active, embedded, systemic and dynamic nature of the concept: "I strongly dislike the term 'schema.' It is at once too definite and too sketchy. The word is already widely used in controversial psychological writing to refer generally to any rather vaguely outlined theory. It suggests some persistent, but fragmentary, 'form of arrangement,' and it does not indicate what is very essential to the whole notion, that the organized mass results of past changes of position and posture are actively doing something all the time; are, so to speak, carried along with us, complete, though developing, from moment to moment. Yet, it is certainly very difficult to think of any better single descriptive word to cover the facts involved. It would probably be best to speak of "active, developing patterns"; but the word "pattern," too, being now very widely and variously employed, has its own difficulties; and it, like "schema," suggests a greater articulation of detail than is normally found. I think probably the term "organized setting" approximates most closely and clearly to the notion required. I shall, however, continue to use the term "schema" when it seems best to do so, but I will attempt to define its application more narrowly. "Schema" refers to an active organization of past reactions, or of past experiences, which must always be supposed to be operating in any well-adapted organic response. That is, whenever there is any order or regularity of behavior, a particular response is possible only because it is related to other similar responses which have been serially organized, yet which operate, not simply as individual members coming one after another, but as a unitary mass. Determination by schemata is the most fundamental of all the ways in which we can be influenced by reactions and experiences which occurred sometime in the past. All incoming impulses of a certain kind, or mode, go together to build up an active, organized setting: visual, auditory, various types of cutaneous impulses and the like, at a relatively low level; all the experiences connected by a common interest: in sport, in literature, history, art, science, philosophy and so on, on a higher level. There is not the slightest reason, however, to suppose that each set of incoming impulses, each new group of experiences persists as an isolated member of some passive patchwork. They have to be regarded as constituents of living, momentary settings belonging to the organism, or to whatever parts of the organism are concerned in making a response of a given kind, and not as a number of individual events somehow strung together and stored within the organism. Suppose I am making a stroke in a quick game, such as tennis or cricket. How I make the stroke depends on the relating of certain new experiences, most of them visual, to other immediately preceding visual experiences and to my posture, or balance of postures, at the moment. The latter, the balance of postures, is a result of a whole series of earlier movements, in which the last movement before the stroke is played has a predominant function. When I make the stroke I do not, as a matter of fact, produce

something absolutely new, and I never merely repeat something old. The stroke is literally manufactured out of the living visual and postural "schemata" of the moment and their interrelations. I may say, I may think that I reproduce exactly a series of text-book movements, but demonstrably I do not; just as, under other circumstances, I may say and think that I reproduce exactly some isolated event which I want to remember, and again demonstrably I do not." (Bartlett, 1932, pp. 201–203).

22. In a similar way, one of the present authors has been involved in depicting the context as the attractor of the intersubjective dynamic of sense-making (Salvatore, Tebaldi & Poti, 2006/2009).
23. This movement is carried out in situations of both external and inner dialogue.
24. It is worth noticing that conceiving the affective context as ubiquitous means that it it cannot be thought of as a kind of structural obstacle/limit of sense-making, as associating them with the situations with strong emotional implication might suggest—on the other hand this vision of the affects as the enemies of thinking is typical of the naïve vision of the emotions. Rather, according to our thesis, the affective context has an essential, constructive role in sense-making that it performs in a constant way.
25. Accordingly the symmetric principle, it is meaningless to decide whether I am living it as the infant or as the mother. The context is the sense of the intersubjective field as a whole.

REFERENCES

Alvarez, A. (1992). *Live company. Psychoanalytical psychotherapy with autistic, borderlines and abandoned children.* London/New York: Tavistock/Routledge.

Austin, J. (1962). *How to do things with words.* Oxford: Oxford University Press.

Bakhtin, M. M. (1981). *The dialogic imagination: Four essays.* (M. Holquist, Ed.; C. Emerson & M. Holquist, Trans.). Austin, TX/London: University of Texas Press. (Original work published 1975; Written during 1930s).

Bakhtin, M. M. (1986). *Speech genres and other late essays.* (Vern W. McGee, Trans.). Austin, TX: University of Texas Press.

Bartlett, F. C. (1932). *Remembering: A study in experimental and social psychology.* Cambridge: Cambridge University Press.

Bickhard, M. H. (2009). Interactivism: A Manifesto. *New Ideas in Psychology, 27,* 85–89.

Billig, M. (1999). *Freudian repression. Conversation creating the unconscious.* Cambridge, MA: Harvard University Press.

Billig, M. (2003). Studying repression in a changing world. *European Journal of School Psychology, 1*(1), 37–42.

Bion, W. R. (1962). *Learning from experience.* London: William Heinemann.

Bowlby, J. (1961). Process of mourning. *International Journal of Psycho-Analysis, 42,* 317–340.

Brenner, C. (1973). *An elementary textbook of psychoanalysis.* New York: International Universities Press.

Brenner, C. (2002). Conflict, compromise formation, and structural theory. *The Psychoanalytic Quarterly, 71*(3), 397–417.

Breuer, J., & Freud, S. (1955). On the psychical mechanism of hysterical phenomena: Preliminary communication. In J. Strachey (Ed. and Trans.), *The standard edition of the complete psychological works of Sigmund Freud* (Vol. 2, pp. 1–18). London: The Hogarth Press and the Institute of Psycho-analysis. (Original work published 1893).

Bucci, W. (1997). *Psychoanalysis and cognitive science*. New York: Guildford Press.

Busch, F. (1993). "In the neighborhood": Aspects of a good interpretation and a "developmental lag" in ego psychology. *The Journal of the American Psychoanalytic Association, 41*, 151–177.

Cabell, K., & Valsiner, J. (2011). Affective hypergeneralization: learning from psychoanalysis. In S. Salvatore & T. Zittoun (Eds.), *Cultural psychology and psychoanalysis. Pathways to synthesis* (pp. 87–113). Charlotte, NC: Info Age Publishing.

Carli, R., & Giovagnoli, F. (2011). A cultural approach to clinical psychology. Psychoanalysis and analysis of the demand. In S. Salvatore & T. Zittoun (Eds.), *Cultural psychology and psychoanalysis. Pathways to synthesis* (pp. 117–150). Charlotte, NC: Info Age Publishing.

Carli, R., & Paniccia, R. M.. (2002). *L'Analisi Emozionale del Testo: Uno strumento psicologico per leggere testi e discorsi [The Emotional Textual Analysis. A tool for reading texts and discourses]*. Milano: Franco Angeli.

Carli., R., & Paniccia, R. M. (2003). *L'Analisi della domanda: Teoria e tecnica dell'intervento in psicologia clinica [Analysis of demand. Theory and technique of the intervention in clinical psychology]*. Bologna, IT: Il Mulino.

Christopher, J. C., & Bickhard, M. (2007). Culture, self and identity. Interactivist contributions to a metatheory for cultural psychology. *Culture & Psychology, 13*(3), 259–295.

Damasio, A. R. (1999). *The feeling of what happens. Body and emotion in the making of consciousness*. Orlando, FL: Harcourt.

De Leo, D. (2009). Intersubjectivity as co-phenomenology: From the Holism of meaning to the being-in-the-world-with-others. *Integrative Psychological and Behavioral Science, 43*(1), 78–83.

Eagle, M. N. (1987). The psychoanalytic and the cognitive unconscious. In R. Stern (Ed.), *Theories of the unconscious and theories of the self* (pp. 155–189). Hillsdale, NJ: The Analytic Press Inc.

Eco, U. (1975). *A theory of semiotic*. Bloomington: Indiana University Press.

Ekman, P., & Rosenberg, E. L. (2005). *What the face reveals: Basic and applied studies of spontaneous expression using the facial action coding system (FACS)* (2nd ed.). New York: Oxford University Press.

Ellenberger, H. F. (1970). *The discovery of the unconsious. The history and evolution of dynamic psychiatry*. New York: Basic Books.

Epstein, S. (1998). Cognitive-experiential self-theory: A dual-process personality theory with implication for diagnosis and psychotherapy. In R. F. Bornstein & J. M. Masling (Eds.), *Empirical perspectives on the pschoanalytic unconscious* (pp. 99–140). Washington, DC: American Psychological Association.

Erdelyi, M. H. (1985). *Psychoanalysis: Freud's cognitive psychology*. New York: Freeman and Co.

Ferro, A. (2003). *Il lavoro clinico [The Clinical Work]*. Milano: Raffaello Cortina Editore.

Fonagy, P., Gergely, G., Jurist, E., & Target, M. (2005). *Affect regulation, mentalization and the development of the self*. London: Other Press LLC.

Fornari, F. (1979). *I fondamenti di una teoria psicoanalitica del linguaggio [Foundations for a Psychoanalytic Theory of the Language]*. Torino, IT: Boringhieri.

Fornari, F. (1981). *Il codice vivente [The Living Code]*. Torino, IT: Bollati Boringhieri.

Fornari, F. (1983). *La lezione freudiana [Freud's Lesson]*. Milano: Feltrinelli.

Freud, S. (1950). Project for a scientific psychology. In J. Strachey (Ed. and Trans.), *The standard edition of the complete psychological works of Sigmund Freud* (Vol. 1, pp. 281–391). London: The Hogarth Press and the Institute of Psycho-analysis. (Original work published 1895)

Freud, S. (1953). The Interpretation of Dreams. In J. Strachey (Ed. and Trans.), *The standard edition of the complete psychological works of Sigmund Freud* (Vols. 4–5). London: The Hogarth Press and the Institute of Psycho-analysis. (Original work published 1900)

Freud, S. (1957). Instincts and their vicissitudes. In J. Strachey (Ed. and Trans.), *The standard edition of the complete psychological works of Sigmund Freud* (Vol. 14, pp. 109–140). London: The Hogarth Press and the Institute of Psycho-analysis. (Original work published 1915)

Freud, S. (1959). Inhibitions, symptoms and anxiety. In J. Strachey (Ed. and Trans.), *The standard edition of the complete psychological works of Sigmund Freud* (Vol. 20, pp. 75–176). London: The Hogarth Press and the Institute of Psycho-analysis. (Original work published 1926)

Freud, S. (1964). New introductory lectures on psycho-analysis. In J. Strachey (Ed. and Trans.), *The standard edition of the complete psychological works of Sigmund Freud* (Vol. 22, pp. 1–182). London: The Hogarth Press and the Institute of Psycho-analysis. (Original work published 1933[1932])

Giannakoulas, A. (1984). I fondamenti di una teoria psicoanalitica del linguaggio: By Franco Fornari.Turin: Boringhieri. 1980, p. 392. *International Journal of Psycho-Analysis, 65*, 218–221.

Gill, M. (1994). *Psychoanalysis in transition*. New Jersey: Hillsdale.

Green, A. (1973). *Le discours vivant: la conception psychanalytique de l'affect* [*Living discourse: The psychoanalytic conception of affects*]. Paris: Presses universitaires de France.

Green, A. (2005). *Key ideas for a contemporary psychoanalysis: Misrecognition and recognition of the unconscious* (Andrew Weller, Trans.). London: Routledge (Original work published 2002)

Greenberg, J. R., & Mitchell, S. A (1983). *Object relations in psychoanalytic theory*. Cambridge, MA: Harvard University Press.

Grossen, M., & Perret-Clermont, A. (1992). *L'Espace thérapeutique [The therapeutic space]*. Lausanne: Delachaux & Niestle.

Harré, R., & Gillett, G. (1994). *The discursive mind*. London: Sage.

Heine, S. (2008). *Cultural psychology*. New York: W. W. Norton & Company, Inc.

Hoffman, I. Z. (1998). *Ritual and spontaneity in the psychoanalytic process*. Hillsdale, NJ: The Analytic Press Inc.

Johnson-Laird, P. N. (1983). *Mental models. Towards a cognitive science of language, inference, and consciousness*. Cambridge, MA: Harvard University Press.

Kernberg, O. F. (1990). New perspectives in psychoanalytic affect theory. In R. Plutchik & H. Kellerman (Eds.), *Emotion: theory, research, and experience* (pp.115–131). New York: Academic Press.

Klein, G. S. (1976). *Psychoanalytic theory: An exploration of essentials* (M. M. Gill & L. Goldberger, Eds.). New York: International Universities Press.

Klein, M. (1967). *Contribution to psychoanalysis, 1921–1945*. New York: Mac Graw-Hill.

Klein, M., Heimann, P., & Money-Kyrle, R. (Eds.). (1955). *New direction in psychoanalysis*. London: Tavistock Publication Ltd.

Klein, N. (1999). *No logo, taking aim at the brand bullies*. New York: Picador.

Lazarus, R. S. (1991). Cognition and motivation in emotion. *American Psychologist, 46*(4), 352–267.

LeDoux, J. E. (1996). *The emotional brain*. New York: Simon & Schuster.

Lichtenberg, J. D. (1989). *Psychoanalysis and motivation*. Hillsdale NJ: Analytic Press.

Linell, P. (2009). *Rethinking language, mind and world dialogically. Interactional and contextual theories of sense-making*. Charlotte, NC: Information Age Publishing.

Marková, I. (2005). *Dialogicality and social representations: The dynamics of mind*. Cambridge: Cambridge University Press.

Marková, I., Linell, P., Grossen, M., & Salazar Orvig, A. (2007). *Dialogue in focus groups. Exploring socially shared knowledge*. London/Oakville: Equinox.

Matte Blanco, I. (1975). *The unconscious as infinite sets. An essays in bi-logic*. London: Gerald Duckworth and Company Ltd.

Matte Bon, F. (1999). Lingua, analisi della lingua e bi-logica [Language, analysis of language and bi-logic]. In P. Bria & F. Oneroso. *L'inconscio antinmico. Sviluppi e prospettive dell'opera di Matte Blanco* (pp. 88–132). Milano: Franco Angeli.

Maturana, M. R., & Varela, J. F. (1980). *Autopoiesis and cognition. The realization of the living*. Dordrecht, Holland: Reidel Publishing Company.

Mitchell, S. A. (1988). *Relational concepts in psychoanalysis. An Integration*. Cambridge, MA: Harvard University Press.

Mitchell, S. A., & Aron, L. (Eds., 1999). *Relational psychoanalysis. The emergence of a tradition*. Hillsdale, NJ: The Analytic Press Inc.

Modell, A. H. (1984). *Psychoanalysis in a new context*. New York: International Universities Press.

Nightingale, D. J., & Cromby, J. (Eds., 1999). *Social constructionist psychology. A critical analysis of theory and practice*. Buckingam: Open University Press.

Noy, P. (1982). A revision of the psychoanalytic theory of primary process. *International Journal of Psycho-Analysis*, 50, 155–178.

Odgen, T. (2004). The Analytic Third. Implications for Psychoanalytic Theory and Technique. *The Psychoanalytic Quarterly*, *73*(1), 167–204.

Peirce, C. S. (1932). *Collected papers of Charles Sanders Peirce* (C. Hartshorne & P. Weiss, Eds.) (Vol. 2). Cambridge, MA: Harvard University Press (Original work published 1897).

Pine, F. (1988). The four psychologies of psychoanalysis and their place in clinical work. *The Journal of the American Psychoanalytic Association, 36*, 571–596.

Rapaport, D. (1960). *The structure of psychoanalytic theory. A systematizing attempt*. New York: International Universities Press.

Ratner, C. (1994). The unconscious: A perspective from sociohistorical psychology. *The Journal of Mind and Behavior, 15*(4), 323–342.

Ratner, C. (2008). Cultural psychology and qualitative methodology: Scientific and political considerations. *Culture & Psychology, 14*(3), 259–288.

Rayner, E. (1995). *Unconscious logic. An introduction to Matte Blanco's bi-logic and its uses.* Hove and New York: Brunner-Routledge Taylor and Francis Group.

Rommetveit, R. (1992). Outlines of a dialogically based social-cognitive approach to human cognition and communication. In A. H. Wold (Ed.), *The dialogical alternative towards a theory of language and mind* (pp. 19–44). Oslo: Scandinavian University Press.

Rosa, A. (2007). Act of psyche. In J. Valsiner & A. Rosa (Eds.), *The Cambridge Handbook of Sociocultural Psychology* (pp. 205–237). Cambridge: Cambridge University Press.

Salvatore, S., Forges Davanzati, G., Potì, S. & Ruggeri, R. (2009), Mainstream Economics and sensemaking, *Integrative Psychological and Behavioral Science, 43*(2), 158–177.

Salvatore, S., Ligorio, M. B., & De Franchis, C. (2005). Does psychoanalytic theory have anything to say on learning?. *European Journal of School Psychology, 3*(1), 101–126.

Salvatore, S., & Pagano, P. (2005). Issues of cultural analysis. *Culture and Psychology, 11*(1), 159–180.

Salvatore, S., Tebaldi, C., & Poti, S. (2009). The discursive dynamics of sensemaking. In S. Salvatore, J. Valsiner, S. Strout & J. Clegg (Eds.), *YIS: Yearbook of Idiographic Science 2008-Volume 1* (39–72). Rome: Firera Publishing. First published 2006, in *International Journal of Idiographic Science* [On Line Journal], Article 3. Retrieved from http://www.valsiner.com/articles/salvatore.htm.

Salvatore, S., & Venuleo, C. (2008). Understanding the role of emotion in sensemaking. A semiotic psychoanalytic oriented. *Integrative Journal of Psychological and Behavioral Science, 42*(1), 32–46.

Salvatore, S., & Venuleo, C. (2010). The unconscious as source of sense: A psychodynamic approach to meaning. In B. Wagoner (Ed.), *Symbolic transformation. The mind in movement through culture and society* (59–74). London: Routledge.

Sandler, J., & Sandler, A.-M. (1978). On the development of object reletionships and affects. *International Journal of Psycho-Analysis, 59*, 285–296.

Sanford, A. J. (1987). *The mind of man. Models of human understanding*. London: Harvester Wheatsheaf.

Saussure, F. de. (1977). *Course in general linguistics* (W. Baskin, Trans.). Glasgow, UK: Fontana/Collins. (Original work published 1916)

Schachter, S., & Singer, J. (1962). Cognitive, social, and physiological determinants of emotional state. *Psychological Review,69*(5), 379–399.

Segal, H. (1991). *Dream, fantasy and art.* London/New York: Tavistock/Routledge.

Singer, J. L. (1998). Daydreams, the stream of consciousness, and self-representation, in R. F. Bornstein, & J. M. Masling (Eds.), *Empirical perspectives on the psychoanalytic unconscious* (pp. 141–186). Washington, DC: American Psychological Association.

Stein, R. (1991). *Psychoanalytic thoeries of affect.* London: Karnac Books.

Stern, D. N. (1985). *The interpersonal world of the infant.* New York: Basic Books.

Stolorow, R. D., Orange, D. M., & Atwood, G. E. (2006). World horizons. A post-Cartesian alternative to the Freudian unconscious. In A. Cooper (Ed.), *Contemporary psychoanalysis in America. leading analists present their work* (pp. 671–689). Washington DC: American Psychoatric Publishing, Inc. [First published 2001: *Contemporary Psychoanalysis, 37*(1), 43–61].

Sullivan, H. S. (1953). *The interpersonal theory of psychiatry*. New York: W. W. Norton & Company, Inc.

Tisseron, S. (2006). *La Honte : Psychanalyse d'un lien social* [The shame: Psychoanalysis of the social linkage] (2nd ed.). Paris: Dunod.

Tomkins, S. S. (1970). Affect as the primary motivational system. In M. B. Arnold (Ed.), *Feelings and emotions* (pp. 101–110). New York: Academic Press.

Valsiner, J. (2001). Processes structure of semiotic mediaton in human development. *Human Development, 44*, 84–97.

Valsiner, J. (2007). *Culture in minds and societies: Foundations of cultural psychology*. New Delhi: Sage.

Valsiner, J. (2009). Integrating psychology within the globalizing world: A *requiem* to the post-modernist experiment with *Wissenschaft*. *Integrative Psychological and Behavioral Science, 43*(1), 1–21.

Valsiner, J., & Rosa, A. (Eds.). (2007). *The Cambridge handbook of sociocultural psychology*. Cambridge: Cambridge University Press.

Visetti, Y. M., & Cadiot, P. (2002). Instability and theory of semantic forms. Starting from the case of prepositions. In S. Feigenbaum & D. Kurzon (Eds.), *Prepositions in their syntactic, semantic and pragmatic context* (pp. 9–39). Amsterdam: John Benjamins.

Vygotsky, L. S. (1986). *Thought and language*. (A. Kozulin, Ed.) (p. 287). Cambridge, MA: MIT Press. (Russian original work published 1934).

Wallerstein, R. S. (2000). Psychoanalytic research: where do we disagree?. In J. S. Sandler, & A.-M. Davies (Ed.), *Clinical and observational psychoanalytic research: roots of a controversy* (pp. 28–31). Madison, CT: International Universities Press.

Weiss, J., Sampson, H., & Mount Zion Psychotherapy Research Group (1986). *The psychoanalytic process. theory, clinical observations, and empirical research*. New York: The Guilford Press.

Winnicott, D. W. (2001). *Playing and reality*. Philadelphia/Sussex: Routledge. (Original work published 1971)

Wittgenstein, L. (1958). *Philosophical Investigations* (2nd ed.). Oxford: Basil Blackwell (German original work published 1953).

Ziemke, T., Zlatev, J., & Frank, R. R. (Eds.). (2007). *Body, language and mind. Embodiment, Vol. 1*. Berlin: Mounton De Gruyte.

Zittoun, T. (2006). *Transitions. Development through symbolic resources*. Charlotte, NC: Information Age Publishing.

PART II

HISTORICAL AND THEORETICAL DIALOGUES

CHAPTER 2

TATYANA ON THE COUCH: THE VICISSITUDES OF PSYCHOANALYSIS IN RUSSIA

René Van der Veer

THE ENCULTURATION OF THEORIES

Psychoanalysis as a doctrine and a worldview has known better times. Although still popular in countries such as France and Argentina, it is now deemed unsatisfactory and even unscientific by many psychologists and psychiatrists all over the world. Books and articles critical of Freud's ideas have appeared in great quantities (e.g., Cioffi, 1998; Eysenck, 1985; Grünbaum, 1986, 1993; Masson, 1985). Experts have called into question psychoanalysis' empirical foundation and testability, its theoretical consistency, and its potency as a psychotherapy. Other psychotherapies, such as cognitive behavior therapy, have taken over its prominent place in clinical practice. In sum, in academia psychoanalysis has lost much of the popularity that it still enjoyed in the first part of the previous century.

The fact that psychoanalysis as a dominant theory along with psychotherapy survives in some countries and not in others points to the fact that the reception of a new theory in a country always depends on the existing

Cultural Psychology and Psychoanalysis: Pathways to Synthesis, pp. 49–65

background culture in that country. Both the general public and the scientific experts may hold ideas that are somehow compatible with the new theory, they may feel that the new theory forms a significant improvement on existing theories, or, on the contrary, they may be under the spell of a rival theory, or may simply find the tenets of the new theory unacceptable. And even if a theory becomes accepted, it may be changed in the process. Different recipient countries may appropriate different variants of the same theory depending on their needs and preferences. On this account, there is no difference with the reception of foreign world views, religions, etc. within a recipient culture. For example, the popularity of some variant of Vygotsky's cultural-historical theory—a variant without any emphasis on his Marxist ideas—in the United States has been attributed to the fact that cultural-historical theory filled a gap which Piagetian theory had left open, that is, supposedly, Vygotsky's ideas were particularly welcome because they showed that individual cognition was socially determined in contrast to Piaget's allegedly solipsistic ideas on that account. Of course, such judgments are only temporary—one may only gradually realize that existing theories are unsatisfactory—which means that the acceptance of a rival theory is critically dependent on the point in time when it appears.

This whole dynamic situation may be illustrated for the fate of Freudian theory at different times and different locations (e.g., Plotkin, 2001, 2003, Roudinesco, 1994) and Piaget's terms of accommodation and assimilation come to mind to conceptualize the whole process. In this chapter, I will sketch a brief history of the reception of psychoanalysis in Russia. On the basis of the still growing literature (e.g., Angelini, 1988; Etkind, 1994a; Fischer, Fisher, Otto & Rothe, 2002; Kätzel, 1987; Marti, 1976; Miller, 1998; Pollock, 1982; Roudinesco, 1994; Van der Veer, 2000a; Van der Veer & Valsiner, 1991; Wharton & Ovcharenko, 1999; Young, 1979), I will describe how Freud's theory and therapy first fell on fertile soil in the Russian empire, then gained momentum during the first years of the Soviet reign, and finally fell into disgrace in the mid-1920s. The Soviet case is somewhat special, because of the strong intervention of the communist regime in scientific affairs, but I believe that the history of the rise and demise of psychoanalysis in the Soviet Union is of more general relevance. Similar histories can be and have been written for other countries and other scientific theories or worldviews (cf. Van der Veer, 1999, 2008).

THE RECEPTION OF PSYCHOANALYSIS: THE PIONEERS

Practically from its inception psychoanalysis was favorably received in Tsarist Russia. Etkind (1993, 1994a, 1994b, 1997) has provided an admirable analysis of the general intellectual climate of that time. He pictures a historical era where artists, poets, writers, philosophers, medical doctors and other intellectuals were fascinated by the hidden world behind apparent reality and devoured the ideas of Henri Bergson, Friedrich Nietzsche, and Rudolf Steiner. Indeed, for some time Steiner's anthroposophy and Freudian psychoanalysis were regarded as rival philosophies. Psychoanalytic ideas were picked up easily and rapidly (cf. Von Wiren-Garczynski, 1967, 1973; Zoshchenko, 1973, 1984), also because many Russian students[1] at the time studied at prominent universities in Germany, Austria, and Switzerland. To be sure, Freud's emphasis on sexuality was considered exaggerated sometimes—this was called Freud's pansexualism—and other psychodynamic figures (Adler, Bernheim, Janet, Jung) became popular in Russia as well. Also, Russian doctors kept relying on hypnosis as a therapeutic mean after Freud had discarded this method. So one could perhaps say that a Russified version of psychoanalysis (with the use of hypnosis and less emphasis on sexuality) gradually developed.

Several of the early students who studied psychoanalysis abroad became prominent figures in the Russian or international psychoanalytic movement. For example, Max Eitingon, Ivan Ermakov, Nikolay Osipov, Tatiana Rosenthal, Sabina Spielrein, and Moshe Wulff were almost all personally acquainted with or underwent analysis by Freud, Jung, or Karl Abraham. With the exception of Eitingon, they all returned to Russia and became instrumental in spreading psychodynamic ideas in their country of origin. A brief account of the careers of these pioneers can clarify the Russian involvement in the early psychoanalytic movement.

Max Eitingon (1881–1943) studied medicine in Leipzig and became intern at the *Burghölzli Hospital* near Zurich. In 1907, the head of the clinic Egon Bleuler, sent him with a patient to Freud in Vienna. Eitingon underwent a training analysis with Freud and they became close friends. Eitingon finished his PhD under the supervision of Jung and moved to Berlin, where he married an actress of the *Moscow Art Theatre*. Over the years, Eitingon published on psychoanalytic themes (e.g., Eitingon, 1912, 1914, 1915) but his reputation is primarily based on his work as an important organizer and administrator for the international psychoanalytic movement. He founded the *Berlin Psychoanalytic Outpatient Clinic*, led the *Internationaler Psychoanalytischer Verlag*, was the president of *The Psychoanalytical Association*, founder and president of the *International Training Committee*, and so on (Jones, 1943). He left for Israel in 1933 and was accused of being a Soviet spy for the NKVD in 1938 and again in 1988, four decades after his death (cf. Draper, 1988).

Ivan Ermakov (1875–1942) was a medical doctor and became director of the *Psychiatric Clinic of Moscow University* in 1911 when his colleagues Osipov and Serbsky resigned. His papers attracted interest in psychoanalysis from about 1913 (Etkind, 1994a, 1994b). When the *Russian Psychoanalytic*

Society was founded in 1922, Ermakov became its president. He was primarily interested in the psychoanalytic interpretation of the creative process (e.g., Ermakov, 1923, 1924), about which he taught courses at the *Psychoanalytic Institute*. He was a driving force behind the *Psychological and Psychoanalytic Library*, which in the 1920s published translations of Freud's books (see below) and several of his own books. Unlike Osipov, he accepted the new regime and tried to make the best of it. He was arrested in 1940 and died two years later (Young, 1979).

Nikolai Osipov (1877–1934) studied medicine at five different German and Swiss universities and returned to Russia in 1904 to work as a psychiatrist in the *Psychiatric Clinic of Moscow University* under the supervision of Vladimir Serbsky. He then learned about psychoanalysis and from 1908, he began publishing psychoanalytic case histories in the *Zhurnal Nevropatologii i psikhiatrii im. S.S. Korsakova*. In 1909, with O. B. Feltsman, he created a book series, called the *Psychotherapeutic Library*, which was to publish translations of books by Freud and his followers (Miller, 1998, p. 34). In 1910, he made a trip to Vienna and met Freud, with whom he kept corresponding over the next decades. Back in Moscow he founded an outpatient clinic at Moscow University where he treated his patients in the psychoanalytic fashion. With Vyrubov, Osipov began a new journal, *Psikhoterapiya*, which primarily published psychodynamic writings. Adler's Russian wife, Raisa Timofeevna, was among those who regularly published in the journal (Etkind, 1994a, 1994b). In 1911, Vyrubov and Osipov also founded the *Moscow Psychoanalytic Society* with Osipov as its president (Fischer et al., 2002). In 1911, Osipov and his colleagues resigned at the university as a sign of protest against the Minister of Education's attempts to curb the autonomy of the universities (Etkind, 1993, p. 211) but retained his private practice. Under the chairmanship of Serbsky, he and his colleagues also kept meeting on Fridays to discuss their patients. After the October Revolution, Osipov fled to the south and eventually left the country to end up in Prague. He there became head of the outpatient clinic of the university and was instrumental in creating Czech style psychoanalysis. He died of a heart disease in Prague in 1934.

Moshe Wulff (1878–1971) studied medicine in Berlin and worked under Karl Abraham. He joined the *Vienna Psychoanalytic Society* in 1911 but returned to his birth town Odessa in that same year. After World War I, he moved to Moscow and with Ermakov founded the *Moscow Psychoanalytic Society* in 1922. Wulff worked as a psychoanalyst at the *Second Medical Clinic of Moscow University*, translated Freud into Russian, and participated in founding the *Detskyj Dom* (see below). He was elected as president of the *Russian Institute for Psychoanalysis* in 1924, which was closed several months later, and left the Soviet Union in 1927 for Berlin and, eventually, after the Nazis came to power in 1933, for Israel. He there founded with Max Eitingon the *Psychoanalytic Society of Palestine* (cf. Wulff, 1912, 1932, 1941).

Tatiana Rosenthal (1885–1921) studied with Jung at the *Burghölzli Hospital* and subsequently became a member of the *Vienna Psychoanalytic Society* and the *Berlin Psychoanalytic Society* (Neiditsch, 1921). She returned to St. Petersburg in 1911 to work at Bekhterev's *Brain Institute* as a neurologist. Bekhterev himself never became converted to psychoanalysis—he was more interested in the phenomena of suggestion and hypnosis (Van der Veer, 2002), which Freud had left behind—but he allowed Rosenthal to treat neurotic patients at the outpatient clinic of his *Brain Institute* with psychoanalysis, and appointed Rosenthal as the head of this clinic. Like several other psychoanalysts, Rosenthal was interested in the psychology of art. Among other things, she published a paper in which she tried to explain Dostoevsky's creative writing from his personal sufferings (Rosenthal, 1919). Rosenthal believed the doctrines of Marx and Freud could be profitably combined, but may have become disillusioned by the course of events in communist Russia. For unknown reasons, she committed suicide in 1921 (Marti, 1976).

Sabina Spielrein (1885–1942) studied medicine at *Burghözli Hospital* in 1904–1905. From 1904 to 1911, she maintained a close personal relationship with her dissertation supervisor and training analyst Carl Jung about which much has been written (Carotenuto, 1982). She returned to the Soviet Union in 1923 and first worked in Moscow at the *Detskyj Dom* (see below) with Vera Schmidt and others. Later on she moved to Rostov-on-the-Don, where she and her family were killed by the Nazi troops. Spielrein is now recognized as the originator of the concept of the death instinct or thanatos (e.g., Spielrein, 1912).

Finally, Vera Schmidt, née Yanitskaya (1899–1937), was a pedagogue by training who married Otto Schmidt, a mathematician and prominent figure in Soviet science. Otto Schmidt (1891–1956) was the leader of several polar expeditions, a vice-president of the *Academy of Science*, and eventually a hero of the USSR discussed in school textbooks. He was also in various periods a member of the *People's Commissariat for Education (Narkompros)*, chief-editor of the *Great Soviet Encyclopedia*, and the director of the *State Publishing House*. In that latter function, he and Vera Schmidt published Ermakov's book series *The Psychological and Psychoanalytical Library*. In 1922, *Narkompros* established the *Russian Psychoanalytic Society* in Moscow with Ermakov as president. Other members were Blonsky, Luria, Kannabikh, Shatsky, and Wulff. Otto Schmidt was the vice-president of the *Moscow Analytical Society* and the *Psychoanalytical Institute*, headed by Ermakov, and head of the *Detskyj Dom* (*Children's Home*), established in the Summer of 1921. The *Psychoanalytical Institute* and the *Children's Home* were housed in the same building. The *Children's Home* was run by Vera Schmidt, together with Wulff, Spielrein (from 1923), and others. It was essentially a psychoanalytic home for the young children (2–4 years old) of the Party nomenklatura, who had no time or inkling how to raise their children. For several reasons (see below) the

Children's Home was closed down in August 1925. Vera Schmidt still managed to publish an account of the project in German (Schmidt, 1924; but afterwards was forced to leave psychoanalysis and began working at the *Institute of Defectology* under the supervision of Vygotsky in 1929. She died of thyroid cancer during the great purge (cf. Van der Veer & Valsiner, 1991).

THE RECEPTION OF PSYCHOANALYSIS: STATE SUPPORT

The work of the pioneers was interrupted by World War 1 and the October Revolution of 1917. Little is known of this hectic period, whether individuals taught psychoanalytic theory or practiced psychoanalytic therapy, but it is certain that after the communists came to power psychoanalysis as a doctrine became quickly visible again. Of course, now the circumstances had fundamentally changed: the regime did not tolerate world views that it regarded as hostile or unhealthy and scientific disciplines now became dependent upon state approval. Some psychoanalysts (e.g., Osipov) did not accept such state interference and left the country but this was relatively rare. Typically, researchers tried to compromise and argue that psychoanalysis either complemented the prescribed Marxist world view or that it somehow coincided with the ideas of Marx, Hegel, and Lenin (cf. Kornilov, 1925). For a while it seemed that such a strategy might work. Indeed, the psychoanalytic movement gained strength and obviously enjoyed state support in the early 1920s. This support became visible in the establishment of the *Russian Psychoanalytic Society*, the *Children's Home*, the *Psychoanalytic Institute*, and the book series *The Psychological and Psychoanalytical Library*. These institutions were funded by the state and subject to its rules. The *Psychoanalytic Institute* and the *Children's Home*, for example, were supposed to cary out scientific research and offer academic courses satisfying certain standards set up and checked by state committees.

The *Russian Psychoanalytic Society* emerged from a fusion of the *Moscow Psychoanalytic Society* and its counterpart in Kazan, which was founded and led by Alexander Luria (1902–1977). The Kazan group consisted of some 15 people, mostly medical doctors and psychologists, of whom Boris Fridman and Rosa Averbukh moved with Luria to Moscow (Van der Veer & Valsiner, 1991). The Moscow group functioned for several years with Luria as its scientific secretary. Among the speakers were Ermakov, Luria, the Schmidts, and Vygotsky. In 1927, Luria resigned as secretary and was replaced by Vera Schmidt. In a climate of increasing criticism of psychoanalysis, the society ceased to exist somewhere around 1930 (Van der Veer & Valsiner, 1991).

As has been said above, the *Children's Home* was essentially a psychoanalytically oriented home for the young children of high Party officials. As such it was unique not just in the Soviet Union but in the world at large. At first an elaborate staff took care of 10–20 children. The personnel also observed the children and took notes,[2] which were to lead to scientific reports about child development. The idea was that the children should lead a life free of bourgeois conventions and follow the inclinations belonging to the psychosexual stage they were in. Thus, children in the anal stage were allowed to play with their feces and children in the genital stage were not discouraged from autostimulation. In order to overcome their prejudices as to these behaviors, the women of the staff followed an obligatory psychoanalytic training where they learned "not to transfer their own complexes to the children" (Osipov, 1922).

The fact that the *Children's Home* was also to function as a research institute led to its first problems. In 1923, an official report judged that the children were treated satisfactorily, that interesting observations had been made, but that no real systematic scientific work was being done (Etkind, 1994b, p. 196). This judgment seriously endangered the existence of the *Children's Home*, but Narkompros chaired by Lunacharsky decided to give the home one more year and to install a committee that would give recommendations to improve its work. This committee reached very favorable conclusions that were accepted by Narkompros, which guaranteed the *Children's Home* existence for some time. After this first crisis had been overcome, Otto and Vera Schmidt made a trip to Vienna and Berlin and met Freud, Abraham, and Rank. It seemed that Freud and his colleagues were very pleased to learn about the *Children's Home* project. However, in July 1924, there was a second crisis: part of the staff, including Vera Schmidt, declared they could not continue working as they lacked sufficient training to cope with the transference phenomena they met. Again, an investigating committee was appointed which reached the conclusion that training of the personnel was indeed needed. In November 1924, Otto Schmidt withdrew his support, Ermakov was replaced by Wulff, part of the personnel was fired, and organizationally the home was separated from the *Psychoanalytical Institute*. In practice, this meant that the home had lost its foothold in the highest circles and had become much more vulnerable to criticism. Rumors about the liberal sexual atmosphere in the home had been around for some time and now it was decided to appoint yet another investigating committee. In January 1925, this committee, chaired by the pedagogue Pinkevitch, observed that the majority of children practiced masturbation and in August of that same year Narkompros liquidated both the *Children's Home* and the *Psychoanalytical Institute*.

THE RECEPTION OF PSYCHOANALYSIS: DEMISE OF THE MOVEMENT

The *Psychoanalytical Institute*, the *Children's Home* and the *Psychological and Psychoanalytical Library* would never have seen the light and existed for several years without support from influential persons in the communist regime. Persons very high in the Communist Party, such as the Schmidts and Stalin, had a child in the *Children's Home*. Otto Schmidt was closely involved with Narkompros and knew such persons as Lunacharsky and Krupskaya intimately. Obviously, then, for some time the Party top was either neutral or positive about the psychoanalytical movement. Etkind (1994) has argued that the great supporter and invisible defender of psychoanalysis in Russia was Leon Trotsky (1879–1940) and that when Trotsky eventually ran into trouble, psychoanalysis lost its support in the Party. Indeed, Trotsky was sympathetic of psychoanalysis—various of his friends and acquaintances had seemingly benefited from psychoanalytic therapy—and had his own ideas about how to combine psychoanalysis with other findings to create a new view of human beings. In 1923, Trotsky—then still a prominent Bolshevik leader and member of the Politburo—wrote a letter to Ivan Pavlov to propose a mixture of conditional reflex theory and psychoanalysis to which Pavlov did not reply (Etkind, 1994, pp. 227–229). Later, he may have been influential in toning down the conclusions of committees who investigated the *Children's Home*. After an internal struggle for power, in November 1927 Trotsky was expelled from the Communist Party and in February 1929 he was forced to leave the Soviet Union. Etkind (1994) has argued that these dates corresponded with, respectively, Wulff's departure for Berlin and Luria's resignation as scientific secretary of the *Russian Psychoanalytic Society* (see above, previous section) and the virtual disappearance of Russian Freudians.

CRITIQUE OF PSYCHOANALYSIS: VOLOSHINOV AND VYGOTSKY

Articles and chapters critical of psychoanalysis began appearing in the Soviet scientific press from about 1924. At the time, the proponents of psychoanalytic theory (e.g., Luria, Zalkind) emphasized the compatibility of Freud's ideas with those of various so-called objective psychologies (e.g., Pavlov's or Bekhterev's reflexology, or American behaviorism). In other words, in their view psychoanalysis offered an objective, biological view of the mind that might be reconciled with the Marxist world view. These so-called Freudo-Marxist theories now came under fire, however. Much has been written about the debate that followed (e.g., Etkind, 1994, Miller, 1985, 1986, 1990, 1998; Van der Veer & Valsiner, 1991) and it can be safely concluded that the only serious criticism of the Freudo-Marxist theories came from Voloshinov (1895–1936), on the one hand, and Vygotsky (1896–1934), on the other.

Voloshinov[3] first move was to argue that psychoanalysis was irreconcilable with Marxism, because its core ideas and method were not objective. The subjects' behavior is not explained by such objective, observable factors as his class, nation, or historical period but by a-historical, a-cultural biological drives. As Voloshinov (1927/1976; 1927/1983, p. 13) wrote: "[For Freud] man's consciousness is determined not by his historical, but by his biological being, the most important part of which is sexuality." One might argue that biological forces and drives belong to the realm of objective facts but according to Voloshinov Freud's biology was based on sheer speculation and the introspective accounts of nervous patients. No attempt was made to situate these hypothetical constructions (e.g., the erogenous zones, the subdivisions of personality) in real physiology or neurology. The whole edifice therefore rested upon the quicksand of introspection and childhood memories of doubtful reliability. In Voloshinov's view, this made Freudian theory akin to the theories of philosophers of life like Bergson, Simmel, and Scheler, who also allegedly undervalued objective biological and socioeconomic factors.

The psychoanalytic method was largely that of introspection: the patient recounts his childhood memories, relates his dreams, and talks in free association. Freud believed that this introspection offered the therapist a unique insight into the patient's intimate inner world. The therapist as it were reveals a world so far inaccessible even to the patient himself. Against this view, Voloshinov argued that introspective utterances are governed by the same rules as other utterances and belong to the social realm. Both "the vaguest idea, even if unspoken, and the most complex philosophical movement equally presuppose the organized communication between individuals" (Voloshinov, 1927/1983, p. 42). That viewpoint implies that we are not dealing with absolutely private experiences of the individual. Freud's mistake was to project the complex relationship between patient and doctor into the patient's mind and regard them as forces in a psychodynamic struggle. However, both conscious and supposedly unconscious commentaries (e.g., in free association) reflect the social situation of communication, of speaking to another person. We cannot step outside this situation and pretend to find private "biological" forces on the basis of these social utterances. As Voloshinov (1927/1983, p. 175) argued: "Experiencing myself, I attempt as it were to look at myself through the eyes of the other person, the other representatives of my social group, my class." The point is, according to Voloshinov, that utterances about both public events and private experiences belong to an ongoing social dialogue. We are always commenting upon our own behavior in terms of our own culture and our most private behavior is constrained by sociocultural rules couched in language.[4] In a characteristic statement that came very close to what Vygotsky wrote at approximately the same time, Voloshinov concluded that "we shall never reach the genuine essential roots of a specific single utterance if we only look for it within the confines of the isolated individual organism, even when the utterance concerns the apparently most personal, intimate aspects of the person's life" (Voloshinov, 1929/1972, p. 174).

By realizing that the patient's utterances are genuinely social and part of the dialogue with the therapist, we avoid positing events of a different epistemological status: for instance, real childhood events, the patient's false memories of them, the therapist's true reconstruction of them, and so on. In reality, what we have are just the patient's and the therapist's different accounts. The therapist tries to persuade the patient to adopt a certain interpretation of events or course of action but there is no need to posit hypothetical entities such as id, ego, and superego. "These utterances are not expressions of the patient's individual psyche. What is reflected in them is not the dynamics of the individual psyche but the social dynamics of the interrelationships between doctor and patient. Here is the source for that dramatism which marks the Freudian construct.... Here indeed, people, not natural forces, are in conflict" (cf. Clark & Holquist, 1984, p. 180). There are no "unconscious forces" which "explain" behavior, the verbal utterances interpreted as "unconscious" are part of behavior itself. It is fully justified to doubt the subject's comments upon his behavior, as do Freudians; they cannot explain it but neither can Freud's unconscious motives qua verbal utterances.

Because our private and introspective comments upon our own behavior—including the comments that Freud saw as originating in the unconscious—are always consciously made in our own language they actually belong to consciousness. What Freud saw as the unconscious are just conscious comments that cannot easily be shared with others. In a way, then, there exists an "unofficial consciousness" whose language is inner speech and an "official consciousness" that makes use of outward speech, but both are thoroughly social. In a "healthy collective," Voloshinov posited, the unofficial and official consciousness might coincide but not so in bourgeois society.

Add to these comments that Voloshinov considered psychoanalysts to form some sort of a sect impervious for criticism and not willing to enter the scientific debate with other psychological theories and we understand that for Voloshinov psychoanalytic theory was no more than a subjective fantastic construction that could in no way be reconciled with the "scientific" world view of Marxism nor with objective biological theories. Moreover, the psychoanalytic attempt to find "primal scenes" and so forth in the patient's early childhood was no more than a projection into the past of current adult bourgeois obsessions.

Just like Voloshinov, Vygotsky began his career as a literary scholar; the first 10 years of his academic career he devoted the analysis of works of art such as novels and plays. Like Volshinov, he was much influenced by Russian formalist theories which stated that aesthetic effects are created by the conscious and skilled use of certain artistic devices. In his doctoral dissertation, Vygotsky (1925/1971) partially agreed with the formalists and argued that it is the artificially created conflict between content and form that created the artistic effect (Van der Veer, 2007). In that same dissertation, he criticized the rival theory of psychoanalysis. Freud himself and such Russian followers as Rosenthal and Ermakov (see above) had used psychoanalysis to explain works of art. Vygotsky granted psychoanalysts that we may have to go beyond conscious processes to understand art, because often neither the producer nor the consumer of artistic products fully grasps the way they evoke aesthetic feelings. But he disliked the idea of art as the sublimation of unconscious drives, namely that both the artist and the connoisseur are satisfying their primitive needs when creating or appreciating works of art. In that conception, the function of artistic form is no more masking their latent (sexual) content, just like the widely varying manifest form of dreams hides their surprisingly monotonous primitive content.

> Communism and totem, the church and Dostoyevsky's creative work, occultism and advertising, myth and Leonardo da Vinci's inventions—it is all disguised and masked sex and sexuality, and that is all there is to it. (Vygotsky, 1926/1997, p. 245)

The problem with that conception is that the different forms and styles of art and their historic development are left without explanation. Why create different styles of writing when the real pleasure is in their hidden content? Works of art may have an unconscious core that is transformed into socially accepted forms but it is that transformation process that needs explaining. In other words, we cannot reduce psychological phenomena to primitive drives and thereby undervalue the conscious processes. Any distinction between the ravings of the madman and the cultural activity of the artist would become blurred. Freud's and Ermakov's explanations of the works of Michelangelo and Dostoevsky were utterly empty in the eyes of Vygotsky.

This is not to say that Vygotsky believed Freud's ideas to be utterly useless. He always had a soft spot for bold, speculative ideas and for a number of years he was active on the edges of the *Russian Psychoanalytic Society*. Together with Luria, he even wrote a preface to the Russian translation of Freud's *Beyond the pleasure principle* in which he praised Freud for his vertiginous ideas such as the concept of the death instinct. Regardless of its factual correctness, this hypothesis—which originated in the work of Spielrein as we have seen—should be valued for its "extraordinary courage and originality" (Vygotsky & Luria, 1925/1994, p. 15). Asking the right questions and advancing new hypotheses were as valuable for Vygotsky as finding answers and empirical verification.

However, with Voloshinov, Vygotsky was very critical of the attempts to combine or merge psychoanalysis with the findings of Pavlov's reflexology or with the tenets of Marxism. In his opinion, such a combination could only be the result of brainless eclecticism. His description of such attempts by his colleagues Luria (1925/2002) and Zalkind (2001) was quite sarcastic:

> We can multiply the number of citizens of Paraguay with the number of kilometers from the earth to the sun and divide the product by the average life span of the elephant and carry out the whole operation irreproachably, without a mistake in any number, and nevertheless the final outcome might mislead someone who is interested in the national income of this country. (Vygotsky, 1926/1994, p. 259)

Vygotsky ridiculed the attempt to fuse two theories, because they were "both scientific," or to combine parts of one theory with parts of another. We cannot leave pansexualism out of psychoanalysis, he argued, because the doctrine of pansexualism is its very core and dismissing it as irrelevant would be like creating "Christianity without Christ" (Vygotsky, 1926/1994, p. 261). What was needed in his view was a careful examination of the core assumptions and basic methods of psychoanalysis to lay bare its fundamental nature, its implicit system. We may then be able to translate certain basic Freudian ideas into our own concepts and verify them with our own methodology. This Vygotsky regarded as the only acceptable way to annex psychoanalysis for positive science. Its results were unclear, however, because Freud was at bottom a subjective thinker and philosophical idealist whose ideas were rooted in the works of such speculative thinkers as Schopenhauer and Lipps (Vygotsky, 1926/1994, p. 263).

TOWARDS A CULTURAL-HISTORICAL PSYCHOANALYSIS

As we have seen, the Soviet thinking about a possible combination of Marxism, positive science, and psychoanalysis came to a full stop in the late 1920s. Even six decades later the leading Soviet historian of psychology Petrovsky still concluded his discussion of Freud's ideas with the following words:

> The bourgeois's animal fear of social turmoil—his distrust of reason and consciousness—was embodied in Freud's theory about the dark unconscious

> forces that allegedly rule the human being from inside and make him into a helpless plaything of the uncontrollable forces of sex and death ... [Freud's doctrine was] the modernist apocalyptic religion of capitalist society. (Petrovsky, 1984, p. 111)

It is somewhat difficult to make complete sense of these two sentences—why would the bourgeois distrust reason? Why would he prefer a theory in which he is described as a plaything of dark forces?—but they made it abundantly clear that any further discussion of Freud's ideas and their compatibility with a Marxist world view was unwise.

That means that if we disregard the numerous non-Russian and post-Soviet attempts to develop Marxist variants of psychoanalysis (e.g., Althusser, Dowrick, Fenichel, Fromm, Kovel, Marcuse, Parker, Reich, Wolfenstein) we are left with the critical remarks of Voloshinov and Vygotsky which did not provide a detailed positive program from which to develop a Marxist, cultural-historically informed psychoanalytic theory. From these remarks we can infer several recommendations for a future cultural-historical psychoanalytic theory.

First, it is clear that the original psychoanalysis methodology left much to be desired. To the extent that Freud offered an account of development, it was largely based on the notoriously unreliable retrospective accounts of neurotic patients. Moreover, these accounts were substantially influenced by Freud's own preconceived ideas about this development. The careful verification and validation of such ideas has proved exceedingly difficult (cf. Grünbaum, 1993).

Second, we must address the hypothesis put forward by Voloshinov that Freud's proposed personality structure consisting of the id, ego, and super-ego is no more than a reification of prevalent motives in specific societies. That is, the supposedly strong urge to seek boundless sexual gratification, the strict social rules against it, and the ego's attempts to negotiate between them, may all be channeled and constrained by society. That would imply that Freud biologized specific (verbal) behaviors that vary by culture and historical era.

Third, we must dismiss the notion that the therapeutic conversation involves the search for some objective hidden truth. Therapy is not about repressed primal scenes and traumatic childhood experiences; it is about changing one's perspective on one's present situation and abilities. Language is a powerful means to establish such changes and it is the therapist who offers linguistic tools to the patient who may or may not accept them. What the psychoanalyst calls "insight" is the acceptance of a new conceptual framework.

Fourth, insofar as psychoanalysis turned into a world view it must tone down its aspirations. Psychoanalysis cannot explain war, the creation of artistic products, or the choice of a profession. Writing scientific chapters may be sublimating sexual or destructive energy—Popper would complain that this claim cannot be falsified—but it remains unclear why such chapters are written in different ways and why some are better than others.

These are only some of the questions that should be answered by a future cultural-historical psychoanalytic theory. It is unclear, however, whether this new theory will resemble classical psychoanalysis any more than a dog resembles the heavenly constellation of that same name (cf. Spinoza, 1677/1955, p. 6).[5]

NOTES

1. A remarkable portion of these students consisted of very able Jewish girls who subsequently left their trace in psychological history. One may think of Gita Birenbaum, Tamara Dembo, Maria Ovsiankina, and Bluma Zeigarnik, all of whom worked with Kurt Lewin in Berlin (cf. Van der Veer, 2000b), and Fanny Chalevsky, Esther Aptekmann, Rosa Averbukh, Tatiana Rosenthal, and Sabina Spielrein, who studied with Carl Jung in Zurich.
2. It has been said that Luria and Vygotsky drew on Vera Schmidt's findings in their scientific writings about children's play, drawing, and so on.
3. With several others, Valentin Voloshinov belonged to the circle of the famous linguist Mikhail Bakhtin (1895–1975). It has been conjectured that works bearing Voloshinov's name were actually written by Bakhtin. As we have no means to resolve this issue of authorship, we here consider Voloshinov to be the author of *Freudianism: A Marxist critique* (cf. Clark & Holquist, 1984).
4. Of course, nowadays our intimate private behavior is possibly more than ever culturally constrained by the countless models provided on the internet.
5. I have borrowed this reference to Spinoza's words from Vygotsky who used it several times in similar cases.

REFERENCES

Angelini, A. (1988). *La psicoanalisi in Russia: Dai precursori agli anni Trenta [Psychoanalysis in Russia. From the precursors to the Thirties]*. Napoli: Liguori Editori.

Carotenuto, A. (1982). *A secret symmetry: Sabina Spielrein between Jung and Freud*. New York, NY: Pantheon.

Cioffi, F. (1998). *Freud and the question of pseudoscience*. Chicago, IL: Open Court.

Clark, K., & Holquist, M. (1984). *Mikhail Bakhtin*. Cambridge, MA: The Belknap Press of Harvard University Press.

Draper, T. (1988). The mystery of Max Eitingon. *The New York Review of Books, 35*(6), 32–43.

Eitingon, M. (1912). Genie, talent und psychoanalyse [Genius, talent, and psychoanalysis]. *Zentralblatt für Psychoanalyse, 2*, 539–540.

Eitingon, M. (1914). Gott und Vater [God and father]. *Imago, 3*, 90–93.
Eitingon, M. (1915). Ein fall von Verlesen. [A case of misreading] *Internationale Zeitschrift für Psychoanalyse, 3*, 349–350.
Ermakov, I. D. (1923). *Etyudy po psikhologii tvorchestva A.S. Pushkina[Studies in the psychology of Pushkin's creativity]*. Moscow: Gosizdat.
Ermakov, I. D. (1924). *Ocherki po analizu tvorchestva N.V. Gogolya[Essays on the analysis of Gogol's creativity]*. Moscow: Gosizdat.
Etkind, A. M. (1993). *Eros nevozmozhnogo: Istoriya psikhoanaliza v Rossii [Eros of the impossible: The history of psychoanalysis in Russia]*. St. Petersburg: Meduza.
Etkind, A. M. (1994a). *Eros nevozmozhnogo: Razvitie psikhoanaliza v Rossii [Eros of the impossible: The development of psychoanalysis in Russia]*.Moscow: Gnozis-Progress-Kompleks.
Etkind, A. M. (1994b). How psychoanalysis was received in Russia, 1906–1936. *Journal of Analytical Psychology, 39*, 191–202.
Etkind, A. M. (1997). *Eros of the impossible: The history of psychoanalysis in Russia*. Boulder, CO: Westview Press.
Eysenck, H. (1985). *Decline and fall of the Freudian empire*. New York: Viking.
Fischer, E., Fischer, R., Otto, H. H., & Rothe, H. J. (2002). Nikolaj J. Ossipow: Le premier émigré politique dans l'histoire de la psychanalyse et sa correspondence avec Sigmund Freud pendant son exil à Prague [Nikolaj J. Ossipow: The first political immigrant of the history of psychoanalysis, and his correspondence with Sigmund Freud during his exile in Prague]. *Topique, 80*, 117–123.
Grünbaum, A. (1986). Précis of the foundations of psychoanalysis: A philosophical critique. *Behavioral and Brain Sciences, 9*, 217–284.
Grünbaum, A. (1993). *Validation in the clinical theory of psychoanalysis: A study in the philosophy of psychoanalysis*. Madison, CT: International Universities Press, Inc.
Jones, E. (1943). Max Eitingon (Obituary). *International Journal of Psycho-Analysis, 24*,190–192.
Kätzel, S. (1987). *Marxismus und psychoanalyse [Marxism and Psychoanalysis]*. Berlin: VEB Deutscher Verlag der Wissenschaften.
Luria, A.R. (2002). Psychoanalysis as a system of monistic psychology. *Journal of Russian and East European Psychology, 40*, 26–53 [Original work: Psikhoanaliz, kak sistema monisticheskoy psikhologii. In K. N. Kornilov (Ed.), *Psikhologiya i marksizm* (pp. 47–80). Leningrad: Gosudarstvennoe Izdatel'stvo, 1925].
Marti, J. (1976). La psychoanalyse en Russie et en Union Sovietique de 1909 à 1930 [Psychoanalysis in Russia and in Soviet Union from 1909 to 1930]. *Critique, 31*, 199–236.
Masson, J. M. (1985). *The assault on truth*. Harmondsworth, Mx: Penguin.
Menegaldo, H. (2004). La psychologie soviétique: Quelques jalons [Soviet psychology: Some highlights]. *Slavica Occitania, 18*, 39–60.
Menegaldo, H., & Breuillard, J. (2004). La psychanalyse russe prise aux mots [Russian psychoanalysis taken at its word]. *Slavica Occitania, 18*, 357–393.
Miller, M. A. (1985). Freudian theory under Bolshevik rule: The theoretical controversy during the 1920s. *Slavic Review, 44*, 625–646.
Miller, M. A. (1986). The origins and development of Russian psychoanalysis, 1909–1930. *Journal of the American Academy of Psychoanalysis, 14*, 125–135.
Miller, M. A. (1990). The reception of psychoanalysis and the problem of the unconscious in Russia. *Social Research, 57*, 875–888.

Miller, M. A. (1998). *Freud and the Bolsheviks: Psychoanalysis in imperial Russia and the Soviet Union*. New Haven: Yale University Press.

Neiditsch, S. (1921). Die Psychoanalyse in Russland während der letzen Jahre [Psychoanalysis in Russia in recent years], *Internationale Zeitschrift für ärtzliche Psychoanalyse*, 7, 381–85.

Petrovsky, A. V. (1984). Voprosy istorii i teorii psikhologii: Izbrannye trudy [Problems of the history and theory of psychology: Selected works]. Moscow: Pedagogika.

Plotkin, M. (2001). *Freud in the pampas: The emergence and development of a psychoanalytic culture in Argentina*. Stanford, CA: Stanford University Press.

Plotkin, M. (2003). *Argentina on the couch: Psychiatry, state, and society, 1880 to the present*. Albuquerque, NM: University of New Mexico Press.

Pollock, G. H. (1982). Psychoanalysis in Russia and the USSR, 1908–1979. *Annual of Psychoanalysis, 10*, 267–279.

Roudinesco, E. (1994). *Histoire de la psychanalyse en France. Vol. 1. 1885–1939 [History of psychoanalysis in France]*. Paris: Fayard.

Rosenthal, T. (1919). Stradanie i tvorchestvo Dostoevskogo [The suffering and creativity of Dostoevsky]. *Voprosy Izucheniya i Vospitaniya Lichnosti, 1*, 88–107.

Schmidt, V. (1924). *Psychoanalytische Erziehung in Sowjetrussland. Bericht über das Kinderheim-Laboratorium in Moskau [Psychoanalytic upbringing in Soviet Russia: Report about the nursery-laboratory in Moscow]*. Leipzig: Internazionaler Psychoanalytischer Verlag.

Spielrein, S. (1912). Die Destruktion als Ursache des Werdens [Destruction as the cause of coming into being]. *Jahrbuch, 4*, 465–503.

Spinoza, B. de (1955). *On the improvement of the understanding. The ethics. Correspondence*. New York: Dover. (R. H. M. Elwes, Trans.; Original work published 1677)

Van der Veer, R. (1999). Piaget in the plural: The story of his reception in Latin America. [review of B. Freitag (Ed.). *Piaget: 100 anos*. Sao Paulo: Cortez, 1997]. *Culture & Psychology, 5*, 217–222.

Van der Veer, R. (2000a). Iwan on the couch. Review of M.A. Miller, Freud and the Bolsheviks: Psychoanalysis in imperial Russia and the Soviet Union. *Journal of Modern History*, 72, 853–855.

Van der Veer, R. (2000b). Tamara Dembo's early years: Working with Lewin and Buytendijk. *Journal of the History of the Behavioral Sciences, 36*, 109–126.

Van der Veer, R. (2002). Bekhterev's social psychology. [Review of V.M. Bekhterev. *Suggestion and its role in social life*. New Brunswick NJ: Transaction]. *Mind, Culture, and Activity, 9*, 72–74.

Van der Veer, R. (2007). *Lev Vygotsky*. London: Continuum.

Van der Veer, R. (2008). The reception of Piaget's early ideas in the Soviet Union. In A. N. Perret-Clermont & J. M. Barrelelet (Eds.), *Jean Piaget and Neuchatel: The learner and the scholar* (pp. 167–185). London: Psychology Press.

Van der Veer, R., & Valsiner, J. (1991). *Understanding Vygotsky: A quest for synthesis*. Oxford: Blackwell.

Van der Veer, R., & Valsiner, J. (1994). *The Vygotsky reader*. Oxford: Blackwell.

Valsiner, J., & Van der Veer, R. (2000). *The social mind: Construction of the idea*. Cambridge, UK: Cambridge University Press.

Voloshinov, V. N. (1976). *Freudianism: A Marxist critique* (N. H. Bruss, Ed., I. R. Titunik, Trans.; final chapter omitted). New York, NY: Academic Press. (Original work published 1927)

Voloshinov, V. N. (1983). *Frejdizm: Kriticheskji ocherk [Freudianism: A critical essay]*. New York, NY: Chalidze Publications. (Original work published 1927)

Voloshinov, V. N. (1972). *Marksizm i filosofiya yazyka [Marxism and the philosophy of language]*. The Hague: Mouton. (Original work published 1929)

Von Wiren-Garczynski, V. (1967). Zoshchenko's psychological interests. *Slavic and Eastern European Journal, 11*, 3–22.

Von Wiren-Garczynski, V. (1973). Sud'ba Pered voskhodom solntsa: Freijd ili Pavlov [The fate of Before the Sunrise]. In Zoshchenko, M. (Ed.), *Pered voskhodom solntsa* (pp. 15–32). New York, NY: Izdatel'stvo Imeni Chekhova.

Vygotsky, L. S. (1971). *The psychology of art*. Cambridge, MA: The MIT Press. (Original work published 1925)

Vygotsky, L. S. (1997). The historical meaning of the crisis in psychology: A methodological investigation. In R. W. Rieber & J. Wollock (Eds.), *The collected works of L. S. Vygotsky. Vol. 3. Problems of the theory and history of psychology* (pp. 233–343). New York, NY: Plenum Press. (Original work published 1926)

Vygotsky, L. S., & Luria, A. R. (1994). Introduction to the Russian edition of Freud's Beyond the pleasure principle (pp. 10–18). In R. van der Veer & J. Valsiner (Eds.), *The Vygotsky reader*. Oxford: Blackwell. (Original work published 1925)

Wharton, C. J., & Ovcharenko, V. (1999). The history of Russian psychoanalysis and the problem of its periodisation. *Journal of Analytical Psychology, 44*, 341–352.

Wulff, M. (1912). Beitragen zur infantilen Sexualität [Contributions to childhood sexuality]. *Zentralblatt für Psychoanalyse, 2*, 6–17.

Wulff, M. (1932). Über einen interessanten oralen Symptomenkomplex und seine Beziehung zur Sucht [About an interesting oral syndrome and its relationship to alcoholism]. *Internationale Zeitschrift für Psychoanalyse, 18*, 283–302.

Wulff, M. (1941). The child's moral development. In K. R. Eissler (Ed.), *Searchlights on delinquency* (pp. 263–272). London: Imago.

Young, D. (1979). Ermakov and psychoanalytic criticism in Russia. *Slavic and East European Journal, 23*, 72–86.

Zalkind, A. (2001). *Pedologiya: Utopiya i real'nost' [Paedology: Utopia and reality]*. Moscow: Agraf.

Zoshchenko, M. (1973). *Pered voskhodom solntsa [Before the sunrise]*. New York, NY: Izdatel'stvo Imeni Chekhova.

Zoshchenko, M. (1984). *Youth restored*. Ann Arbor, MI: Ardis Publishers.

CHAPTER 3

FREUD AND CULTURAL PSYCHOLOGY

Tania Zittoun

This chapter fully assumes a sociocultural perspective, and proposes to reread the work of Sigmund Freud from this perspective. This position highlights how much Freud had a deep sense of humans as "being of culture." His enquiry has many more similarities with current enquiry than is usually admitted. I then explore some consequences of this proximity.

CULTURAL PSYCHOLOGY AND PSYCHOANALYSIS

Today, the field of cultural psychology is interested above all in how human life is enabled through, and by culture. Cultural psychology has its origin in the work of the Russian psychologist Lev Vygotsky, and in some other pragmatist authors, such as William James, Dewey and Charles Peirce, as well as German *Ganzheit* psychologists (Diriwaechter, 2004). It was introduced to North America and Europe through the works of Jerome Bruner (1990), Michael Cole (1996), James Wertsch (1998) and Jaan Valsiner (1998). This psychology can be said to examine the *person,* actively constructing meaning and sense; this person is embedded in his/her social and cultural

Cultural Psychology and Psychoanalysis: Pathways to Synthesis, pp. 67–85

environment; he/she changes through time; and as the environment is itself also changing, cultural psychology attempts to identify the transactions taking place between the person and the environment.

So what about Freud's work today? There have been debates on what constitutes the foundation of Freud's work: the attention he paid to unconscious processes, his theory of libido, his topology of mind, his death instinct, or his work announcing neurosciences.[1] Here I want to emphasise another, rarely discussed aspect of Freud's work: his underlying conception of the human person in its world of culture. Freud can be said to have developed a new approach to the human person, seen in all its uniqueness. On the one hand he attempted to account for the complexity and richness of human interior life—the sort of richness described by authors such as Shakespeare, Dostoyevsky, or Goethe. On the other hand, Freud was interested in the way in which a specific person deals with the constraints of shared reality, interprets daily events, and struggles to make free choices, on the basis of the history of her past interactions. And this is the reason I want to examine Freud's work here: the psychoanalysis he defined can be seen as an attempt to consider the person as a unique, changing, culturally situated individual, in all his/her richness and contradictions.

In that respect, cultural psychology and Freud's work can be seen as two approaches with a similar goal: accounting for the complexity of humans in their world of culture. However, cultural psychology and psychoanalysis develop different methods, examine very different observables, and have radically different theories. So what is the interest in examining the two approaches together?

I see two main reasons to propose such a reading. First, the evolutions of cultural psychology and psychoanalysis have often been intertwined and have enriched each other. Second, the two approaches share a deep theoretical assumption. Consequently, beyond their differences, the two traditions can enrich each other.

Historical Reasons

I will be very brief on the historical proximity of the two approaches. Firstly, historically, both cultural psychology and psychoanalysis can be seen as reactions to the dominant approaches to the human psyche.

Freud was trained as a medical doctor in Vienna, at the turn of the twentieth century. He was interested in neurology. He visited Charcot in France around 1885, where he encountered cases of hysteric people. Unsatisfied with both the treatment they received and the theorization of their symptoms, he was to develop his conceptions of repressed affects and representations that would constitute the basis of his theory of the unconscious.[2] Freud's model of mind differed radically from the theories of his time. On the one hand, it differed radically from medical science of his time. On the other hand, it also diverges from current German speaking psychology. European psychology was moving on one side towards a *Völkerpsychologie*, a sort of cultural anthropology, and on the other side, towards a physiological, behavioral experimental psychology. Freud seems never to have been very interested in these two lines of research. For example, according to Farr (1988), *Totem and Taboo* might have been seen as a reaction to Wundt's work in *Völkerpsychologie*. Also, he might have been led to define a "meta-psychology" to talk about the unconscious, because Wundt strongly stated that experimental psychology was studying only conscious processes.

One way to see the proximity between cultural psychology and psychoanalysis is therefore to see them as proposing alternatives to a dominant paradigm more or less at the same historical time. On the one hand, one of the origins of cultural psychology can be found in *Ganzheitpsychologie*, which happened to concur and object to the dominant *Völkerpsychologie* and experimental approaches that were dividing psychological life. On the other hand, the main roots of cultural psychology lie in the work of Vygotsky, who was also in opposition with some over positivistic approaches to the human psyche (Vygotsky, 1926/1997).

Another way is to examine the way in which Vygotsky—as one of the key figures in cultural psychology—was actually reading Freud. Vygotsky read Freud, and edited some translations of his texts; he quotes full sentences and ideas—often without mentioning their origins (Van der Veer & Valsiner, 1991). Sabine Spielrein, who personally knew Vygotsky, Freud and Piaget, might also have facilitated the circulation of ideas (Santiago-Delefosse & Delefosse, 2002). Vygotsky seems to have officially renounced Freud's ideas as being bourgeois and individualistic, yet many lines of that thinking remain in his work, even if they are not explicitly acknowledged as such.

Theoretical Reasons

The second reason to bring cultural psychology and psychoanalysis together is grounded in theory. Fundamentally, cultural psychology and psychoanalysis are theories assuming the semiotic mediation of mind and behavior (see also Salvatore, 2004, 2006). They consider that the development of the person requires the progressive acquisition of signs that enable the world where people live to be represented, distanced and created. Both of them also consider that culture can be transmitted through generations thanks to the objects and languages that encapsulate past people's experiences. In turn, these collective signs will become what constructs each person, in what is common to human beings, as well as in what makes each of us unique.

Of course, beyond this basic assumption about the nature of human life, cultural psychology and psychoanalysis have developed different methods and theories. As we know, they have also concentrated on different aspects of the phenomena involved; the facts thus examined and explained are quite incommensurable. As a result, the two approaches can usefully complement each other. Because of the logic of disciplines, some issues addressed by one approach have been forgotten by the other one. Bringing the two approaches together reveals the blindspots of each approach. For example, issues related to *conflicts* (see Zittoun, 2005), *nonverbal meaning-making*, *emotional* and embodied life, which are the daily bread of psychoanalysis, have been overlooked by cultural psychology. Psychoanalysis can thus play the role of a mirroring other in order to reflect the limits of cultural psychology (Gillespie, 2006), and invite it to develop its theory so as to address these issues in its own terms. For example, recent developments of cultural psychology thoroughly explore issues such as emotions and their transformations (Valsiner, 2007), ambivalence (Abbey & Valsiner, 2004) and conflict (Zittoun, 2005).

THEORETICAL CONTRIBUTIONS OF FREUD FOR A CULTURAL PSYCHOLOGY

In the rest of this paper, I will highlight Freud's view on culture, and then identify four themes in Freud's work which are all relevant for a cultural psychological enquiry. Some have been addressed by it, other still wait to be addressed.

I thus first examine how Freud understood the specificity of *man as a being of culture*. I do so by examining the text *Civilization and its discontent* (Freud, 1930/1961), which, in German, was called "*Das Unbehagen in der Kultur*" ("the uneasiness in culture"). Note then that in the Standard Edition, the notion of "Kultur" has been at times translated by "civilization" and at times by "culture." Hearing them both as translation of the term "Kultur," we see that Freud identifies three aspects of human culture:

1. Culture is the total sum of the realisation and settings through which our lives are distinct from these of animals and which have two goals: the protection of humankind against nature, and the regulation of human relationships. Here Freud includes agriculture, and the mastery of fire, and then all the tools, which extend the power of the human body: from microscopes to telephones and planes.
2. Culture includes useless things: playgrounds, flowers at windows — everything which has to do with order, cleanliness and aesthetics, which do not exist in nature; here, I assume we can include arts, poetry, literature, etc.

3. Culture finally includes higher mental functions (let us read "civilization" as "culture" as in the original edition and other translations):

> No feature, however, seems better to characterize civilization than its esteem and encouragement of man's higher activities—his intellectual, scientific, and artistic achievements—and the leading role that it assigns to ideas in human life. Foremost among those ideas are the religious systems, on whose complicated structure, I have endeavored to throw light elsewhere. Next come the speculations of philosophy; and finally what might be called man's "ideals"—his ideas of a possible perfection of individuals, or of peoples or of the whole of humanity, and the demands it sets up on the basis of such ideas. (Freud, 1961, p. 94).

Here, then, Freud considers culture as the mental representations, or mental mediations, through which people fix goals, support intentions, canalize goal-directed attention; human activity is thus understood as a hierarchic system of semiotic regulation, with some "higher mental behaviors" that channel or constrain lower ones.

Freud's work explores these three aspects of culture. Firstly, he examined the condition and the use of tools and rules which enable humans to survive and live together. We can see Freud's analysis of everyday tools and discourses as extensions of ourselves, for example, in *The Interpretation of Dreams* (Freud, 1900/1953), *The psychopathology of everyday life* (Freud, 1901/1960), *Jokes and their relation to the Unconscious* (Freud, 1905/1960). Secondly, Freud was an active "culture consumer"; he read literature, poetry, collected sculptures and antiquities. This is reflected in his work, where he examines specific cultural artifacts, such as novels, poems, sculptures, and so on, as cultural production, representing and crystallizing some aspects of the human condition. See for example, in *The Moses of Michelangelo* (Freud, 1914/1960), the *Delusion and dream in Jensen's Gradiva* (Freud, 1907/1959), his studies on Da Vinci, Dostoyevsky, etc. Thirdly, Freud follows political and social events closely. This is reflected in some of his writings, such as *Thomas Woodrow Wilson, Twenty-eighth President of the United States: A psychological study* (Freud & Bullitt, 1967). Complex symbolic and religious systems are examined in studies such as *Totem and taboo* (Freud, 1913/1955), *The Future of an Illusion* (Freud 1927/1961), *Civilization and its discontent* (Freud, 1930/1961), *Moses and the monotheism* (Freud, 1939/1964), etc.

This suggests that the work of Freud—the discovery of the unconscious, the analysis of the human person—is deeply rooted in analysis of cultural production, be these political and religious systems, works of art, or everyday action. I will now focus on Freud's understanding of humans as beings of culture. On the basis of these texts, I will explore four lines in Freud's work which, I will argue, correspond to four core questions in cultural psychology.

Freud and Cultural Tools

In cultural psychology, we speak about the "use of tools" to designate different sorts of mediation of human action and thinking. We say that computers, language or toys are tools for thinking. The notion of tool comes mostly from Vygotsky. We are often unaware, however, that Freud had a very interesting sense of the way objects, textiles, images, artworks, become part of our thinking and our emotions: as mentioned above, Freud problematized the question of material and symbolic objects as tools to extend our power over nature and to enable life in society. In his clinical work, Freud also seems to see objects as tools mediating some forms of thinking. Freud is very attentive to the objects mentioned by his patients when they tell him dreams or phobias. Freud identifies these objects, and reflects on their psychological function. He seems to ask, what meaning do they have for that person, what thinking or emotions do they convey? Here an example taken from the *Interpretation of Dreams* (chap. VI, section D, pp. 347–348, emphasis in original text):

> She was descending from a height over some strangely constructed palisades or fences, which were put together into large panels, and consisted of small squares of wattling. It was not intended for climbing over; she had trouble in finding a place to put her feet on and felt glad that her dress had not caught anywhere, so that she stayed respectable as she went along. She was holding a BIG BRANCH in her hand; actually, it as like a tree, covered with RED BLOSSOMS, branching and spreading out. There was an idea of their being cherry-BLOSSOMS; but they also looked like double CAMELLIAS, though of course those do not grow on trees. As she went down, first she had ONE, then suddenly TWO, and later again ONE. When she got down, the lower BLOSSOMS were already a good deal FADED.

Freud's commentary is identifying the reported objects: fences, flowers, branches, white, and red. He sees them as "hieroglyphs" that have two levels of meanings. At one level, there is an explicit meaning (a woman climbing a fence, etc.). At the other level, each of the objects, their perceptual qualities, and their geographical organization, designates other thoughts and emotions. To find them, Freud will ask the dreamer to freely associate around each of the objects mentioned in the dream. Through these associations, other webs of meaning will emerge; these constitute the "latent" discourse.

This latent discourse can be more or less dissimulated. One can dream about eating strawberries because one wants to eat strawberries. There can also be some formal correspondence between the object of the dream and some desired object—for example, a hat can represent the phallus. And sometimes the processes that link the objects of the dream to the objects of the thoughts are more complex. In this example, the association of the dreamer goes from the flower, that the dreamer identified as a camellia, to the paintings representing the Annunciation; yet the flowers are red, as in Alexandre Dumas' *Dame aux Camellia*. There is here the juxtaposition of ideas of virginity, and of menstruation—and to the end of purity, here the number of flowers referring to the number of her fiancés. Thus, Freud has a subtle theory of symbolization. Objects have the symbolic function of designating very complex ideas that are difficult to master. They have this function thanks to their double anchorage in culture and in individual life. Take the white flower. On one hand, it belongs to a complex culture, in which the flower is used by religious painting to represent virginity; on the other hand, each of us has been exposed to these flowers and someone has explained to us why it is so. Now every time we think about that flower we can at once mobilize this network of ideas, feelings, representation, etc. Thanks to their double cultural and personal anchorage, using objects for their symbolic function is thus a very economical tool for thinking.

This idea thus rejoins one of the core themes of cultural psychology: the importance of tools, objects and signs in mediating thinking and human action. It however proposes other routes for exploring how objects might convey parts of thinking. Cultural psychology focuses on complex artifacts or culturally constituted sign systems. Psychoanalysis calls our attention to trivial objects that can become important for a given person. It also tries to examine how objects from the environment can contain and convey some of a person's thoughts and emotions. Objects can thus convey feelings and thoughts, and by reflecting these to the person, can be part of new forms of understanding. The role of trivial objects in thinking and feeling has been explored in current psychoanalytical work (e.g., Tisseron, 1999) but not in cultural psychology.

The Constitution of Signs

If we examine objects as carrying parts of thinking, we are moving towards a theory of signification, or of semiotic mediation. In such fields, one question is at the heart of current research in developmental and cultural psychology. How it is that children start to use an object for another, a doll for a mother, a word for an internal state? How does the ability to use signs emerge, and thus the ability to use the white flower?

Freud proposes an explanation in the *Interpretation of Dreams*. He proposes an ontogenetic explanation for the emergence of thinking through signs, starting with a model of mind as a reflex apparatus—a stimulus-response structure. At a certain point, internal needs appear in the organism of the infant, causing an internal modification (e.g., the experience of hunger). To account for the fact that the hunger is perceived, one must postulate the existence of some intermediary between stimulus and response. Because of this internal modification, or need, the infant will be looking for satisfaction: she will make a noise or enter into a state of agitation. The mother, then, provides the child with some food (e.g., milk) which satisfies the need. The infant can now retain a perception of the satisfying object thus provided, and thus a mnesic trace of the object is united with the mnesic trace of the satisfaction of the need. Because of this mnesic trace, the need will now appear to the infant as a wish (for a certain satisfaction). The wish could be satisfied though the memory of the previous satisfaction, which would create a hallucinatory satisfaction (the real need, the hunger, is not satisfied by a memory of food). In contrast, the mother could acknowledge the need, and provide the child with an object to satisfy it. The real food would thus be united with the hallucinated food, the wish and the need would be satisfied at once. A sign is born here, at the meeting of wish and reality, thanks to the acknowledgement of the mother.

This might be now put into a triangle, the corners of which are the subject (the child), the other (the mother), and the object by which the mother satisfies the need she recognizes in her child. The mother recognizes and feels the needs of the child (and reciprocally), the object satisfies them; but as it becomes a sign, it re-presents these experiences. Then, the other replaces the object with a name or a sign, and the child learns to use the sign to act on the other to cause her to provide the object. This leads us to a second triangle, a subject-other-sign triangle. Finally, the subject is able to regulate him/herself thanks to signs, in a subject-sign-subject triangle (see Zittoun, Gillespie, Cornish & Psaltis, 2007).

Freud thus has a theory of the genesis of the ability to use signs or represent, a recurrent question of cultural approaches to development. We find a very similar structure in Vygotsky's account of the emergence of symbol in the early 30's (1978). It is only relatively recently that sociocultural approaches to development have proposed similar accounts elaborated through observational and experimental techniques (Nelson, 2007; Moro & Rodriguez, 2005), thus joining current development in cognitive-psychoanalytical research (Fonagy, Target, Gergely & Jurist, 2002). Such strong similarity in theorization might be seen as another call to examine possible contribution of psychoanalysis to cultural psychology.

A Theory of Art and Play

A third important issue in the modern study of humans in their world of culture is their relation to cultural artifacts and imaginary experiences, such as that enabled by computer games, virtual worlds, films and fiction. We painstakingly try to describe the specific nature of these experiences. One way to explain them is to see them as an extension of children's play. But in doing so, researchers have been often confronted with Piaget's (1951) rather negative judgement on imaginative play. To go beyond this, authors have rediscovered Vygotsky's analysis of children's play and the arts, and also Winnicott (1971/2001)'s idea of the transitional area. Yet, these two authors were drawing on Freud's accounts of play and the arts.

Freud developed some important insights into children's play, and as mentioned, has a huge interest in the visual arts, literature and cultural creation. In a text called *Creative writers and day-dreaming* (Freud, 1908/1959), Freud is interested in the poet and writer's work. He announces that he sees the origin of the artists' creation in child's play:

> Might we not say that every child at play behaves like a creative writer, in that he creates a world of his own, rather, rearranges the things of the world in a new way that pleases him? It would be wrong to think he does not take that world seriously; on the contrary, he takes his play very seriously and he expands large amounts of emotion on it. Then the opposite of play is not what is serious but what is real. (Freud 1908/1959, p.143–144)

Freud adds that the child knows perfectly well the difference between reality and the world of the play. The child uses objects coming from the material world and makes them enter his imaginative play-world; he then mobilizes affects coming from his inner life. We could say that the child deploys his inner life and emotions outside, on the scaffolding offered by the objects-in-the-play. Finally, the playing child satisfies needs, gains pleasures, and sometimes endures unpleasant experiences.

Freud will insist on the relationships between play and the elaboration of emotions. In *Beyond the pleasure principle* (Freud, 1920/1955), he develops the often-quoted example of the child playing with a spool tied to a string in the absence of his mother; he throws the object away in anger, and pulls the string to bring it back, saying alternatively "O-ooo," that Freud interprets as "Fort" (away), and A-a-a-a, understood as "Da" (here). Freud proposes two interpretations linking the play with the going-and-coming of the mother—the play itself is aimed at facilitating the child's acceptance of her departure, and simulating his desire for her to return (he plays happily at that moment). According to an initial hypothesis, the child moves from a passive attitude of suffering a painful abandonment to an active creation—he creates the object-mother's going away. In a second hypothesis, with that movement the child satisfies his aggressive drive against the mother (he throws her out).[3] On the basis of this text and

Freud's text on creation, we can say that play has mainly four emotional functions:

1. Child's play is guided by his desire "to be big and grown up. He is always playing at being 'grown up,' an in his games he imitates what he knows about the life of his elders" (1908/1959, p. 146)—it is related to socialization, and to the child's frustration of being excluded from the adult world.
2. Play is dream-like—it is a space to live and actualize fantasies.
3. In play, the child can live and experiment strong emotions that would find no room in real life, such as his aggressive feelings against the mother (here we are in a sort of "cathartic function");
4. In play, such as in the string example, an active manipulation and a repetition of a movement allow a progressive elaboration of painful experiences related to a human relationship (separation): it is active (vs. passive), and repetition allows a progressive assimilation, a "digestion," of the experience.

This fourth function has to be highlighted. Freud distinguishes between repeating past experiences, and remembering. One can only remember what has not been traumatic, what has been worked through—which is, related to images or representations that which can be symbolized, notably through language. Inversely, what is too strong emotionally, or too shameful to be digested will be repeated (Freud, 1914/1958): one re-enacts the same choices of object, identifications and actions, or one can become ill. This tendency to repeat would be the "death drive" in *Beyond the pleasure principle* (Freud, 1920/1955)—a sort of negative assimilation. Here, we see that it is possible to transform a repeatable item into one that can be remembered through play and active manipulation (in children and adults). Play allows the child to link and connect mnemonic traces and discontinuous images and emotions; it allows the transformation of something haunting primary process into secondary process, it facilitates a linking process.

So if there is some continuity between children's play and adult's cultural experiences, how are these described? In *Creative writers and daydreaming* (Freud, 1908/1959), Freud distinguishes between children and adults as follows. In play, the child actualizes and explores his fantasmatic life[4]; he does so overtly, publicly, without shame. For Freud, from adolescence on, the person learns to hide his/her imaginary life and impossible desires. He/she can live these out in her dreams and private fantasies. Only artists have the privilege, like children, to have direct access to their desires and the complexity of their self—and to share it consciously with others. This is what makes the richness of the experience for which they account. For example, in a classical novel, the writer shows us a representation of complex emotions and desires and of their dynamics. He acknowledges the complexity and the multiplicity of the parts of his psyche; he often represents and distributes these among the characters and all through the imaginary scenario.

Freud then emphasizes the reader's experience. Thanks to the writer's work and disposition, a reader has the possibility of living experience quite close to his own earlier, childhood play. In effect, knowing that this experience is "unreal," that it is offered by another (who takes the responsibility for it, with a public assessment), that it is still experienced in a private way, the reader can involve himself in the experience with confidence. He/she can feel the most violent emotions, knowing that he/she will later be able to stop (by stopping reading); he/she will be able to see part of him/herself with the support given by the text; all kinds of things happen to this part in the fiction-world, even the most dreadful and reprehensible; he/she knows that in most cases, all this will find a happy resolution, with the hero's victory, and he/she also directly enjoys the esthetic pleasure from it. The experience is therefore extremely advantageous: the person can experience as an adult what was possible in play; and on the imaginary level, she can satisfy some narcissistic needs and be successful.

Thus, here there is a strong similarity, and I would suggest, continuity, between child's play and adult's cultural experience. The main difference between play and cultural experience is the shared, social dimension of the latter, and the fact that is anchored in past experiences. Their main similarities are that they give access to unconscious experiences, and enable their active elaboration. In other words, Freud's account of a cultural experience is therefore very far from what is often mentioned about his account—that it enables catharsis, that it is a form of regression.

So what remains of these rich descriptions in cultural psychology? Vygotsky (1931/1994) knew these texts very well; he emphasized the social dimension of any imaginative, culturally based experience (both in terms of mediating structure and because of its embeddedness in a specific sociocultural context) (Van der Veer & Valsiner, 1991; Vygotsky 1925/1971). Additionally, thanks to his developmental orientation, he would enable cultural psychologists to see play and imagination as part of self-generated zones of proximal development.

One of the current challenges of cultural psychology is to understand the role of virtual experiences all life long: for example, the way we interact through computer with absent others; the way in which we push the limits of our possibilities by engaging in culturally mediated actions; the experience we have at the movies or in a traditional celebration. I think that Freud, and after him Vygotsky, give us basic keys to approach the specificity of these phenomena. The great power of such cultural experiences is firstly due to the fact that they take place precisely where the collective meets the individual. They thus enable the personal to be mediated with cultural tools. Yet, there is a specificity to these imaginary experiences, that they are part of the *transformation* of human experience (Zittoun, 2006). To show this, I now have to turn to a fourth aspect of Freud's thinking: the way he conceptualizes the progressive elaboration of human experience through signs.

A Theory of Higher Mental Function

One core issue in human and social sciences has always been the following—that of the link between embodied, organic processes, and high-level phenomena. People refer to it as the body-mind problem and often go back to Descartes. Yet, non dualistic views would see the body and thinking as continuous, or as two emergent aspects of deeper common processes. Such ideas go back to Antiquity, have been beautifully supported by Spinoza, and are at the core of Freud's work. They are also central in current cultural psychology.

So let me present the problem simply: let's see human experience as a potato-shaped closed form. One of its sides is made out of embodied impressions and perceptions; the other side contains differentiated and precisely articulated thoughts. How does it go from here to there? In other words, how can embodied fears inhibit thinking and action (higher processes)? How can rules prescribed by others (parents, priests, and the social world)—become internalized and organize one's actions and feelings?

The answer given by cultural psychology as well as Freud is that it is precisely signs, or representations, or symbolic processes that enable these transformations.

A post-Freudian psychoanalyst, André Green, (Green, 1973, 2000) has developed Freud's theory of the psychic apparatus. I will follow his presentations. For Green, from a "topical" perspective, six zones of experience can be identified: (1) the body, where sensations, needs, drives are experienced—and also called the id; (2) the unconscious; (3) the preconscious; (4) the conscious; and (5) the real (the external reality) given through perceptions. (6) The *Ego* is the part of the psychism that the person experiences as being him/herself. It encompasses the zones of consciousness, the preconscious, and part of the unconscious. These three parts are, in some conditions only, accessible to consciousness.

Note that the *unconscious* designates all psychic activities that are beyond the direct apprehension of the person. It is not to be confused with the "cognitive unconscious" evoked by Piaget and by some approaches in cognitive psychology, where the unconscious designates the invisible and noncontrollable work of automatic information processing (see also Wilson, 2002).

It is also understood as a set of processes and dynamics that have dynamic relationships with the body, drives, and consciousness. Furthermore, it admits that it is partially constituted by repressed drives that have not accessed consciousness. It can be the locus of conflicts, which may have consequences on thought, behavior, relationships to oneself or the real, also *in the long term*. Unconscious psychic activity is regulated on one hand by factors linked to reality (the Freudian reality-test) and, and on the other hand by a sort of originary fanstamatic structure.

The idea is here that any psychic formation—any idea, representation—is an intermediary between the body and the real. Two movements are at the origin of psychic images (representation). One movement comes from the external world, what is not the person, through perceptions; the other movement comes from the body, and is constituted by sensations and drives. Drives can be defined as embodied (somatic) desires or needs, tending to seek satisfaction in the world; affects are their visible aspects.

Drives tend to diffuse through different layers of the psyche where they are transformed, before eventually finding a form that can bring conduct within the socially shared reality. From the soma, they access the unconscious under the form of *psychic representation of the drive*, where they can be connected to *representations of things* (conscious or unconscious mnemonic traces linked to interactions with objects-in-the-world), and progressively, be linked to *representation of words* (allowing reflectivity). Such doubly linked emotional experiences can thus enter consciousness, under a symbolic form (Green, 1973, 2000, 2002/2005). In this model, then, the transformation of embodied motions to higher-level thinking is a question of progressive semiotic linking; it is a model of *gradients* (in Green's words, 2002/2005).

Comparable models, depicting the progressive move of ideas through various layers of elaboration, can be found in current psychology. This "topic" organization is seen as a hierarchy of psychic processes, in which we differentiate more or less distanced modes of thinking, several layers of representations (Nelson, 2007), or lower level and higher psychic functions.

To finish here: very often our cultural experiences are interesting because they "map out" various parts of this gradient, and transform them. For example, we might hear a folk tale which awakes unconscious fears of being abandoned; yet, the fears are expressed in words understood by consciousness; and the tale goes towards a nice, moral ending, which becomes here a high-level, abstract mediation (Green, 1992; Zittoun, 2005, 2006). In that sense, the folk tale that we are reading can transform embodied experiences into conscious, verbalized ones. In other words, Freud's models can help us to see that many cultural experiences have a developmental function, or play an important role in our lives, because they might bring unconscious and invading emotional and representational processes into consciousness.

CONCLUSION

Freud's work has often been said to have modified our western culture: it has transformed common sense, philosophy as well as clinical practice. [5] In this presentation, I had a limited purpose: I have tried to show that one possible contribution to current cultural psychology was due to Freud's often overlooked analysis of the dynamics of culture in the mind or of the mind in culture. I have explored four aspects of this analysis:

1. The idea that human thought is mediated or enabled by the use of various cultural tools for thinking.
2. Such mediation is possible, because humans have the ability to use signs, and Freud developed a convincing account of the emergence of signs in children, confirmed by current research.
3. Freud then explored people's relationship to two types of cultural activities, children's play and adults' artistic and cultural experiences; he showed their commonalities and the communities of the processes involved. I have suggested that such ideas might be very helpful for those of us who try to understand the role of different culturally mediated activities in human development.
4. Freud's work is based on a nondualistic understanding of humans functioning. Note that his model of the psychic apparatus, might give us a way to understand how various cultural experiences are part of the elaboration of our experiences.

Freud's work has many meeting points with current cultural psychology, which can be defined as a psychology of human meaning-making, as the meeting of the social and the individual, in time. One core similarity is that cultural psychology and psychoanalysis are models trying to capture semiotic processes in meaning-making. One core difference is that Freud's work is mostly interested in unconscious processes, while psychology tries to avoid addressing these. My reading suggests that, if there are so many overlaps between psychoanalytical investigation and that of cultural psychology, then we might also gain something on reflecting on these unconscious dynamics. But I will leave this here and go back to a more general observation.

Freud has often been criticized—or admired—for getting us to understand that people are prisoners of their unconscious and of acting out beyond their control. However, it might also be argued that Freud proposed a theory of human emancipation. Freud certainly shows us how deeply our thoughts are rooted in our affects and emotions. He also shows us, quite extensively, what might happen when individuals, politicians and large groups of people ignore these powerful forces, which might then govern us. Yet, Freud also showed us how we might become aware of these constraints and of our own fears, and use the tools provided by the culture in which we live to recognize these energies, channel them, and use them as agents, fully aware of their limits.

ACKNOWLEDGMENTS

This chapter is based on a lecture presented at the University of Nicosia (Cyprus) for the 150th birthday of Sigmund Freud in November 2006, invited by Charis Psaltis, and further discussed at the 2007 ISTP conference in Toronto (Canada).

NOTES

1. Each time one aspect has been emphasized by some commentator, others have risen to show the inanity of the notion. Freud's work has often been rejected as a whole on the grounds that this, or that aspect, appears too poetic to be true. Yet, Freud' work represents over fifty years of clinical observations, the systematic attempt to analyze, the enrichment of case study with theory, and daring interpretations, etc. It was produced in a specific context, and Freud had to account for his observations with the theoretical models and metaphors at his disposal. Contemporary critics of Freud are often unaware of the historical context of the production of Freud's idea, or use it to discredit these ideas; they are also often unaware of the most creative explorations of contemporary psychoanalysis. This paper goes beyond partisan quarrels, and my perspective on Freud is informed by recent evolutions of psychoanalysis and cultural psychology.
2. The idea of an active unconscious is, in brief, the following: people have wishes and desires, for example they want to have strawberries in the winter, or to marry a handsome but poor young man; these wishes and desires are not possible, or not socially acceptable; they thus have to be hidden or repressed. The idea of the active unconscious is that these ideas are not frozen, but are dynamic; their emotional load pushes these ideas forward, so that they might be heard in various ways. A person not able to have strawberries might thus dream of them; or a woman whose love is forbidden might start to hear her young man's voice ...
3. Later authors would add that, by manipulating the string, the child reinforces his own ability to symbolize, through his manipulation of the space between the mother and herself (Winnicott, 1971/2001), or thanks to his manipulation of the string, as a concrete link, facilitating the ability to symbolize the notion of relationship and to master it, and therefore to have access to an understanding of the notion of separation (Tisseron, 1999).
4. Play therefore has some affinity with the dream; Anna Freud will thus use child's play as another Royal road to the child's unconscious.

5. Freud's influences on our society are deep and numerous. They all follow from his identification and theorization of unconscious processes, as they are explored systematically in the *Interpretation of the Dreams* (Freud, 1900/1953). On this basis, Freud's work has affected the medical treatment of psychopathology; it has questioned the border between health and disorder in mental life, and the reflection on the doctor–patient relationship (Major & Talagrand, 2006, p. 37). It has then also questioned the teacher–student relationship. It has made people think differently about their choices—of partners, of activities—and about their everyday mistakes—since every slip of the tongue is now "revealing" some hidden discourse. Serge Moscovici's (1961/2007) important work on the social representation of psychoanalysis examines how French people in the '60s started to use Freudian notions in their everyday life, for example, they came to say things like "This guy has an inferiority complex." In the USA, psychoanalysis met a huge success. In some spheres of the society, it was a must to undertake a personal psychoanalysis; in the '40s and '50s most people working in the arts and entertainment underwent personal analysis. This has made a certain sensibility to unconscious processes widespread. Woody Allen is a caricature of that sensitivity. More radically, authors such as Thomas Mann, then Paul Ricoeur (1965/1970) and many postmodern theorists have seen in the idea of "the unconscious" a fundamental challenge to people's illusion of mastering their lives. Freud would thus have introduced "suspicion" about human's freedom.

REFERENCES

Abbey, E., & Valsiner, J. (2004). Emergence of meanings through ambivalence [58 paragraphs]. *Forum Qualitative Sozialforschung/Forum: Qualitative Social Research [On-line Journal], 6*(1), Art. 23. Retrieved from http://www.qualitative-research.net

Bruner, J. S. (1990). *Acts of meaning*. Cambridge, MA: Harvard University Press.

Cole, M. (1996). *Cultural psychology. A once and future discipline*. Cambridge (MA)/ London: The Belknap Press of Harvard University Press.

Diriwaechter, R. (2004). Ganzheitpsychologie: The doctrine. *From past to future, 5*(1), 3–16.

Farr, R. (1988). The shaping of modern psychology and the framing of historical accounts. *History of the human sciences, 1*(1), 113–121.

Fonagy, P., Target, M., Gergely, G., & Jurist, E. L. (2002). Affect regulation, mentalization, and the development of self (1st ed.). New York: Other Press.

Freud, S. (1953). The interpretation of dreams. In J. Strachey (Ed. and Trans.), *The standard edition of the complete psychological works of Sigmund Freud* (Vols. 4–5). London: The Hogarth Press and the Institute of Psycho-analysis. (Original work published 1900)

Freud, S. (1955). Totem and taboo: Some points of agreement between the mental lives of savages and neurotics. In J. Strachey (Ed. and Trans.), *The standard edition of the complete psychological works of Sigmund Freud* (Vol. 13, pp. vii–162).

London: The Hogarth Press and the Institute of Psycho-analysis. (Original work published 1913)

Freud, S. (1955). Beyond the pleasure principle. In J. Strachey (Ed. and Trans.), *The standard edition of the complete psychological works of Sigmund Freud* (Vol. 18, pp. 7–64). London: Hogarth Press and the Institute of Psycho-analysis. (Original work published 1920)

Freud, S. (1958). Remembering, repeating and working through. In J. Strachey (Ed. and Trans.), *The standard edition of the complete psychological works of Sigmund Freud* (Vol. 12, pp. 145–156). London: Hogarth Press and the Institute of Psycho-analysis. (Original work published 1914)

Freud, S. (1959). The Delusion and Dream in Jensen's Gradiva. In J. Strachey (Ed. and Trans.), *The standard edition of the complete psychological works of Sigmund Freud* (Vol. 9, pp. 1–96). London: The Hogarth Press and the Institute of Psycho-analysis. (Original work published 1907)

Freud, S. (1959). Creative writers and day-dreaming. In J. Strachey (Ed. and Trans.), *The standard edition of the complete psychological works of Sigmund Freud* (Vol. 9, pp. 141–153). London: Hogarth Press and the Institute of Psycho-analysis. (Original work published 1908)

Freud, S. (1960). The psychopathology of everyday life: Forgetting, slips of the tongue, bungled actions, superstitions and errors. In J. Strachey (Ed. and Trans.), *The standard edition of the complete psychological works of Sigmund Freud* (Vol. 6, whole volume). London: The Hogarth Press and the Institute of Psycho-analysis. (Original work published 1901)

Freud, S. (1960). Jokes and their relation to the unconscious. In J. Strachey (Ed. and Trans.), *The standard edition of the complete psychological works of Sigmund Freud* (Vol. 8, whole volume). London: The Hogarth Press and the Institute of Psycho-analysis. (Original work published 1905)

Freud, S. (1960). The Moses of Michelangelo. In J. Strachey (Ed. and Trans.), *The standard edition of the complete psychological works of Sigmund Freud* (Vol. 13, pp. 209–238). London: The Hogarth Press and the Institute of Psycho-analysis. (Original work published 1914)

Freud, S. (1961). The future of an illusion. In J. Strachey (Ed. and Trans.), *The standard edition of the complete psychological works of Sigmund Freud* (Vol. 13, pp. 1–56). London: The Hogarth Press and the Institute of Psycho-analysis. (Original work published 1927)

Freud, S. (1961). Civilization and its discontents. In J. Strachey (Ed. and Trans.), *The standard edition of the complete psychological works of Sigmund Freud* (Vol. 21, pp. 59–148). London: The Hogarth Press and the Institute of Psycho-analysis. (Original work published 1930)

Freud, S. (1964). Moses and the monotheism. In J. Strachey (Ed. and Trans.), *The standard edition of the complete psychological works of Sigmund Freud* (Vol. 23, pp. 1–138). London: The Hogarth Press and the Institute of Psycho-analysis. (Original work published 1939)

Freud, S., & Bullitt, W. C. (1967). *Thomas Woodrow Wilson, Twenty-eighth President of United States: A psychological Study*. London: Weindelfeld & Nicolson.

Gillespie, A. (2006). *Becoming other: From social interaction to self-reflection.* Charlotte, NC: Information Age Publishing.

Green, A. (1973). *Le discours vivant: la conception psychanalytique de l'affect [Living discourse: The psychoanalytic conception of affects]*. Paris: Presses universitaires de France.
Green, A. (1992). *La déliaison. Psychanalyze, anthropologie et littérature [Unlinking: psychoanalysis, anthropology and literature]*. Paris: Hachette Littératures/Les belles lettres, Pluriel.
Green, A. (2000). *André Green at the Squiggle Foundation*. (J. Abrams, Ed.). London: Karnac Books.
Green, A. (2005). *Key Ideas for a Contemporary Psychoanalysis: Misrecognition and Recognition of the Unconscious* (Andrew Weller, Trans.). London: Routledge (Original work published 2002)
James, W. (1890). *The principles of psychology* (Vol. I). New York: Dover publications.
Major, R., & Talgrand, C. (2006). *Freud*. Paris: Gallimard.
Moro, C., & Rodriguez, C. (2005). *L'objet et la construction de son usage chez le bébé. Une approche sémiotique du développement préverbal [The object and the construction of its usage by the infant. A semiotic approach of preverbal communication]*. Berne: Peter Lang.
Moscovici, S. (2007). *Psychoanalysis* (G. Schott, Trans.). New York: Blackwell. (Original work published 1961)
Nelson, K. (2007). *Young minds in social worlds. Experience, meaning, and memory.* Cambridge, MA/London: Harvard University Press.
Piaget, J. (1951). *Play, dreams and imitation in childhood* (Trad. C. Gattegno & F. M. Hodgson). Melbourne/London/Toronto: William Heinemann Ltd. (Original work published 1945)
Ricoeur, P. (1970). *Freud and philosophy: an essay on interpretation* (D. Savage, Trans.). New Haven/London: Yale University Press (Original work published 1965)
Salvatore, S. (2004). Inconscio e discorso, inconscio come discorso [Unconscious and discourse, Unconscious as discourse]. In M. B. Ligorio (Ed.), *Psicologia e cultura. Contesti, idenitità ed interventi* (pp. 129–158). Rome/London: Firera Publishing Group.
Salvatore, S. (2006). Steps toward a dialogical and semiotic theory of the unconscious. *Culture & Psychology, 12*(1): 124–136.
Santiago-Delefosse, M. J., & Oderic Delefosse, J.-M. (2002) Spielrein, Piaget and Vygotsky. Three Positions on Child thought and Language. *Theory & Psychology, 12*(6), 723–747.
Tisseron, S. (1999). *Comment l'esprit vient aux objets [How mind comes to objects]*. Paris: L'Aubier.
Valsiner, J. (1998). *The guided mind. A sociogenetic approach to personality.* Cambridge (Mass) & London: Harvard University Press.
Valsiner, J. (2007). Human development as migration. Striving towards the unknown. In L. M. Simao & J. Valsiner (Eds.), *Otherness in question. Labyrinths of the self* (pp. 349–378). Charlotte, NC: Information Age Publishing.
Van der Veer, R., & Valsiner, J. (1991). The role of psychoanalysis. In Van der Veer, R., & Valsiner, J. *Understanding Vygotsky: a quest for synthesis* (pp. 78–111). Oxford & Cambridge (MA): Blackwell.
Vygotsky, L. S. (1997). The historical meaning of the crisis in psychology: A methodological investigation. In R. W. Rieber & J. Wollock (Eds.), *The*

collected works of L. S. Vygotsky. Vol. 3. Problems of the theory and history of psychology (pp. 233–343). New York: Plenum Press.

Vygotsky, L. S. (1994). Imagination and creativity of the adolescent. In R. Van der Veer & J. Valsiner (Eds). *The Vygotsky reader* (pp. 266–288). Oxford/Cambridge (Mass): Blackwell.

Vygotsky, L. S. (1971). *The psychology of art* (Scripta Technica Inc. Trans.). Cambridge, MA & London: MIT press. (Original work published 1925)

Wertsch, J. V. (1998). *Mind as Action.* New York/Oxford: Oxford University Press.

Wilson, T. D. (2002). *Strangers to ourselves. Discovering the adaptive unconscious.* Cambridge, MA/London: The Belknap Press.

Winnicott, D. W. (2001). *Playing and reality.* Philadelphia/Sussex: Routledge (First published 1971 by Tavistock Publication Ltd).

Zittoun, T. (2005). *Donner la vie, choisir un nom. Engendrements symboliques [Giving life, choosing a name. Symbolic begetting]*. Paris: L'Harmattan.

Zittoun, T. (2006). *Transitions. Development through symbolic resources.* Charlotte, NC: Information Age Publishing.

Zittoun, T., Gillespie, A., Cornish, F., & Psaltis, C. (2007). The metaphor of the triangle in theories of human development. *Human Development, 50*, 208–229.

CHAPTER 4

AFFECTIVE HYPERGENERALIZATION: LEARNING FROM PSYCHOANALYSIS

Kenneth R. Cabell and Jaan Valsiner

There is much to learn from psychoanalysis. This is possible, even if its premises are limited by the uncritical borrowing of master narratives from Occidental mythology and an exaggerated focus on sexuality. Psychoanalysis may be based on limited general axioms in its way of construing the human *psyche*—yet, it does so in sophisticated ways that lead to new theoretical models that are adequate to the complexity of phenomena. What psychoanalysis has accomplished since its emergence in the consulting rooms of Viennese doctors is to keep our attention persistently on affective processes and their social regulation. In line with that focus cultural psychology can benefit from the sophistication of the sensitivity to phenomena that abound in psychoanalytic discourse. Hence, the focus of this chapter—what can a semiotic cultural psychology learn from psychoanalysis?

Cultural Psychology and Psychoanalysis: Pathways to Synthesis, pp. 87–113

FEELINGS IN FOCUS: SENSIFIED GENERALIZATION

From the discourse of psychoanalysis, cultural psychology can learn where to look for relevant phenomena of affect. It might be time to rephrase Descartes in a significant way—*we feel, therefore we are*. Or—more precisely—because we can reflect upon our feelings—*we feel that we feel*. It is affective relating to the world that allows us to feel, feel that we feel, and to continue the recursive notions of reflective feeling. Daily experiences provoke flows of affective kind that lead to the emergence of a generalized feeling state. Generalized feeling states allow for the emergence—through semiotic means—of associated memories. The reconstruction of associated memories yields a reflective analysis, allowing recursive feeling about feelings. The reflective analysis of feeling then produces microchanges in the person's self-reflection.

Human subjective experience, or the memory of it, is always built on affective relating to the world. That relating is a totality—a combination of past, present, and future felt simultaneously as one. An example of such affective processes of relating can be found in an introspective account of female orgasm—a rare find of direct account of affect in psychoanalytic literature:

> In intercourse, the transcending of physical limits means that I am conveyed to a strange world where feelings of time, as I know them here, do not exist, where feelings of space, as I am bound in by space here, become meaningless. *Time itself is stretched out, not in the sense where extension implies a conception either of beginning or end, but in the sense that I may drift along forever in a sort of time-river; drift, yet remain in the same place.*
>
> As far as space feelings are concerned, intercourse presents a paradox: a feeling of expansion into infinity, a blending into the universe about one, a melting and fusing—yet also a feeling of infinite contraction, of an intense focusing to a minute part of space and even into a small part of one's physical self as it ordinarily is. There is another paradox in the *identification's loss with one's partner, and yet a realization that I am myself, unalterable.*
>
> Apart from a sense of the unreality of time and space, I have been acutely aware of form and colors—a strange, half-mad constellation of circles black and blue and red and gold, expanding, contracting, merging, converging—*coming close, infinitely large, then receding to the thin point where awareness fades and they are forgotten*. (Matte Blanco, 1998, p. 442, *italics added*)

This retrospective account of the psychological phenomena at the moment of orgasm includes the arrival at the subjective moment of timelessness. This is achieved by the rapid dynamics of the subjective flow of affective images. Affective relating yields generalized feelings that are described as if the self and the other merge—yet in ways that fortifies the self. The paradoxical merging and fortification of the self and other provides a reflective analysis—a feeling about ones feelings—producing the *sense of unreality*.

Similar phenomena of affect, feeling and sense are within part of our everyday ordinary encounters. Psychoanalysis and the cultural-semiotic framework converge with the theoretical role of affects as communicators, signals, and regulatory phenomena within hierarchies. It is within this domain that we can study the manifest content of small phenomenological features of ordinary conduct as central to the extraordinary *Psyche*. This is possible through *sense-making* processes, or of *sensifying*, as Welby indicated:

> ... "to sensify" must share the uncertainty of reference which belongs to sense itself. It might mean e.g. the attributing of our "senses" to a tree or rock, when we suppose to hear, feel, see, etc. like ourselves ... we may perhaps be allowed to use "sensification" for that fundamental tendency to "assign sense" and "give meaning" without which Attention, Imitation and even Adaptation itself would either not exist or would be deprived of all their practical value. (Welby, 1896, p. 31)

In cultural psychology, we axiomatically assume that all human beings are unstoppable sensifiers. They do not need any unconscious impulse to become involved in the sense-making process. Sense-making grows out of the need to pre-adapt to the future (i.e., currently not yet known) environmental conditions. The role of the social others in that process is that of guidance of the processes of *Aktualgenese* (usually known as *microgenesis*—Abbey & Diriwächter, 2008; Valsiner & van der Veer, 2000, Chapter 7). This sensifying process organizes both lower (subconscious) and higher (hyperconscious) psychological functions—we arrive both at our generalized personal values and our little conduct peculiarities through that process. Here—again—history of psychoanalysis from its very beginning gives cultural psychology rich material for further elaborations.

THE FIRST CASE—ANNA O—AND ITS RE-INTERPRETATION

Josef Breuer's early case history of Anna O. has been a staple intellectual food for psychoanalysts and its critics. For our purposes it is instructive to re-visit the case. Notably, the case was depicted in the medical literature with a delay—the clinical events happened in 1880–1881 while its debut in the emerging psychoanalytic discourse took place only in 1893 (*Über den psychischen Mechanismus hysterischer Phänomene,* Breuer & Freud, 1893/1955) and finally—as the starting point of psychoanalysis—in 1895 (Freud & Breuer, 1895/2004). In a general description, Freud—who in the case of Anna O. was a secondary source—described the phenomenon:

> Dr Breuer's patient was a girl of twenty-one, of high intellectual gifts. Her illness lasted over two years, and in the course of it she developed a series

> of physical and psychological disturbances .... She suffered from rigid paralysis, accompanied by loss of sensation, of both extremities on the right side of her body; and the same trouble from time to time affected her on her left side. Her eye movements were disturbed and her power of vision was subject to numerous restrictions. She had difficulties over the posture of her head; she had a severe nervous cough. She had an aversion to taking nourishment, and on one occasion she was for several weeks unable to drink in spite of a tormenting thirst. Her powers of speech were reduced, even to the point of her being unable to speak or understand her native language. Finally, she was subject to conditions of "*absence*" of confusion, of delirium, and of alteration of her whole personality, to which we shall have presently to turn our attention. (Freud, 1910/1961, pp. 4–5)

Recently, historians have retraced Anna O.'s case study and historical roots, resulting in multiple discrepancies. For one, Ernest Jones revealed the true identity of Anna O. as Bertha Pappenheim in the 1950s—a woman of many constructive contributions to society over the decades (until her death in 1936) after her encounters with emerging psychoanalysts in her youth. Historians have also since revealed that Sigmund Freud had confided in Carl Jung that the patient had never actually been entirely cured. Objective research and historical accuracy have partly separated myth from reality in the foundation of psychoanalysis (Ellenberger, 1972/1993). Another view of Anna O. will allow for not only a reinterpretation according to cultural psychology, but will allow for the analysis of old ideas to develop new ideas. The locus of such move into the classic case is that of *overdetermination*—which has been a concept well developed in psychoanalysis, and—from a different angle—is crucial for cultural psychology.

Multiple determination, or overdetermination, (*Überdetermination* as Freud sometimes used it) is the concept that a psychological or behavioral event (and its emergence) could be explained by multiple (but redundant) organizing qualities. Its relevance in the late nineteenth century scientific thought was paralleled by Hans Driesch's introduction of the notion of *equipotentiality* in 1898. Overdetermination in psychoanalysis entails a layering principle. Through redundant layering, conscious and unconscious processes can reach either (1) the same ends by different means or (2) different ends by the same means. In the former, the overdetermination of the ends is the result of the qualitative organization of redundantly layered means. This is analogous to the overdetermination of the hysterical symptom, or the dream symbol. In the latter, the overdetermination of the means results in a qualitative organization of multiple ends that are redundant options of one another. This is analogous to the production of multiple dreams symbols that represent the same latent dream thought. This became relevant in many of Freud's psychoanalytic phenomena such as hysteria, dreams, everyday errors (Parapraxes), jokes, etc. In dreams, overdetermination was described in many ways, but can best be explained in Freud's (1901/1953) *On Dreams* when he says,

> A good portion of what we have learned about condensation in dreams may be summarized in this formula: each element in the content of a dream is "overdetermined" by material in the dream thoughts; it is not derived from a *single* element in the dream thoughts, but may be traced back to a whole number. These elements need not necessarily be closely related to each other in the dream thoughts themselves; they may belong to the most widely separated regions of the fabric of those thoughts. (p. 32)

The principle of overdetermination in psychoanalysis was built on a more prominent axiom—the axiom of determinism. Freud believed in mental causality and therefore psychological events could not be overdetermined if they were not determined in the first place. Freud shows the relationship between determinism and overdeterminism when he says (Freud, 1910/1961) in his *Five Lectures On Psychoanalysis,*

> ... psycho-analysts are marked by a particularly strict belief in the determination of mental life. For them there is nothing trivial, nothing arbitrary or haphazard. They expect in every case to find sufficient motives where, as a rule, no such expectation is raised. Indeed, they are prepared to find *several* motives for one and the same mental occurrence ... (p. 40)

Psychoanalysis can be credited to consistently remind us of the multiple layering within systems. But it is precisely within the redundant layering of means and ends that systems of meaning and the meaning making process is illuminated. Overdetermination is a catalyst for meaning making that produces high variability in the domain of psychological phenomena. The numbers of ways in which meanings may become constructed is in principle infinite.

Yet, there is microgenetic order—the process of development from the potential meanings to the manifest ones implies not only a multilinear framework of development, but also shows that multilinear development converges at different equifinality points (Sato, Yasuda, Kido, Arakawa, Mizoguchi, & Valsiner, 2007; Valsiner, 2007). Psychoanalysis uses the notion of *latent* meanings—which contradicts the developmental focus of cultural psychology. The meanings are constructed on the move—not being brought out from the reservoir of the unconscious.

To give an example where cultural psychology and psychoanalysis may find a phenomenon in common let us troddle into the sacred grove of psychoanalysis. Multilinearity in sensifying is shown in case of hysterical symptoms and their overdetermination. Freud wrote in *Studies on Hysteria* that he "... knows the main characteristic in the etiology of neuroses, that their genesis is on the whole *overdetermined* and that several factors must coincide for this to take effect ..." (Freud & Breuer, 1895/2004, p. 264). Undergoing investigation in the case of Anna O., overdetermination is seen in the psychophysical symptom of the repeated and redundant inability to hear. This symptom took the following forms as described in Anna O.'s case study (Freud & Breuer, 1895/2004, p. 40):

1. Not hearing someone coming into the room. Absent mindedness. One hundred and eight separate and detailed cases of this, indicating the people, circumstances, and often the date. The first instance was not hearing her father come in.
2. Not understanding when several people speak at once. Twenty seven times. The first again involved her father and an acquaintance.
3. Not hearing when alone and spoken to directly. Fifty times. The origin: her father had asked her in vain for wine.
4. Becoming deaf through shaking (in the carriage or similar such circumstances). Fifteen times. The origin: her young brother shook her angrily when he caught her listening at the door of the sickroom.
5. Becoming deaf when frightened by noise. Thirty-seven times. The origin: her father had a choking fit when swallowing.
6. Becoming deaf during a deep absence. Twelve times.
7. Becoming deaf as a result of long periods of listening and eavesdropping so that she would not hear when spoken to Fifty-four times.

There is blatant redundancy in the recurrence of the inability to hear. The overdetermination in meaning rests with the multiple layers of associations to Anna O.'s affective experiences. Multiple meaning construction pathways are used (different affective phenomena related to hearing) to express the same end (hysterical symptoms related to non-hearing or hearing impairment).

Ambivalence in Sensification

The notion of overdetermination has been relevant and developing in cultural psychology (Obeyesekere, 1990—overdetermination of meaning by multiple levels of symbolization; Valsiner, 2007—the same objective or goal includes redundant and multiple meanings). Together, cultural psychology and psychoanalysis rely on a layering principle that exemplifies sensification. The sensifying process may ascribe multiple meanings—to an object or distal phenomena. The regulation and organization of redundant meanings is a function of affective processes. Therefore, we can see the relevant notions of overdetermination do not just lie within the domains of action and motivation, but also affects, feelings, and emotions. The "layering" and redundancy of affects can be seen best within the psychoanalytic view of hysteria. The very specific conditions of affective ambivalence—inability to drink while thirsty—took a very particular form in the case of Anna O.:

> The first time that—by chance and quite unprovoked—talking things through during the evening hypnosis caused a long standing disturbance to disappear, I was very surprised. There had been a period of intense heat during the summer and the patient had suffered from a terrible thirst, for, although she could give no explanation for it, it had suddenly become impossible for her to drink. She would pick up the glass of water she was longing for, but as soon as it touched her lips she would push it away as if she were hydrophobic. At the same time it was clear that during these few seconds she was in an absence. She lived only on fruit and melons, etc., so as to ease her excruciating thirst. This had been going on for about six weeks, when, *in her hypnosis, she grumbled about her English lady-companion, whom she did not like, and then, giving every sign of disgust, recounted how she had gone into her companion's room and seen her small dog, the revolting animal, drinking out of a glass. She explained that she did not say anything, for fear of being impolite.* Having given vent to the irritation that had been there inside her, she asked for a drink, drank a great quantity of water without any inhibition and woke up form the hypnosis with the glass at her lips. At this the disturbance disappeared forever. (Freud & Breuer, 1895/2004, p. 38, *italics added*)

Ambivalence to drinking from a glass linked with a reported experience in the context of a disliked other person led to the establishment of an *affective block of drinking from glass* (in general). The generalization was catalyzed by the fear of being impolite. The semiotic block could be removed by Breuer when Anna O. was under hypnosis. In Freud's interpretation,

> In the episode of her lady-companion's dog, *she suppressed any manifestation of her very intense disgust*, out of consideration for the woman's feelings; while she watched her at her father's bedside she was constantly on the alert to prevent the sick man from observing her anxiety and her painful depression. When subsequently she reproduced these scenes in her doctor's presence *the affect which had been inhibited at the time emerged with peculiar violence, as though it had been saved up for a long time*. Indeed, the symptom which was left over from one of these scenes would reach its highest pitch of intensity at the time when its determining cause was being approached, only to vanish when the cause had been fully ventilated. (Freud, 1910/1961, pp. 14–15, *italics added*)

As can be seen, in Freud's account, the affect is strangulated when it is blocked from a normal outlet where a discharge of affect can succeed (Freud & Breuer, 1895/2004). The discourse is clinically focused—If discharge fails, illness occurs because the affect is put to abnormal and pathological use in various (displaced) activities (Freud, 1910/1961). This *reactive* model is contrary to our *constructive* model in cultural psychology—where affect is the starting ground for semiotic organizers that—by their function—can generate "illness" and "resiliency" at the same location. Overdetermination allows for multiple meanings to be ascribed to the same event. This is possible because all meaning-making involves overdetermined *signs of dual nature*—that consist of the core (A) and its immediate interdependent context (non-A). The {A & non-A} complex is surrounded by the wider environment that has no functional connections with it ("not-A"—Josephs, Valsiner & Surgan, 1999). Both components of the complex are best considered in terms of fields.

Dynamics of Sensifying: Dialectics of the fields Heimlich and Unheimlich

The internal dynamic relation of A and non-A leads towards a dialectical synthesis along the lines of Hegel. It entails the differentiation of the opposites within the same whole, their relationship of contradiction, and—as a result—the overcoming of the previous opposition by creating a new whole.

The existence of the core and its immediate interdependent context as a complex whole can be illustrated even further through phenomena described by psychoanalysis. We have illustrated the signs of dual nature with the ambivalence of the thirst <> nonthirst dynamics in Anna O's symptoms. From this emerges the question of the simultaneously existing A and its negation or opposite non-A, as well as the relationship between the two.

In Freud's (1925/1997) essay on *Negation* he notes that a negation—or the claim of nonexistence—actually acknowledges existence. The internal dynamics of A and non-A by can be exemplified by discussing the relationship of existence and nonexistence observed in Anna O. (and other psychoanalytic phenomena). In hysteria, content is forced to be unknown by the mechanism of repression, and yet simultaneously forced to be known through the return of the repressed. For example, symbolic psycho-physcal symptoms in hysteria are a disguised conversion and reappearance of the repressed content. We can now see the connection between the thirst and nonthirst. Although Anna O. was thirsty, she developed an inability to drink as a result of a hysterical symptom. The latent content behind the symptom (the affect of disgust and repulsion in relation to the dog drinking from a glass) had been repressed. However, the same latent content is forcefully acknowledged by the presenting symptom—the return of the repressed as affective disgust with and repulsion of thirst. The opposites in tension (A and non-A: thirst and nonthirst) acknowledges both sides—and gives rise to the meta-level mechanisms in opposite processes of denial and nondenial (which equals the acknowledgement)—simultaneously.

Repulsion, as seen in the repulsion of thirst, can rise to the realm of affective aesthetics—which is a field of affective hypergeneralized relating to the world. Freud comments,

> On this topic we find virtually nothing in the detailed accounts of aesthetics, which on the whole prefer to concern themselves with our feelings for the beautiful, the grandiose and the attractive—that is to say, with feelings of a positive kind, their determinants, and the objects that arouse them—rather than with their opposites, feelings of repulsion and distress. (Freud, 1919/2003. p. 123)

Freud again brings up the duality—A and its negation (a mutually generated opposite) non-A—in the realm of aesthetics. Affective relating to a painting can be one of hypergeneralized love or beauty. Freud discusses the opposite side of affective relating to the world. He discusses affects such as repulsion or disgust. This is illustrated further in Freud's (1919/2003) essay on the feeling of the discomfort about something that feels nonhome-like (*Unheimlich*). Discomfort and repulsion are a generalized "feel" (of affect) associated with nonpositive affective relating. The feel of nonpositive affective relating brings us to the analysis of the word *Unheimlich*, which Freud states is in opposition of "*Heimlich,*" "*Heimisch,*" and "*Vertraut*" (Freud, 1919/2003, p. 124).

Freud writes that he gets the impression not many words in other languages fully capture the "feel" of *Unheimlich* since it denotes a particular "species" of the feelings "eerie," "mysterious," and "frightening" (Freud, 1919/2003, p. 124). Freud's survey of the languages results in the following:

Latin

1. locus suspectus—an eerie place
2. intempesta nocte—in the eerie night hours

Greek

1. xénos – foreign, alien

English

1. uncomfortable	4. dismal	7. haunted
2. uneasy	5. uncanny	8. a repulsive fellow
3. gloomy	6. ghastly	

Spanish

1. sospechoso
2. de mal aguero
3. lúgubre
4. siniestro

French

1. inquiétant
2. sinister
3. lugubre
4. mal à son
5. aise

(Freud, 1919/2003, p. 125)

None of the dictionary accounts of any of the languages sufficiently cover the feeling associated with *Unheimlich*. The starting contrast here is the feeling about "being at home" (in a house that is a home) in contrast to being away from home. The feeling of course can occur independently of the physical object (house that is one's home)—one can feel "at home" in a previously unknown place, as well as feel discomfort in one's own home. Freud defines *Heimlich* as "belonging to the house," "not strange," "familiar," "tame," "dear and intimate," "homely," etc (Freud, 1919/2003, p. 126). In opposition, *Unheimlich* is defined through the use of a passage—from fiction—that emphasizes the unity of the opposites. Freud quotes,

> "Die Zecks sind alle heimlich." "Heimlich? ... Was verstehen Sie unter Heimlich?" ... "Nun ... es kommt mir mit ihnen vor, wie mit einem zugegrabenen Brunnen oder einem ausgetrckneten Teich. Man kann nicht daruber gehen, ohne dass es Einem immer ist, als konnte da wider einmal Wasser zum Vorschein kommen." "Wir nennen das unheimlich; Sie nennen's heimlich. Worin finden Sie denn, dass diese Familie etwas Verstecktes und Unzuverlassiges hat?"
>
> ["The Zecks are all 'heimlich.'" "Heimlich? ... What do you mean by 'Heimlich'?" "Well, I have the same impression with them as I have with a buried spring or a dried up pond. You can't walk over them without constantly

> feeling that water might reappear." "We call that unheimlich; you call it 'heimlich'. So, what makes you think there's something hidden and unreliable about the family?"] (Gutzkow as quoted in Freud, 1919/2003, p. 129, our correction of translation)

The mutually generated relationship *Heimlich<>Unheimlich* begins to emerge in Freud's analysis. The Gutrzkow quotation implies that the feeling of *Unheimlich* is something that was once *Heimlich* (known, homely, familiar), and has returned. Consequently, the feeling associated with both is an issue of the boundary. The boundary issue is that of transformation of one into the other (or a new feeling—B—emerging from the non-A:

B becomes dominant over A

B emerges from non-A

A generates non-A

A

Or in specific terms:

UNHEIMLICH dominates over HEIMLICH

UNHEIMLICH emerges from non-HEIMLICH

HEIMLICH generates non-HEIMLICH

HEIMLICH

Something that evokes feelings of *Unheimlich* was once *Heimlich*. This can be displayed through a look at how the boundary between the opposites is allowing the emergence of the *Unheimlich* from the whole field of non-*Heimlich*. Here we combine the "unhomely" or "unfamiliar" nature of *Unheimlich* with the "homely" or "familiar" nature of *Heimlich* by showing the emergence of *Unheimlich* from *Heimlich* and its dominance over the other parts. In this sense, the discomfort about the unfamiliar is in some way a "species" of the familiar (Freud, 1919/2003). Water *that once filled* the dried up pond yields to *Heimlich*—reconstruction of a memory from the past. However, it has since disappeared—and this creates the distance of the discomfort of the here-and-now setting. Yet, there is a possibility it might appear again—and this feeling of its *possible* reappearance leads to the growth of the *Unheimlich* feeling. Unheimlich *is then an affect that is pre-adaptive to the future.* The (possible) reappearance of a phenomena gives way to the feeling of the *Unheimlich*—the eerie, mysterious, uncanny and frightening possibility—that is discomforting.

But why do we experience *Unheimlich* for something familiar? For Freud, the uncomfortable was content that had been repressed, and for whatever reason, has reappeared in association into the sensifying field (Freud, 1919/2003). Therefore, originally frightening to the self, repression "marks" or "signals" the content as such. The detection of this signal constitutes manifest *Unheimlich* phenomena. As part of the familiar, the *Unheimlich* is part of the *Heimlich* whole. Yet—at the same time—it is the opposite of—or from—the *Heimlich*. The feeling is—in seemingly paradoxical sense—comfortably discomfortable. The ambivalence present in part<>whole relationships in the psychological field is the never-ending source for such transformations.

From the perspective of semiotic cultural psychology, the *Unheimlich* is a hypergeneralized affective field—an overwhelming feeling within the realm of the frightening. The *Unheimlich* evokes feelings of fear and dread. For Freud, this unique hypergeneralized notion is due to its "... specific affective nucleus, which justifies the use of a special conceptual term" (Freud, 1919/2003, p. 123). In cultural psychology, the sensification field is set up by its borders—constraints—rather than any specific nucleus. The hypergenealized affective state of *Unheimlich* allows for the ability to feel overwhelming eeriness and fright—without the possibility to identify the source of the feeling. It results in the conscious proposition "I am feeling something and yet I am unable to specify what it is."

It is this propositional statement that was the initial cause of Anna O.'s hysterical illness. Hysteria, and the affects that cause it, present themselves in a hypergeneralized state. The hysterical illness began when Anna,

> ... woke up one night in a state of great anxiety about the patient's high fever and under the strain of expecting the arrival of a surgeon from Vienna for the operation. Her mother had gone away for a while and Anna was sitting at the patient's bedside with her right arm resting over the back of the chair. She fell into a daydreaming state and saw a black snake coming from the wall towards the patient in order to bit him ... she wanted to fend off the creature, but was as if paralysed. Her right arm hanging over the back of the chair had "gone

> to sleep," becoming anesthetic and paretic, and when she looked at it, her fingers turned into tiny snakes with skulls (her nails) .... *When the snake had disappeared, she tried in her terror to pray, but every language failed her, she could speak none at all until finally she came upon a nursery rhyme in English and then found that she could also think and pray in this language.* (Freud & Breuer, 1895/2004, p. 42, *italics added*)

The reappearance of snake like symbols, the hysterical paralysis, the symbolic symptom of an inability to speak, and affects of terror and fright elicited a hypergeneralized sensifying field of which was *uncomfortable*. Its conscious proposition manifested as "I am feeling something and yet I am unable to specify what it is, but it is uncomfortable and unhomely."

Not only does the hypergeneralized feeling field present itself in the A, non-A dynamics with hysteria, but the affective process itself requires vertical growth. By vertical growth, the A <> non-A relationship must develop a new level B, and its mutual opposite, non-B. The quality (A, non-A) is being changed if the local extended quantity reaches a threshold—boundary—and is either reversing its dominance (non-A becomes the core and A the context, and vice versa) or generating a new sign (B) with its context (non-B). In the latter case, we are witnessing the process of abstraction—and with it—generalization and further hypergeneralization.

ABSTRACTION, GENERALIZATION AND HYPER-GENERALIZATION

In the processes of human mental activity the central issue for thinking is that of *abstraction*. Abstraction entails mental operations with mental tools that are distanced from the specific referents they represent. Abstraction leads the way to *generalization*—the abstracted general features of the representation become applicable to new specifics via extension of the abstracted features to phenomena that were previously not considered as the basis for abstraction. Finally, generalization can lead to a state of hypergeneralization (see Figure 4.1).

Hypergeneralization is the process of escalation of the abstract generalized meaning through the whole of the psychological system. Its boundaries can be infinite. Yet, generalization can proceed further—towards loss of clearly definable features of the abstracted concepts. Our most general meanings go through such process—meanings of *love* or *beauty* in English, or *amae* in Japanese, or *prem* in the Hindu meaning system—may begin from specific lived-through experiences, lead to abstraction and generalization of those, and reach at a state where these overgeneralized notions become basic personal or human values. Such values then permeate human conduct at all levels—from immediate reactions to new situations to processes of long soul-searching and life-philosophical contemplation.

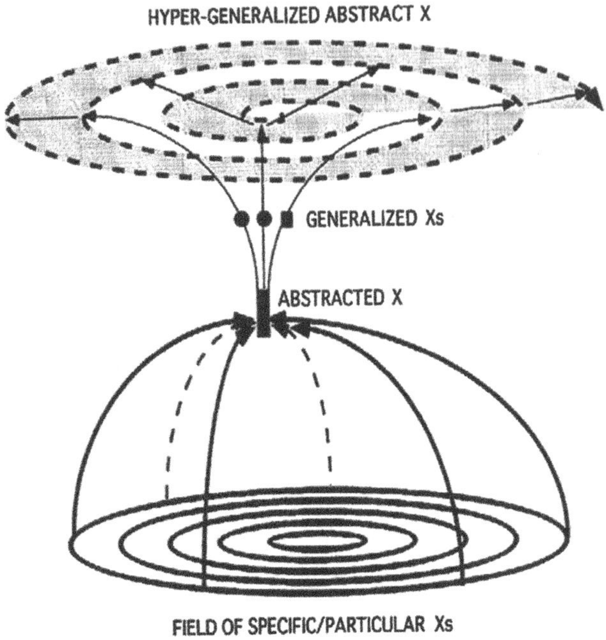

Figure 4.1. From the Particulars to Abstraction, Generalization, and HyperGeneralization

They guide human conduct—in ways that are not accessible to human verbal presentation (Valsiner, 2005, 2007).

How does generalization of meanings (and their hypergeneralization or overgeneralization) work? Any concept used in our social lives is already a result of generalization—it rises above the here-and-now situation by way of abstraction. Any concept entails the construction of mental "sameness" on the basis of various kinds of similarities in experiencing over time. The process of hypergeneralization entails synthesis of new qualities that are not present in the elements. Concerning *beauty*, Charles Sanders Peirce remarked:

> ... when we hear a sonata of Beethoven's the predicate of beautiful is affixed to it as a single representation of the complicated phenomena presented to the ear. The beauty does not belong to each note or chord but to the whole. We have not therefore *heard* the beauty for we have heard only single chords successively. What we have heard is therefore only the *occasion* of the feeling that it is beautiful, only the data to reduce which to unity the sense of beauty serves (Peirce, 1866/1982, pp. 471–472)

As human experience is constantly directed towards the future—in pre-adaptation to the uncertainty of that future—the evaluation in the feeling is diffuse, yet directed. Feelings play their role in human adaptation precisely because of their "fuzzy" character—their "aboutness" rather than certainty. Such aboutness comes through semiotic mediation. It is the human invention—creating and using signs—that makes such transfer of generalized experiences possible (Valsiner & Rosa, 2007).

Hypergeneralization entails turning an abstracted generalized finite set $X = \{X_1, X_2, \ldots X_n\}$ into an abstract *generalized field of meanings*—which by its size surpasses the range of the particulars. The process of hypergeneralization extends the boundary of the meaning field—expanding the horizon. A horizon is a moving border—it constrains the field accessible for us, and moves further as we explore the field—always remaining the limit to the present state of accessible environment. It is thus through sense-making that the person can transcend the here-and-now setting and create omniscopous hyper-generalized meanings that can be transferred to any particular situation to cover any particular situation (e.g., "justice," "patriotism," "love," etc.).

Constructing Semiotic Hierarchies: Unity of Escalation and De-Escalation

Processes of semiotic self-regulation operate through temporary hierarchies of signs (Valsiner, 2001). Generalized and hypergeneralized feelings, as well as differentiated emotions—all encoded as signs—operate as parts of such hierarchy. Signs operate upon signs, and become regulators in respect to one another. The multifunctional nature of signs guarantees the emergence of flexible hierarchical systems of semiotic regulation. The move of a sign into a regulator's role creates the minimal case of a hierarchical dynamic system of semiotic regulators—a superior sign regulates its underlying process. Thus, the person's self-awareness "I am angry" leads to constraining of the primary feeling field.

The hierarchy of semiotic regulation is dynamic—a constructed regulator can immediately be superseded by another level of hierarchical semiotic regulation. Thus, the person who has just entered the regulation of the primary field through the labeling of anger, can generate yet another sign of higher generality that regulates the use of that emotion label—"it is UNFAIR for me to be ANGRY". The regulation by signs includes—recursively—constraining (enabling) the generation of a super-ordinate organizer from the field of possible signs. We may encounter potentially ever-increasing and ever-generalizing growth of the semiotic regulatory system (Figure 4.2).

Here we see a linear unconstrained growth of a sign hierarchy that regulates the flow of the lower psychological process. A person is feeling something (but it is not yet clear to oneself what that some*thing* is). In reality,

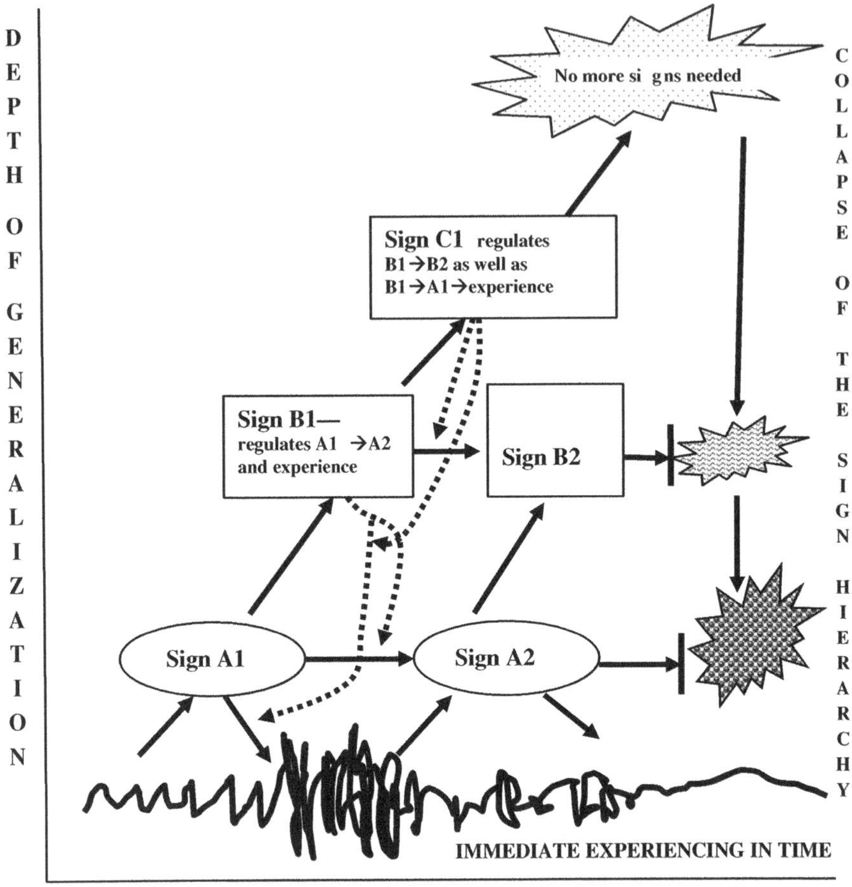

Figure 4.2. The Semiotic Regulatory Hierarchy

it is a field (range) of affective phenomena, not clearly specified. It is not clear what the various manifestations of the feeling are precisely like, it is only clear that the feeling is moving (by the person's introspective) towards becoming narrowly focused. Then, at some instant, the person realizes "I am *angry*" (i.e., creating a sign—A(1) to reflect upon the feeling process).

From the instant of the recognition "I am angry," the feeling realm becomes redirected. The previous feeling becomes now as part of the system of anger, and widens to include other feeling-phenomena through the sign of "anger." This widening guides redefining the range of senses at the sign level. It can lead to the emergence of *unfairness* (A(2)), so the person creates a sign hierarchy:

It is ***unfair*** (A2) →

→ that I am ***angry*** (A1) →

→ feeling **this all** (base level)

A further level—can be added onto the top of that hierarchy—**A(n + 1)** —that introduces constraints upon the previous levels (including the primary feeling field) as well as set the limits for further growth of the hierarchy. As is obvious from the example, the levels of hierarchy entail generalization (and hypergeneralization). The notion *unfair* is a hypergeneralized field-like sign that "captures" the generalized notion of *anger* and neutralizes its feeling at the base level.

The development of affect emerging within a topographic model of the mind sets the basis for a dynamic theory of abstraction, generalization, and hyper-generalization within a hierarchy. The excitation and inhibition of affect is a result of experience—whether it is an internal psychological precipitating agent, or an external stimulus of the environment. This differentiates into general immediate presemiotic feeling, subjective experience, and its natural *Gefühston* (Valsiner, 2007). The immediate presemiotic feeling starts at the base of a hierarchy within the depths of the unconscious. Such affect has not been differentiated or articulated to the point where semiotic markers can identify whether the nature of the affect is of a quality and degree that merits its allowance or prevention from preconscious or conscious levels.

Affective processes burst into an overwhelming flow that can be described as "restless." This allows us to realize that "*I am feeling something,*" *and yet be unable to specify what it is*. Both the affect and its precipitating psychical phenomena (or memory of it) are unconscious and therefore we cannot consciously identify or express what we feel.

PAST PROCESSES AT THE BORDER OF THE PRESENT WITH FUTURE POSSIBILITIES

Hysterical conversions to Freud were overdetermined in meaning. As Freud famously stated, "*hysterics suffer for the most part from reminiscences.*"—multiple (but redundant) associated memories (Freud & Breuer, 1895/2004, p. 11). Freud suggested that the fixation of powerful affects on associated memories inhibited future actions. The fixation of the past in the present, in terms of regulatory mechanisms, means the blocking of the future possibilities.

According to Freud, there are two ways in which the traumatic "seed" of hysteria emerges:

1. A traumatic affective state is present and a thought emerges within the state that is independent from the affective state, but becomes associated with the affective state. The thought and affect becomes interrelated and together marked as "traumatic" Freud & Breuer (1895/2004).
2. A thought emerges but brings about contingent affect of a traumatic quality. As Freud puts it, "Any experience which gives rise to the distressing affects of fright, anxiety, shame, or psychical pain can have this effect ...." (Freud & Breuer, 1895, p. 9). The interrelation of the newly associated thought and affect becomes marked as "traumatic."

According to psychoanalysis, such "traumatic" experiences are normally dealt with in one of two ways: abreaction or associative processing. It is possible, with the failure of abreaction, that repression can occur—a pathological mechanism of "dealing" with traumatic affect. Abreaction is a discharge of the quantity or "quota" of affect associated with the thought (Green, 1999). The discharge of affects leads to the erosion and fading of the thought (Freud & Breuer, 1895/2004). Freud gives the example of both voluntary and involuntary abreactions in which someone can either "cry their eyes out" or seek "acts of revenge" (Freud & Breuer, 1895/2004, p. 11). Freud writes an example of the process of abreacting by confession of *an individual's tormenting secret* (Freud & Breuer, 1895/2004). This example is most notably in the case of Anna O.

> Now it happened, at first by chance, then intentionally, that someone in the house would let slip one of these key words while the patient was complaining about her "torment"; she would soon join in, and begin to paint in a situation or recount a story, at first hesitantly in her paraphasic jargon, but becoming more fluent as she went along, until finally she was speaking perfectly correct German .... These stories were always sad but sometimes very pretty, in the style of Hans Christian Andersen's Bilderbuch ohne Bilder [Picture-book Without Pictures] and this was probably her model: the starting or central point was usually the situation of a girl sitting anxiously at an invalid's bedside, but other quite different motifs were also worked into the composition. A few minutes after the story had been completed she would wake up, and was clearly relieved or, as she called it, "bomfortable" (comfortable). (Freud & Breuer, 1895/2004, pp. 32–33)

We have touched upon abreaction earlier in the chapter with Anna O.'s release from the symptom of the inability to drink when thirsty. The current example of Anna O.'s produces abreaction by imagination and constructions of her stories is in a more common "everyday" way not associated with Breuer's method of hypnosis. Fictional story construction allowed Anna, in her own personal and contextualized way, to release in the present, her powerful affect of the past.

The model that Freud presents for affective relating is one of past-to-present orientation similar to that of a dynamic figure-ground model. In a figure-ground model, part of the model is paid attention to in the here-and-now (the figure), while the other parts are neglected (the ground). Quite similarly, Freud proposes that there are certain affects, which we are paying attention to and that occupy our minds until it can be abreacted and released. Therefore, the affects we pay attention to in the here-and-now are analogous to the figure, and when they are abreacted, becoming faded, and eroded into the past, they become analogous to the ground. The addition of time suggests that the present is represented in the figure and the past in ground.

For hysterical patients, the affect has not been properly transformed from figure to ground—the affect is inhibited from normal discharge in abreaction. Therefore, it remains in the figure, in the here-and-now. This provides a constant disturbing effect on the present. This affect can be repressed if it cannot be abreacted. This is the pathological mechanism of "dealing" with affect of a traumatic quality. Yet, again we see the past-to-present orientation in the Freudian model. Past affects and thoughts repressed into the unconscious effect the present by the construction of hysterical symptoms. The past-affecting-the-present in the Freudian model is also an affective blocking of future possibilities.

Moving Towards a Future-Orientation

Eventually the main determinant of Anna's hysterical conduct was resolved by abreacting the very first pathogenic experience—full of traumatic affect. This episode was one described earlier, where Anna had fallen asleep and dreamt/hallucinated about snakes and paralysis. This fear became associated with her father's illness and the two became interrelated from there after. Nevertheless, abreaction (the erosion and fading away of affect) eventually released Anna from a multiplicity of symptoms.

> And so the paralytic contractures and anesthesias, a number of quite different visual and auditory disturbances, neuralgias, coughing, shaking, etc. and, ultimately even the speech disorders were "told away. (Freud & Breuer, 1895/2004, p. 39)

The disappearance, erosion, and fading of affect can also be observed in the association complex—the second method of normal, everyday affect discharge.

> After an accident, for example, the memory of the danger and the (diminished) repetition of the fright are joined by the memory of what happened next, the rescue, the consciousness of being safe again. A memory of a hurtful statement is corrected *by putting the facts right, by considering one's own worth and so on, such that, through the work of association, the normal person succeeds in causing the accompanying affect to disappear.* (Freud & Breuer, 1895/2004, p. 12)

From the cultural-psychological perspective, the affect does not "disappear," erode, or fade. Affect becomes transformed through sensifying process. The issue is not of "cure" but of development—and that development occurs at the intersection of past and future. The Trajectory Equifinality Model (TEM—Sato et al., 2007, Sato, Hidaka, & Fukuda, 2009) outlines the map of the processes that are involved (Figure 4.3).

First of all, each feeling is a feeling-*forward* process—facing the future—not an irritable pathogenic quality of the past-affecting-the-present. Yet, in this feeling-forward process there is a coordination with the past of two kinds—what actually happened and what could have happened (yet did not) takes place. The TEM models also shows the possible trajectories of the future—potentialities and possibilities. In the cases described by Freud & Breuer (above) the coordination with the future possibilities is blocked,

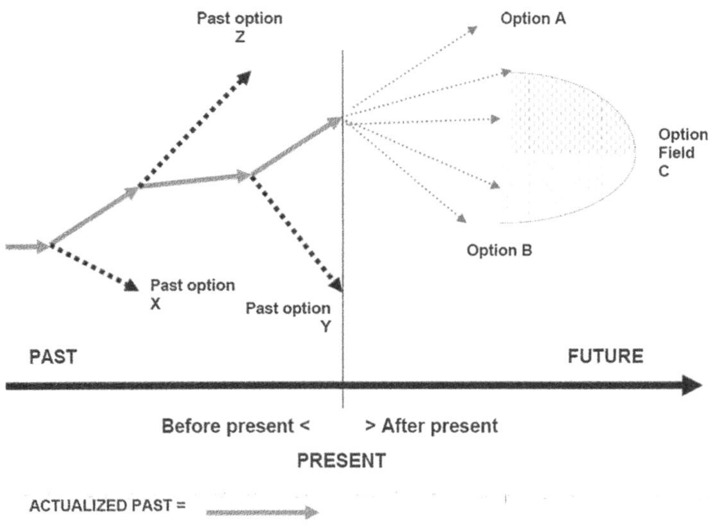

Figure 4.3. TEM model of constructing development

and on the basis of coordinating merely past events the action in the present can be blocked. Freud corroborates that point, saying,

> It may therefore be said *that ideas that have become pathogenic have been preserved with such freshness an affective strength* because they are *denied the normal erosion* that occurs through abreaction and reproduction in states of uninhibited association. (Freud & Breuer, 1895/2004, p. 14, *italics added*)

Again, the metaphors used by Freud are those focusing on the past-to-present, not to past-to-future orientation. This preservation of the affective strength as discussed in the quote is a result of the same condition(s) by which abreaction and associative processes are inhibited. The suppression and repression of the traumatic experience allows for the dissociation of the imagery of (or for) the future from that oriented towards the past.

Freud and Breuer emphasized that the "causes" and "determining quality" of hysterical symptoms are of

> ... either memory of a single major trauma, which we find par excellence in what is called traumatic hysteria ... or of a series of closely related partial traumas, such as underlie in common hysteria. Or, in the final instance, the attack may bring back events which have been raised to the level of trauma by coinciding with a moment which is so disposed. (Freud & Breuer, 1895/2004, p. 16)

The psychoanalytic lens allows for ways of overcoming the past—but not construction of the future. If future were to occur in that case, it has the focus on repetition.

REPETITION COMPULSION: A RESULT OF HYPER-GENERALIZATION

Cultural psychology is focused on future-orientation and the development along the lines of pre-adapting to the future. Such future-oriented models can be constructed from the psychoanalytic quality of repetition of the repressed—a compulsion to repeat. In her case study, Anna O. had lost the ability to talk and became mute for approximately two weeks. However, mute does not mean catatonic. Anna tried to communicate but all efforts fail. This symptom—lacking the ability to speak when wanting to speak—is a particular set of overdetermined dual meanings that display a repetitive nature to them. The symptom was recurring. It was almost as if Anna had a compulsion to repeat—but not a voluntary act to do so.

As presented earlier, the thought by which she was offended was resolved by saying nothing of it—by negating it through repression. Yet, the negation (repression) forces the mind to acknowledge the thought and affect in the transformed expression of the presenting symptom—the inability to speak. Its repetitive quality allowed the experience of the past to not only control the present but shapes the future. Anna O. was,

> ... unable to speak: (a) for fear, since first she had hallucinated at night; (b) since she had once again stopped herself from saying something (active inhibition); (c) since she was once unfairly scolded; (d) in ever similar circumstance (in which she was offended). (Freud & Breuer, 1895/2004, p. 43)

The overwhelming affect of fear (and the *Unheimlich*/uncomfortable) produces a state of affective hypergeneralization. Here, the compulsion to repeat guides future action to quell the overwhelming and hypergeneralized feeling of affect. The affect involved in each experience above is negative—fear, disgust, impoliteness, etc. Therefore, affective relating becomes a regulatory and organizing process that pre-adapts to possible experiences in the future, and prevents them from occurring in the imminent present-to-future by directly inhibiting speech in the here-and-now. The repetition to inhibit speech is not voluntary, but an involuntary compulsion. Future action guided by affective processes is one of hypergeneralized notion.

Order, cleanliness, beauty—they are all hypergeneralized affects that occupy special requirements of society. However, to maintain these hypergeneralized affects, individuals and societies employ the use of repetition compulsions. Freud writes in *Civilization and its Discontents*,

> Order is a kind of compulsion to repeat which, when a regulation has been laid down once and for all, decides when, where and how a thing shall be done, so that in every similar circumstance one is spared hesitation and indecision. (Freud, 1930/1989, p. 793)

The important part here is to realize the implications of the compulsion to repeat with civilization. Civilization is a set of mediated repetitions. With the socially mediated rules, regulations, and repetitions, we are spared the unpleasure that we receive from hesitation, indecision, and the burden of the overwhelming. It is a way of mediating what we need to do, when we need to do it. If we were to stop and think, we would be presented with an overwhelming flood of affect, indescribable to the friend, and unknown to the self. An excellent example of such semiotically regulated pleasure out of unpleasure is the introduction of increased airport security regulations under the hyper-generalized sign-field of *security*. People who travel through airports are subjected to all kinds of un-pleasures—taking off shoes, belts, throwing away one's desired liquids, being hand searched—while gaining the pleasure of "feeling secure"—or at least such feeling is suggested to them.

Repetition compulsion is a way in which we are involuntarily forced to act to overcome an overwhelming feeling of indescribable affect. When such hyper-generalizations occur, we unconsciously and involuntarily force ourselves (a compulsion) to create and construct something known to the individual—a repetition of previously known behaviors. In terms of the {A & non-A} meaning complexes it entails a previously fixed version of B to arise from the non-A region. Freud comments,

> The patient cannot remember the whole of what is repressed in him, and of what he cannot remember may be precisely the essential part of it. Thus, he acquires no sense of conviction of the correctness of the construction that has been communicated to him. He is obliged to repeat the repressed material as a contemporary experience instead of, as the physician would prefer to see, remembering it as something belonging to the past. (Freud, 1920/1989, p. 602)

By repeating we can anticipate what is to come, reducing anxiety produced by the overwhelming feeling of repressed affect. Again the "return of the repressed" has come back to haunt the mind. This time it is not in the form of a hysterical symptom, or a feeling of uncanny, but rather, a repetition compulsion.

Abdin's Problem—and its Solution

Abdin's story in Obeyesekere's (1990) book, *The Work of Culture* exemplifies person's individual repetition compulsion mediated by an overdetermined symbol. Abdin is a 44-year old man who every year hangs on hooks and cuts his tongue in ritual for the great Hindu-Buddhist god, Skanda (see Obeyesekere, 1990, pp. 3–10). If such a ritual was a one-time occurrence, then we would be back to Freud's theory of abreaction and the past control of the present. However, because Abdin is repeating this every year, there is a future-orientation—the quelling of an anticipated overwhelming hypergeneralized feeling. If this were not anticipated, the hypergeneralized state, and all its overwhelming affect, can take control of Abdin. This in fact happened. When Abdin ceased his ritualistic penance, no longer wanting to hang on hooks, he fell victim to hysterical symptoms. When Abdin resumed his ritual of penance—hanging on hooks—the hysterical symptoms disappeared. Obeyesekere (1990) writes,

> Abdin's experience led me to reflect once again on the nature of the personal symbols he employs: they have a repetitive character and possess a compulsive motivation for him. In other words, these symbols operate very much like neurotic symptoms and fit Freud's neat characterization of neurotic behavior as "repetition compulsion" owing to the "return of the repressed." Furthermore,

> even his penances entail body mutilation, bringing them, on the gross phenomenological level at least, close to the symptom. It is certainly possible to express notions of mutilation and castration in a totally indirect symbolic idiom radically different from actual acts of mutilation. I believe that symbolic formation can occur on various levels and in various degrees of remove from psychic origins. The symbolic idiom in Abdin's case is phenomenologically close to its counterparts in symptom formation; they share common features so that under certain conditions of psychic stress, symbol can revert to symptom and vice versa. (p. 10)

The "return of the repressed" and its multilinear development through hysteria, feelings of discomfort, and repetition compulsion operates on the regulatory level of personal symbol. It is these symbols, and their corresponding counterparts, signs, that regulate and organize mental life in a past-to-future oriented framework.

CONCLUSION: CONSTRUCTIVE OVERDETERMINATION OF MEANING

Regulation and organization of mental life, both in cultural psychology and psychoanalysis, are mainly the result of affective processes. As seen in his essay on *Resistances to Psychoanalysis* (1925/2002) Freud emphasized,

> The powerful resistances against psychoanalysis were not of an intellectual nature, then, but stemmed from emotional sources .... The greater part of them came about because the theory offended powerful human feelings. There was the same reaction to Darwin's theory of evolution, which tore down the dividing wall between man and animal that arrogance had created. (p. 91)

To Freud, there were three devastating revelations to humankind's self-image (and possibly even narcissism) resulting in affective responses. The first was Copernicus' theory that the earth was not the centre of the universe. The second, was Darwin's theory of evolution, showing continuity between man and animal. The third was psychoanalysis, positing that humankind does not even know their own mind—they were not always in control of their behaviors and cognitions. It is the common belief that the "intellectual nature" (the quality of thoughts, ideas, etc.) actually organize and regulate our psychic life. However, the implications from Freud's statement reveal that affective processes are not something that "bring us down" from our highly rational intellectual states to primitive and disorganized states, but rather, that affects are actually highly regulating and *organized in their ability to signal the individual to past, present, and future "feelings."* Extracting from the quote by Freud, the offence and "powerful human feeling" is a result of affective regulation and indication of feelings and feeling states towards certain thoughts, ideas, and beliefs. This is how we see them in cultural psychology. Affective processes do not only "*postdict*" or explain how we feel about phenomena, but also *predict*. This gives affect pre-adaptive functions.

Psychoanalysis is not wrong—but limited. It is limited by time—not only its own time (nineteenth century Vienna) but by its assumption of models of time. It builds on a narrow cultural myth. By expanding its dynamic focus and eliminating its master one can arrive at a reasonable theoretical framework that links well with the notion of culture's role in psychical self-organization. Gananath Obeyesekere has laid the foundation for such move:

> If psychoanalysis focused on the overdetermination of motive, one must, in a psychoanalytic anthropology, balance this with the overdetermination of meaning (i.e., polysemy). Thus, overdetermination as I use it, and I think it is not a departure from Freud, refers to either the multiple motives that go to make the symbolic form, or the multiple meanings in a symbolic form or sequence that are determined by a variety of motives; or combinations of both. (Obeyesekere, 1990, p. 56)

This is a classic many-to-many (rather than isomorphic, i.e., one-to-one) relationship. Obeyesekere concentrates on the levels of symbolic remove of the meanings from deep motivations. All cultural symbols are removed from their motivational beginnings—some may remain isomorphic to these (Freud's focus), while others may move faraway from the origin, losing the original link. The symbolic remove requires the *principle of substitutionability*—a sequence of replacement of earlier symbols by new ones (at the same level of symbolic remove—*horizontal substitutionability*), and by way of abstracting generalization (arriving at the hyper-generalized semiotic fields)—*vertical substitutionability*. The latter entails the emergence of qualitatively new symbolic levels that may emerge on the basis of unconscious motives, but as a result of the symbolic remove process acquire autonomy and start to serve as up-conscious regulators of the conscious mental processes.

NOTE

1. Consider examples such as "the night feels dangerous"—there is no specifiable reason for the person who experiences the feeling to be cautious—yet the feeling provides the "this is about danger" kind of flavor to the setting.

REFERENCES

Abbey, E. A., & Diriwächter, R. (Eds.). (2008). *Innovating genesis*. Charlotte, NC: Information Age Publishers.

Breuer, J., & Freud, S. (1955). On the psychical mechanism of hysterical phenomena: Preliminary communication. In J. Strachey (Ed. and Trans.),

The standard edition of the complete psychological works of Sigmund Freud (Vol. 2, pp. 1–18). London: The Hogarth Press and the Institute of Psycho-analysis. (Original work published 1893)

Ellenberger, H. (1972). The story of "Anna O": A critical review with new data. In Micale (Ed.). (1993), *Beyond the unconscious. Essays of Henry F. Ellenberger in the history of psychiatry* (pp. 254–272). Princeton, NJ: Princeton University Press.

Freud, S. (1953). On dreams. In J. Strachey (Ed. and Trans.), *The standard edition of the complete psychological works of Sigmund Freud* (Vol. 5). London: The Hogarth Press and the Institute of Psycho-analysis. (Original work published 1901)

Freud, S. (1961). Five lectures in psychoanalysis. In J. Strachey (Ed. and Trans.), *The standard edition of the complete psychological works of Sigmund Freud* (Vol. 11, pp. 1–56). London: The Hogarth Press and the Institute of Psycho-analysis. (Original work published 1910)

Freud, S. (1989). Beyond the pleasure principle. In P. Gay (Ed.), *The Freud Reader*. (pp. 594–625). New York: W. W. Norton & Company, Inc. (Original work published 1920)

Freud, S. (1989). Civilization and its discontents. In P. Gay (Ed.), *The Freud reader*. (pp. 722–771). New York: W. W. Norton & Company, Inc. (Original work published 1930).

Freud, S. (1997). Negation. In P. Rieff (Ed.), *General psychological theory: Papers on metapsychology* (pp. 213–218). New York: Touchstone Simon & Schuster, Inc. (Original work published 1925).

Freud, S. (2002). Resistance to psychoanalysis (A. Bance, Trans.). In A. Phillips (Ed.), *Wild Analysis*. (pp. 81–92). New York: Penguin Books. (Original work published 1925)

Freud, S. (2003). The uncanny (D. McLintock, Trans.). In A. Phillips (Ed.), *The Uncanny* (pp. 121–162). New York: Penguin Books. (Original work published 1919)

Freud, S., & Breuer, J. (2004). *Studies on hysteria* (N. Luckhurst, Trans.). New York: Penguin Books. (Original work published 1895)

Green, A. (1999). *The fabric of affect in the psychoanalytic discourse*. London: Routledge.

Josephs, I. E., Valsiner, J., & Surgan, S. E. (1999). The process of meaning construction. In J. Brandtstätdter and R. M. Lerner (Eds.), *Action & self development* (pp. 257–282). Thousand Oaks, CA: Sage.

Matte Blanco, I. (1998). *The unconscious as infinite sets* (2nd ed.). London: Karnac Books.

Obeyesekere, G. (1990). *The work of culture*. Chicago, IL: University of Chicago Press.

Peirce, C. S. (1982). Lowell Lecture IX. In M. Fisch (Ed.), *Writings of Charles S. Peirce*. Vol. 1 (pp. 471–488). Bloomington, IN: Indiana University Press. (original lecture delivered in November 1866)

Sato, T., Yasuda, Y., Kido, A., Arakawa, A., Mizoguchi, H., & Valsiner, J. (2007). Sampling reconsidered: Idiographic science and the analyses of personal life trajectories. In J. Valsiner, J., & A. Rosa, A. (Eds.), *Cambridge handbook of sociocultural psychology* (pp. 82–106). New York, NY: Cambridge University Press.

Sato, T., Hidaka, T. & Fukuda, M. (2009). Depicting the dynamics of living the life: The trajectory equifinality model. In J. Valsiner, P. Molenaar, M. Lyra and

N. Chaudhary (Eds.), *Dynamic process methodology in the social and developmental sciences* (pp. 217–240). New York, NY: Springer.

Valsiner, J. (2001). Cultural developmental psychology of affective processes. Invited Lecture at the 15. Tagung der Fachgruppe Entwicklungspsychologie der Deutschen Gesellschaft für Psychologie, Potsdam, September, 5.

Valsiner, J. (2005). Affektive Entwicklung im kulturellen Kontext [Affective Development in cultural context]. In J. B. Asendorpf (Ed.), *Enzyklopädie der Psychologie. Vol. 3. Soziale, emotionale und Persönlichkeitsentwicklung* (pp. 677–728). Göttingen: Hogrefe.

Valsiner, J. (2007). *Culture in minds and societies*. New Delhi: Sage.

Valsiner, J., & Rosa, A. (Eds.) (2007). *The Cambridge handbook of sociocultural psychology*. New York, NY: Cambridge University Press.

Valsiner, J., & van der Veer, R. (2000). *The social mind: Construction of the idea*. New York, NY: Cambridge University Press.

Welby, V. (1896). Sense, meaning and interpretation. *Mind, 5* (17), 24–37.

PART III

OVERCOMING BARRIERS

CHAPTER 5

A CULTURAL APPROACH TO CLINICAL PSYCHOLOGY: PSYCHOANALYSIS AND ANALYSIS OF THE DEMAND

Renzo Carli and Fiammetta Giovagnoli

PSYCHOANALYSIS AND RELATING

This paper is based on the theory, proposed by Matte Blanco (1975), about the psychoanalytical notion of unconscious; the aim of our work is to apply this theory to social relations. But it will be difficult to understand this paper without having any knowledge of the theoretical basis of the psychoanalytical approach to the unconscious as an explication of emotional life.

Psychoanalysis is a psychological theory of the social bond, conceiving the latter as an emotional relationship with real objects which are transformed, by means of affective symbolization, into elements endowed with significant affective intentionality. In the psychoanalytical perspective therefore every aspect of reality assumes a specific emotional intentionality and calls for the activation of an adequate relationship. Even the absence of a "good" object can take on the significance of the presence of an object that

Cultural Psychology and Psychoanalysis: Pathways to Synthesis, pp. 117–150

is "dangerous, being oppressive"; the transformation of the "good—absent" object into an oppressive object is one of the ways the child learns to re-evoke the presence of the gratifying object. But this transformation of a good object's absence into an oppressive object also "works" with the adult: it can help for instance in learning to tolerate frustration.

In psychoanalytical theory, emotion is formed from the process of generalization and symmetrization, governing the mind's unconscious mode of being; it is an authentic mental logic, capable of constructing broader and broader classes, supported in their cohesion and homogenization by a specific "glue," provided by the objects' emotional coloring (see Salvatore & Zittoun, 2011). The "bags" of symmetry that Matte Blanco (1975) talks about, is what is left of the heterogeneous reality, subdivided into numerous interrelated parts, when the various components are "lumped" into emotional classes, such as those that divide reality in black-and-white terms, into the reductive friend/foe dichotomy. The unconscious mode of being, therefore, constructs relations as emotional responses fitting the affective symbolization of the objects encountered in reality.

The notion of collusion—as one of the present authors, working with colleagues, has established (Carli, 1987, 1992, 1993, 1994a, 1994b, 1995, 1997; Carli & Paniccia, 1981, 1999, 2002, 2003, 2005), elaborates this psychoanalytic view of the social bond. Collusion is the unconscious way of experiencing the social bond—that is, the sharing of the affective symbolization of the relationship performed by the persons involved in it. Collusion, therefore, produces an emotionally shared context, as the space of the social exchange organized by the symbolizations of the other persons and of the objects present in the context, which are known by means of the symbolizations themselves.

Clinical analyses that we (with other colleagues) have been carrying out on individual cases as well as on organizations and institutions for the last thirty years (*inter alia,* Carli, 2004; Carli, Guerra, Lancia, & Paniccia, 1984; Carli & Paniccia, 1981, 1999, 2002, 2005; Carli, Paniccia, & Lancia, 1988; Carli & Salvatore, 2001; Guerra & Paniccia, 1987) have led us to elaborate a "hierarchical" model of the symbolizations organizing collusive processes, starting from the emotional dichotomy of friend/foe. This is the most primitive emotional distinction that can be used to symbolize a context: it is a dichotomy which, to paraphrase Matte Blanco (1975), brings us out of the homogeneous indivisible universe into which our mind would plunge if we were not able to make this initial classification, serving on an emotional plane to orient our behavior towards survival-oriented functions. If we think for instance of the basic assumptions put forward by Bion (1961), it is easy to see their connection with the friend/foe pattern: *fight/flight* as the essential principle when faced with a reality symbolized as foe; *dependence* and *pairing* as principles organizing the relationship with the reality symbolized as friend. These dimensions can also be associated with the three motivations for social relations put forward by Atkinson's school, summed up by McClelland (McClelland, Atkinson, Clark, & Lowell, 1953) as: *affiliation*, in close connection to the principle of dependence; *power*, closely related to fight/flight; *achievement*, which can be linked to pairing. However, Bion and McClelland's typologies are descriptive. Only if one considers them as springing from the original dichotomic dynamics of collusive symbolization do they enhance the sense of models of interpretation of the psychological processes nourishing the social bond.

A more complex vision of the differentiation of the friend/foe pattern shows three possible areas of affective symbolization, which we can call *inside/outside*, *high/low* and *in front/behind*.

If we think of the friend/foe pattern applied to the inside/outside dichotomy, it can be seen that the things "brought inside" can be good and friendly, while the things "put outside" are bad or hostile.

This emotional category area can involve great extensions: for instance the feeling of belonging as a reassuring "inside," against which is placed the feeling of foreignness as a dangerous threatening "outside." In view of this emotional categorization it is possible to understand the collusive dynamics governing the rejection of diversity, in all its manifestations, as a dangerous aspect of reality insofar as it negates the expectation of the reproduction of the system of membership which it is hoped will always remain the same. The same applies to the category of the reassuring "bringing inside" in contrast to "putting outside," in the sense of losing, and feeling deprived and threatened by the loss itself. Hence, the dynamics of possession seen as enveloping in a greedy limitless way, in contrast to holding, as the fear of losing what one possesses. The reference to the "body" in this dichotomy of emotional symbolization is clear, as is its infinite metaphorical extension.

We could continue with the high/low dichotomy which implies symbolic emotional dynamics of power, of subjugating or dominating. Or with the in front/behind dichotomy that enables us to range over the very broad area of symbolic emotional dynamics of true and false, of showing and concealing, of supposing and suspecting (what lies "behind" it?).

These few comments are not intended to examine the individual organization of collusive dynamics in depth, but to point out that, thanks to the process of emotional symbolization of objects, the unconscious mental system is able to construe most of the modalities of social relating found in the area of sociality. Starting from the relationship, one can develop a clinical knowledge of psychological events; this path is certainly more useful and fruitful than seeking the defining characteristics of single individuals. On this point, clinical psychology, in the sense of the *psychology of relationships*, differs from psychiatry and the individualistic approaches to social problems, enriching the role that the clinical psychologist can play, with a specific, innovative vision.

The categories proposed for the reading of collusive dynamics enable us to deal not so much with individuals "affected by psychopathology," but rather with problems that people, social groups or organizations present to the clinical psychologist. This approach leads to "diagnosis of the problem" rather than "diagnosis of the individual."

THE RELATIONSHIP AS CLINICAL OBJECT

In psychoanalytical theory, the relationship with emotionally symbolized objects represents the original condition upon which the relationship with reality is organized. The construction of an "inner world" comes about thanks to these experiences of relating emotionally. It is only with a deformation of the psychological problems, and of the relationship within which these problems are brought to the psychologist, that a particular problem can be defined as a psychopathological characteristic of the person. This deformation consists of the fact that the person is "clinically" characterized without the slightest reference to the context in which his/her problem arose and developed.

An example may help to understand this statement better. A woman with serious bulimia problems, overweight according to the clinical medical point of view, tells of an unpleasant episode that she experienced—the previous event that enables the episode to be understood is that, by making great sacrifices, the woman and her husband have managed to buy back, from a government body, the house they have been living in for many years, in the old centre of a town in Lazio. She is glad to have contributed to this "feat," which is important for her husband and herself since their very low wages give them little to live on, and since the cost of living is constantly going up. The woman invites relatives and friends for a drink to celebrate the event. A nephew comes up to her and says, smiling, "Aunty, now you're rich you'll have to make a will to leave something to all us relatives." The woman feels a sudden wave of anger with her nephew, a very strong, uncontrollable anger which triggers one of her usual bouts of gorging. Talking about the episode during a psychotherapy session, she appears to be indignant, offended and angry about her nephew's unpleasant, rude remark. She gets even angrier when she is told that her nephew probably wanted, in a good-humoured way, to underline the "wealth" she had achieved by buying the house; a wealth that "deserved" a will, a new idea for her seeing that up to then she had never had any material possessions to "hand down." The ironic sense of the "guilty" comment was clear to the onlookers, even at the time of the episode, says the woman bitterly;

and her own violent reaction seemed incongruous to her, at least to a "part" of her.

Let us look at the possible reasons for the rage. One factor could be the nephew's unfortunate expression, talking about the will and therefore about death. However, this would not justify such a degree of rage, but rather a rebuke such as "What are you talking about?!". No, rage in the "infinite" sense can only be understood if we look at the emotional elaboration of specific "stimulations." The comment, in its narrative sense, does not justify the anger. But if we look at the two words loaded with emotional meaning "will" and "leave," perhaps we can get closer to the meaning of the emotionally intense reaction. "Will" (or 'testament') refers to a document drawn up before witnesses who attest (from the Latin verb *testari*), and therefore to a document that will be valid after death. "Leave" [in Italian "lasciare" from the Latin *laxus* (relaxed, loosened)], refers to losing, not being able to hold onto, as for instance when the sphincters are loosened. In buying the house, the woman has just made a purchase, and she finds herself having to face the fear of loss, and of *dying in the loss*; this losing is seen as having to leave it to others; hence the anger and the compulsive need to "put in" food, as an apotropaic act (i.e., an act having the power to contrast the undesired event), designed to ward off loss by acquiring. But fear of loss is also "fear of losing weight" or of losing parts of her body, seeing that the house can be symbolized as the enveloping body. The two emotionally dense words evoke an emotional response that has nothing to do with the meaning of the comment uttered by the nephew, but instead is connected to the fantasies the woman associates with the two emotionally significant words. This reconstruction is possible if the nephew's remark is treated like a dream, listening to the woman's reaction as she talks about her anger and the feelings evoked by the comment, as if they were connected to a dream episode. This dream episode is organized as phantasmatic emotionality evoked by the emotionally dense words in the nephew's comment. The woman's associations have in fact been polarized on the two words remembered. These words have been transformed into a forced, duty-bound relationship where the nephew plays the role of all those who disapprove of the woman's obesity and want to force her to lose weight, to lose a part of herself, to let go of what she possesses to become attractive again and to let herself be possessed by others, particularly her husband. The woman's obesity began when the man with whom for many years she had had a clandestine relationship, made her his wife. During the illicit relationship, the woman experienced her own beauty as a seductive power, therefore, as the power to keep the man she was having the affair with. When they got married, the woman experienced a profound change in symbolizing her affective sexual relationship with her husband: from an active seductiveness that was always new, the woman felt she had been plunged into conjugal duty, a sort of obligation to satisfy her husband's desire. Hence, the fantasy of a relationship in which seductive activity (from the Latin *secum ducere,* leading with oneself) was transformed into the passivity of letting herself be possessed. Hence, the defensive response of gorging as if "holding" within her, as the opposite response to feeling that she was "losing" parts of herself, in letting herself be possessed. The calls to lose weight, real or metaphorical like the one made by the nephew with the joking request for a will, are seen by our woman as invitations to accept promptly the passivity to which marriage "condemns" the woman. Hence, the anger and the defensive response of gorging. Without an analysis of the relationship with her partner and with family members and friends, and without an analysis of the emotional symbolizations that these relationships entail, it is difficult to grasp the sense of the problem presented by the woman in psychotherapy, when she tells her story of the event.

We think that the relational perspective in clinical psychology and in psychoanalysis practised with the limits of psychiatric training, is difficult because it seems that there are no models for a useful interpretation of relationships. We put forward the notion of collusion to overcome this lack. From our psychoanalytic point of view, collusion does not have the commonsense meaning of a deceitful allegiance. Rather, it is the process of affective symbolization that organizes the relationship.[1] In the example given above, it can be supposed that the nephew has a predatory fantasy towards the aunt who has "become rich" by buying the apartment; a joking predatory fantasy, as we have underlined, but one that is collusively perceived as dangerous and threatening by the woman who transforms it symbolically into an invitation to "leave," to "lose," to assume a passive attitude that she sees as an irreparable defeat of her seductive power. The transference relationship itself takes on a deeper and more useful clinical meaning if read in the category of the collusive process.

At the same time, the relational perspective involves a profound change of models in the theory and in the objectives of psychoanalytical work. There is the shift from the correction of the individual deficit to the identification of lines of development in people's process of adaptation in their context. This also entails a critical reading of the individual deficit reduction approach: a reading that cannot avoid critical consideration of the notion of psychological "normality" at which deficit correction explicitly or implicitly aims (Grasso & Stampa, 2011). This normality, in turn, is inexorably linked to social conformism, to the norms of a society without problems for the ruling social groups, and therefore, for psychotherapy as the standard-bearer of constituted power and of the normality that every strong social power sets out to establish.

If one pursues development in the relationship between people and context, on the other hand, the psychotherapist cannot foresee and establish the parameters of such development: psychoanalysis thus becomes a tool in motivating an adequate use of resources, rather than an opportunity to correct disorders. In the case of the woman in the example, it is not a question of bringing her back to a "normal" weight and to a "normal" passive behaviour towards her husband, with both things being closely tied to a conformist vision of the marriage bond. In the culture in which the person in question lives, this conformism involves the woman's duty to be attractive and to submit to conjugal duties, and therefore to forget the fantasy of seducing the man in an illicit situation. Perhaps, it means reconstructing the competence to live out a relationship of exchange in marriage, valorizing the reciprocal motives to build a gratifying relationship together.

THE INDIVIDUALIST STEREOTYPE AND THE LACK OF ATTENTION TO THE CONTEXT IN CLINICAL PSYCHOLOGY

The vast majority of clinical psychologists in Italy seem to have little interest in constructing knowledge and intervention models that can respond to the needs of the specific context where they work. It is as if, unlike other professions, the ability to respond to society's demands were not the criterion to legitimate and develop clinical psychology. This lack of interest in the social demand is attested by the limited amount of research designed to discover the image of the psychology profession among the population, the potential customers of this profession. At least in Italy, psychologists do not seem particularly interested in knowing the expectations that "others" have of the profession; they seem scarcely interested in knowing the social demand, the modality of representation or, if you like, the image of clinical psychologists and of the professional service they offer.

Various authors underline the low social profile of clinical psychology.

> The psychology profession is in a critical condition: the mismatch between training and professional activity; quantitatively and qualitatively low levels of employment; fragmentation and progressive lowering of competence levels and profiles; (...) confusion between the practice of the profession and imitative practices with low or inexistent ethical and competence levels (ranging from card-reading to talk-show psychology); lowering of the social prestige of the role; political, cultural and institutional weakness compared to other professions (in particular, in the public health field, but also in that of organizations, schools, and social services); an essentially absentee attitude on issues of national interest (Salvatore, 2006, p.121).

In these words, Salvatore describes the Italian situation of the psychology profession. It is a profession bound up in models of knowledge-getting and intervention that have trouble meeting the demands of the social system.

If one considers research in clinical psychology, one finds the same mismatch between the knowledge gathering phase and the intervention phase. We see a type of research that has left no mark on the history of our culture, on the history of our "convivence" in society, while this same history and culture of convivence stimulate the scholars and researchers in other fields of human sciences to apply themselves in order to bring improvement.

Underneath the lack of cultural importance of clinical psychology, we see its entrenchment in models that treat the individual as an object for knowledge-getting and intervention. Clinical psychology considers the behavior of the single person, his belief system, his motivations or his emotionality, as if the single person existed, characterized by this set of variables, independently of the context in which he or she lives. No heed is taken of the space–time coordinates within which the individual is placed: space in the sense of context (cultural, emotional, symbolic, cognitive) of which the individual is part; time in the sense of the individual's historical, diachronic dimension. The *individualist stereotype* is capable of permeating most of the scientific production and the theoretical proposals of clinical psychology.

The Individualist Stereotype and Clinical Psychology as The Science of Intervention

The various psychological theories can be grouped into two broad areas.

The first sees psychology as a science designed to formulate hypotheses on specific laws governing human behavior and to prove them empirically. The second sees psychology as a science of intervention (clinical, social, educative), designed to pursue changes in individuals, considered in relation to the context in which they live and work.

The first deals with the individual as the object of study; the second is interested in the individuals' relationship with the contexts where they live with others, as the area for intervention.

The first bases its verification on the possibility of experimentally testing the statements made, on the experimental operationalization of hypotheses about human behavior. In the second, the verification of psychological practice is related to the aims of the stakeholder commissioning the intervention and to the social function of the intervention.

In this paper, we wish to pose a question. Has experimental psychology enabled general laws of human behavior to be identified, capable of influencing people's life together, the well-being of individuals, communities, and social groups?

To answer this, let us think of some of the best-known examples of experimentation in psychology. Asch's research into social pressure (Asch,

1955); the experimental situation known as *strange situation* adopted in the study of the attachment styles (Ainsworth, Blehar, Waters, & Wall, 1978); Festinger's research into cognitive dissonance (Festinger, 1957); Witkin's work on the field dependent–independent cognitive style (Witkin, 1950). How does experimentation work in the research cases mentioned? We think that, in general terms, the following hypothesis can be made: certain individuals are chosen, responding to criteria of representativeness of the population being studied, in terms of preestablished variables, such as sex, age, area of residence, socioeconomic class and so on. This "group" of people are subjected to standardized stimuli, chosen to serve the hypothesis that is to be proven experimentally (Here we will ignore the problem of the control group, serving for the demonstration of the null hypothesis). The responses to the stimuli offered to the experimental subjects are then recorded, and, based on a classification of these responses, the hypothesis is considered proven or not proven.

Solomon Asch's well-known experiment can be used as an example. The author had designed a specific experimental situation. The aim was to study the conflict evoked by social forces on individual people, to make them act against their convictions and values; to show the forces that the individual can activate in order to resist coercion and threats directed at their integrity. The experimental situation consists of 7–9 people who have to decide which of the three different length lines is the same as the "standard" line, presented alongside the other lines. The experimenter asks the participants to sit on the chairs in the front row (as often happens with college students) in the experiment (described as a perception test); he asks each person to announce his/her own decision, starting from the first in the row. At the end of the row, in the second last seat, there is the only experimental subject; the others are all "accomplices" of the experimenter and have been trained to give the wrong answer unanimously, without exception. The experimental subject's response behavior is revealed, in conflict between the phenomenic, perceived evidence, comparable to "individual integrity" and the pressure of the group of accomplices, comparable in turn to social pressures that aim to undermine beliefs and values. Well, in the responses given by one third of the experimental subjects, their decision "caved in" to the pressures of the majority, at the expense of the perceived evidence. In the comments on the experiment, a lot is said about conformism, independence, and the problem of consensus. The conclusion reached is that there are great individual differences in response to the experiment: the experimental subjects can be divided into two groups: the independent ones on the one hand, the submissive ones on the other. Each group, moreover, also shows internal variability in motivations for the independent or submissive behavior adopted during the test.

Let us think about the experimental set-up: it is designed to discover the single individual's response to social pressure, artificially prepared by the experimenter and acted out by the experimenter's accomplices, as if in a theatrical performance. The phenomenic evidence is used as the expression of the individual's integrity, and the pressure of the people present in the experiment, with the experimenter's agreement, is considered to represent the threatening coercion of social pressures. There is no mention of relations between the experimental subject and his companions, who are also his college-mates; no mention of the relationship between the experimental subject and the experimenter, who is however a professor at his college. There is no analysis of the social sense of the "trick" carried out with the experiment: where social pressure is exerted on the basis of an "experimental" agreement between people, so as to place one of them in a situation of artificial conflict, the result not of social pressure but of the false agreement. Let us now try to take a position outside the experimental situation and look critically at the interaction between experimenter, accomplices and experimental subjects in the specific historical and cultural situation where the experiment was carried out. To do this, one obviously cannot use "empirical" methodologies like the experimental situation used by the researcher in question. And yet, we think we can get a deeper knowledge of what is called social pressure by looking at the experiment as a whole; this includes the result of the experiment in its empirical mechanism. Other models concerning the relationship, just to take one example, that of the "double bind," could give the experiment and its results a more interesting meaning than the "individualist" classification into "independent" and "submissive."

The examples could go on, considering those cases where the subjects are classified beforehand according to specific psychological dimensions, and where the response to the environmental stimulus they receive makes it possible, in terms of the experimental variable, to differentiate the subjects previously classified with other variables. In psychology, the scientific literature is full of experiments of this type. What has all this research shown? The connection between attachment styles and defences most commonly used in psychotherapy by adult subjects; the connection between attachment styles in adult subjects and success levels in the most varied social tasks (obviously, the most mature defences and the highest success rate are characteristics of the subjects with "secure" attachment styles); the connection between different cognitive styles (field dependence—independence) and the behaviour of subjects in tasks such as group decisions in situations of uncertainty, or performance on intelligence and aptitude tests.

What use has the social system made of these results? It can be stated, with some caution, that the psychology of general laws, the psychology that has claimed to describe the individual's behavior, attitudes, interests, response to controlled environmental stimuli in the logical structure represented by the statement, "if.... then....," has not produced results of great significance.

This is far different from economics, sociology, biology, physics and chemistry, which with their laws, have created opportunities and tools to exert an innovative influence on the social system of convivence.

Failure of Empiricism in Psychology

We think there are essentially two reasons for this failure of empiricism in psychology: the laboratory condition required for the formulation of general laws on the psychology of the individual, which is an artificial state, different from reality[2]; the specific decision to study the single individual regardless of his context, and therefore of the relationship between them and of the cultural dimension underlying the story. This second reason, in our view, is the most problematic.

The individualist stereotype is cogent in the psychotherapeutic field too. We are referring to the psychotherapy approaches that place the individual at the centre of their model, split from his coordinates of time and space, that is, from his specific cultural context.

The literature dealing with psychotherapy research abounds with references to psychotherapy models oriented to modifying the individual's behavior. If there is no framework of reference on normality and pathology, this behavioral modification is equivalent, as we have said, to conforming to the social norm. We see a growing deference to the common way of thinking or to the positions of the majority.

> If we consider recent history, we see that various factors contribute to clinical psychology assuming a corrective, medicalized form. This form is increasingly evident in its psychotherapeutic expression, which moreover tends to take on an emphatically conformist guise and a dominating position in the clinical psychology intervention. (Paniccia, Giovagnoli, & Giuliano, 2008, p. 57)

Concerning the area of clinical research nowadays considered most significant by the scientific community, Massimo Grasso writes,

> Clinical research aiming to measure the efficacy of the psychotherapies sets out to record and measure the patient's "progress." What models of "psychological normality" or of "mental health" is this "progress" oriented by? If one explores some of the work that sums up the issue (...) one comes up with some paradoxical outcomes, simply by considering the extreme consequences of an intrinsically ideological vision of the problem (...). This ideological

> vision could be expressed as a formula equating conformism to normality and normality to health: the feeling of subjective psychological and/or physical well-being corresponding to embracing current values and life-styles, or to recognizing one's membership of a sector of society, is assumed a-critically and in a linear way as a fundamental parameter of clinical judgement. (Grasso, 2006, p. 7)

Also in the case of the individual's psychotherapy, we find the same neglect of the demand for psychotherapy intervention on which it would seem to be quite obvious that psychotherapy should base itself. This mismatch between demand and intervention practice is clear to other disciplines, ready to occupy the client spaces neglected by psychotherapy. An example is philosophical counselling, presented by the professionals who practise it as an alternative to psychotherapy. The latter is seen as an intervention which is unable to treat the demand of those who are not represented as having a deficit or being maladjusted and needing to be brought back to the norm, but who, as Galimberti (2006) argues, want to benefit from their investment in life. In criticizing the capacity of psychotherapy to respond to its clients' needs, the philosophical point of view gives no chance of appeal: psychology is defined as a self-centered discipline, closed in on itself, taking refuge in preestablished criteria of normality and pathology, more interested in becoming part of the club of the so-called exact sciences than in responding to its clients' needs (Achenbach, 2004; Lahav, 2004; Mace, 2001; Pollastri, 2005; Ranchetti, 2003, Sini, 1993).

To become one of the so-called exact sciences, psychotherapy has adopted medicine's working model: a patient informs his doctor of a symptom (this part of my abdomen hurts), the doctor passes from symptoms to signs (semeiotics structures the medical examination) and lastly to tests (in the laboratory, increasingly specific and sophisticated) so as to link the symptom to an etiological diagnosis and therefore to a therapy. The therapy, one has to remember, is strictly dependent on and consistent with the causes of the pathology diagnosed and the specificity of the illness in the individual person who has presented the symptoms. This procedure cannot be used by the psychotherapist: in psychotherapy there is no framework of reference on the normality and pathology of the problems that are to be dealt with. It follows that the problem presented by the patient has to be reinterpreted in the light of the form of psychotherapy practised by the particular psychotherapist and defined by the theory of technique underlying that specific psychotherapy. This is why a person with a specific problem may undergo psychoanalysis, systemic or cognitive psychotherapy, depending merely on whether he went to a psychoanalyst, a systemic therapist or a cognitive psychotherapist. In this case, the demand of the person asking for an intervention is assessed in relation to the applicability of the therapeutic technique to the patient's case. The problem presented by the patient is seen in this perspective.

The way of interpreting the demand involves significant consequences for the aim of the psychotherapy work. If the demand is taken literally, the goal of the person intervening is to modify the situation which is presented as problematic, in the demand. When the demand is taken literally, what happens can be read in terms of the *collusion model:* collusion between the psychologist who intervenes and the "party," implicitly the one making the demand, with the power to get the psychologist to intervene. This party with power may be the person with whom the psychologist will carry out his psychotherapeutic intervention, or someone commissioning the psychologist to intervene psychotherapeutically with a client. Otherwise, the demand can be considered a pretext for understanding the problem—that is, the demand itself can be considered as not clearly expressing the problem but alluding to it in ways and forms that can be interpreted and analyzed. In this case, the goal is to establish an idea of the demand itself. This is therefore a goal that can be called methodological.

Taking this kind of goal as criterion, the different forms of psychotherapy can be divided into two broad groups. On the one hand, there are the psychotherapies whose objective is to modify behavior; on the other, those that have methodological objectives designed to stimulate thought about the emotionality that characterizes the onset of the problem, once working conditions have been set up that can suspend the emotional acting out of the person presenting the problem. Modifying behaviour means thinking that the problem lies in the behavior of the person asking for the psychotherapist's intervention; one is therefore faced with an operation, with various options, designed to change the behavior or the cognitive structures of the problematic person. It is obvious that if one intervenes on the individual, and if one takes the demand literally, one cannot avoid intervening on behavior or attitudes that seem at odds with normality, in order to bring them back to the norm.

Setting up emotional thinking on the emotions, on the other hand, means hypothesizing that change, if it is possible, is a modification of the "culture" in which the problem is posed that leads to the demand being made on the psychotherapist. What is hypothesized is a symbolic mind, based on the emotional symbolization of reality. The latter is conceived of as the driving force of the mental representation of the shared context, and therefore of the action. This means that the action is always collusive action, being necessarily part of a social and cultural dimension.

One may wonder about the reasons for the persistence of the individualist stereotype as the anchorage of professional clinical psychology. Why do psychologists forego models of psychological intervention and leave space to other disciplines that are better able to free themselves from the hegemony of scientist culture? The answer is to be found in the specific local culture of psychotherapy.

> This tendency can be explained by the hope of having greater collusive success, responding to the expectations of control typical of a society that, engaged in the difficult task of trying to integrate diversity, seeks reassurance in conformity. (Paniccia, Giovagnoli, & Giuliano, 2008, p. 56)

Psychotherapy's anchorage to some form of distress and its individualistic orientation mean that conformist models are implicitly taken as the intervention goals. Clinical psychology, seen in this way, risks becoming the "long arm" of the social power whose interest is to control and standardize behaviors and cognitive systems. The advantage of taking the intervention demand "literally," comes from the fact that it is enough for something to be reported as "not working" for the person making the intervention to be given total responsibility for diagnosing, finding the causes of the problem and identifying the best strategy for the intervention itself. By means of the medical model, the demand implies a profound passivity, a de-responsibilization on the part of the person presenting the problem; once the problem has been "reported," it is no longer in the province of the person making the demand, but is taken on totally by the person that will do the intervention. A further advantage, if it can be called so, is that the problem is limited, one could say bottled up, in the person presenting the problem, and so all involvement of the context in which the problem arose is excluded. Power, as the symbolic emotional organizer of clinical psychology, hinders the ability to deal with the social demand addressed to our profession. For professional relationships not to be based on power, an alternative model is needed. We will deal with this model in the next section.

Analysis of the Demand and Local Culture

Let us start from the premise that even when the demand for intervention presented to the psychologist comes from single individuals, it always refers to their process of adapting to the context. The object of the psychologist's intervention is the relationship between the individual and the context where he lives, not the individual taken in isolation. What is needed is obviously a model to consider the demand in this analytical perspective.

About fifteen years ago, Carli and Paniccia put forward a model for the possible analysis of the demand for intervention. This model takes different modes and types of demand that the psychologist may receive into account: demands that may come from single individuals, from family groups or from specific organizations, as well as from complex organizations or social systems with various roles. We will briefly outline this model.[3]

The idea underlying the two authors' model is that of *collusion*: our mind in its unconscious working can be identified with the affective symbolization of the emotionally important aspects of the context. Affective symbolization follows specific rules, the most important of which is, as we have pointed out above, the attribution of emotional intentionality to all the objects involved in the symbolization. This means that through the affective symbolization of the context, one triggers an emotionally involving relational modality that it a source of implications not only on the level of emotional fantasy but also on that of adaptive action. All the people who share a context actually share its affective symbolization; we call *collusion* the symbolic-affective sharing of the context by the people who live in that context. Collusion can therefore refer to the affective symbolization defined by specific contexts.

There can be different ways of affectively symbolizing a context on the part of the various components of the context; these symbolic-affective modes will, moreover, be related to each other, due to the sharing of the context by such components. We use the expression "local culture" to indicate the set of different collusions that the various components of a context set up within the context.

Along with the notion of collusion, that of *Local Culture* originates with the aim of offering a model for the collection and analysis of social relations in the psychoanalytical theory of the emotions. Local Culture refers to the *collusive emotional symbolization of specific "objects" of reality by the people who share a specific context.* In a recent work, we studied the representation of the neighborhood of San Lorenzo, in Rome, and its relations with the Faculty of Psychology situated in that area; the representation of the CSM (Mental Health Centres)—of its roles in the professional population working in these centers was also studied; as was the representation of the psychologist's professional image among the population of Tuscany; the representation of the Italian banking system in a representative sample of the Italian population; the representation of the new information technologies among the same Italian population, and that of traffic and traffic rules among the population of Rome. We could go on at length, in view of the different uses our research group has made of this data. The recording of Local Culture is possible, and useful, in many situations, when it can give information and general strategies to adopt in carrying out a clinical-psychological intervention. The idea of Local Culture contains the intersection of the theory of *emotional symbolization* of specific objects and that of *the context*; constructs that are well suited to defining both the objects to be studied as well as their collusive symbolization.

In the research on the San Lorenzo neighborhood, as we said, the object of the collusive dynamics analyzed was the representation of the neighborhood and its relationship with the Faculty of Psychology, as they are symbolized in the group of heads of the associations operating in the neighborhood on the one hand, and in the population of the area, on the other. What was studied was the representation of the neighborhood,[4] of its changes, of its evolution, also in connection to the presence of the Faculty of Psychology, its university activities and its students. We thought about the population participating in the research and the illustrative variables characterizing it: groups of different ages, sex, educational level and occupational situation. We are also thinking about the emergence of different attitudes towards the neighborhood: for example, the *acceptance* or *rejection* of San Lorenzo and its "liveability," to mention the two extreme attitudes. Now, considering the illustrative variables alone, we might find (just as an example) that the young and the students accept the neighborhood, while the pensioners and the elderly reject it. What information could we draw from this finding? Little, very little. In fact, we would not have any element to explain the phenomenon recorded: we would not be able to formulate any hypothesis on the reasons for the acceptance or rejection on the part of specific groups of the population living in the area. This is due to a reason that is as simple as it is obvious: in the theories underlying studies on the "liveability" of a neighborhood, there is no hypothesis about the relation between acceptance–rejection of one's place of residence and the illustrative variables we have just mentioned. There are no hypotheses on the relation between acceptance–rejection of the neighborhood and the sex, age group, and whether one is a student or a pensioner. Once the data has been collected, we could certainly hypothesize a connection between the acceptance expressed by the young and the rejection on the part of elderly men: for example, the fact that the neighborhood is undergoing a great transformation, with a greater range of evening and night-life; but they would be *hypotheses based on stereotypes found in the researcher or in the information sporadically given by the mass media, not on the interpretation of information deriving from the data*.[5]

To collect data on the local culture, more complex studies are needed on attitudes and on the cultures that give rise to them. Opinions, assessments of objects, and their emotional symbolization are aspects that never refer merely to one side of reality, and they are never the characteristics of one single person.

The multiplicity of objects and the multiplicity of people: these are the typical elements that organise a local culture.

The problem is that of understanding the interactions between this double multiplicity and source of variability, of showing its articulations and differentiations, knowing that what is found has to be situated at a specific point in time. We must stress that the "multiplicity" we are talking about has nothing to do with a sum total of elements (the objects of symbolization and the people who symbolize), but has connection with the interaction between the elements themselves. Regarding the objects, as we have said, it is not a matter of finding the symbolizations of, for example, the neighborhood *and* of its various aspects, the traffic *and* the efficiency of the services *and* the reliability of the institutions *and* the main factors of growth. From a point of view focusing on the sum total of the findings, we would obtain numerous opinions on the most varied fields and topics, without any criterion for connecting the data. Let us suppose, instead, that people are asked to assess the best ways to be successful in Rome and in the neighborhood of San Lorenzo; let us suppose that two alternatives emerge: *being part of a power group* or *planning strategies for growth and foreseeing changes*. Let us also suppose that each of the two modalities proposed is correlated to a specific validated model of the *vision* of social life: belonging to power groups as social opportunism and the hope of gaining contacts to help improve one's position; planning in order to anticipate changes as the capacity to strategically guide one's development. We therefore have an important anchorage for an understanding of which symbolic dimension people use to represent their own development. Let us now ask whether the people of San Lorenzo *are interested only in themselves and their own family*, or *follow the rules* or *are trying to improve convivence*: this is an item that explores the incidence of familism,[6] compared to following the rules for its own sake or to an involvement that takes *others* into account in a dynamics of convivence in society; from familist commitment, to rule-following, to the effort to develop sociality. We now have two types of information: it will be important to understand how these kinds of information interact, in order to make hypotheses on the culture, they can give rise to. If, for example, we have a grouping of the type *belonging to power groups only interested in themselves or in their own family*, then we can legitimately make inferences differentiating this grouping from another of the type *anticipating changes/ improving convivence in society*. We now take that acceptance of the neighborhood is manifested by the second group, while the rejection is a feature of the first. Now, we would thus have some elements on which to base the analysis of the culture of acceptance and of rejection of San Lorenzo and of its "liveability."

If multiple aspects are proposed in asking the inhabitants about their neighborhood, we could identify different groups, constituted by different variables inserted in the questionnaire; it would then be possible to hypothesize different models of local culture.

Similar considerations can be made regarding the people participating in the research. If they are considered "one by one," their function will only be that of adding to the number of responses: with 100 subjects, we might find the following distribution: 40 of them state that familism dominates in the neighborhood; 37 say that rule-following prevails; 23 the promotion of convivence. It will not be easy to use this information. But if the responses of the various subjects are linked to the multiplicity of questions asked, then the interaction between subjects and answers given to the various questions may provide *groupings of subjects/responses* that are easier to interpret for the purposes of recording the cultural components.

IOD Methodology

In order to reveal and measure the Local Cultures our research group elaborated the IOD methodology (IOD: Indicators of Organizational Development). This is a methodology that, in a questionnaire prepared *ad hoc* for the different areas of investigation, poses questions about the opinions and attitudes towards the Italian and local social system, towards the various institutions and the most varied professional figures, along with questions related to the subject of the research: in our case, the image of the neighborhood in relation to the city of Rome and the presence of the Faculty of Psychology. It is important to underline that the construction of every question or group of questions comes about on the basis of *specific models of interpretation of the collusive dynamics in the system of social relations.* With IOD, it is not a matter of knowledge-getting questions whose meaning is made explicit and defined by the question itself: scales of approval or acceptance of specific objects of reality (such as opinions on the Limited Traffic Zone in San Lorenzo), collection of opinions or of indicators concerning reputation, assessments of one's past or of one's experience and so on. Instead, with IOD the questionnaire serves to analyze a complex series of dimensions and psychosocial models that can investigate important components of the culture characterising the research participant's group.

The statistical processing of the data envisages the analysis of *all the responses* to the various questions *produced by all the participants* in the research. All the data obtained are *processed together*, so as to identify the connections between responses to the different questions and individuals: these connections serve to *reduce the variability of the individuals' responses* and to reveal specific clusters of responses/individuals that give clues on the collusive culture underlying the clusters themselves. There are good reasons for hypothesizing a close connection between collusive processes characterizing the different cultures (in relation to the aim of the research) and the statistical process leading to the identification of clusters of responses/individuals within the factorial space of the data.

Local culture therefore originates from the reduction (statistical and clinical psychological) of individual variability. We know that social interaction produces collusive emotional symbolizations; we know that such symbolizations, shared by those living in the same context, allow for a reduction of the original emotional *ambiguity* towards the objects of reality with which the group relates. The reduction of the ambiguity towards the objects of reality, on the other hand, is a process concerning "groups" of objects or "groups" of individuals. Objects that have a close symbolic-emotional relationship are carried along "together" into dimensions of the friend/foe type, and this occurs in the social relationship, therefore, as a result of various individuals relating together. The "social" reduction of ambiguity is the result of a collusive process and generates an (emotional) sharing of specific affective symbolizations for those participating in this collusive process. This is how Local Cultures are generated. The term "culture" implies for us the shared emotional participation on the part of a group of people, in a collusive process; the term "local," in turn, stands for the specificity of the set of objects of reality that are transformed, from the original ambiguity, into shared emotional symbolizations and the specificity of the set of people collusively symbolizing these objects. Local Culture and organizational goals.

In the model proposed, the importance of collusion can be understood only in relation to the demand for reality posed by the limits of the context; collusive processes are therefore conceived in relation to the actors' interpretation–construction of the limits of the context they belong to. As we shall see below, collusion can also be acted out as denial of the context; this is what we call *denial of the extraneous*.

Think for instance of a technical high school in the Lazio area: the teachers in this school symbolize the school context as a place of discipline and order, while the pupils symbolize it as a place where the young transgressively challenge adults. This implies a conflict established within the school, caused by the two contrasting symbolic-affective dynamics. This conflict, and the collusive dynamics that led to its emerging among teachers and pupils, can be considered the local culture of the school in question. Due to the pragmatic implications of the local culture (continual acting out of conflicts in teacher–pupil relations; learning difficulties created by the conflictuality; families' dissatisfaction with their sons' school experience) the school principal contacted the psychologist, originally asking for a reduction in the teacher–pupil, adult-youth conflict that was spoiling school operations. In the case we are briefly mentioning, the psychologist did not take the demand literally, but set out to analyze the collusive dynamics underlying the "conflictuality" event; to do so, he tried to shed light on the local culture underpinning the relationships between groups and between generations. The interpretation of the local culture, which the psychologist sees as the initial phase of his intervention, is not designed to reduce the symptom presented as the pretext for the demand (the conflictuality); the aim is to identify lines of possible development of the structure in which the intervention is being made. In its connection with the goals typical of a specific context, the local culture actually constitutes the driving force of functionality and development. The local culture, in the sense of the integrated set of the different symbolic-affective modalities of the context, makes a major, decisive contribution to the construction of the achievement function and to the pursuit of the objectives typical of the context.

In the example, we have given, think of the symbolic aspect—"the teenagers' challenge to the adults": if this challenge is able to free itself from the emotional acting out of pupils versus adults, and construct a relationship between the emotional dynamics of the challenge and the school's learning goals, then the local culture will be able to establish an innovative and transformational form of learning, as a critical defeat of the orderly, repetitive – disciplined—learning style advocated by the teachers-adults. The teacher/adult—pupil/youth conflict can be freed of the reciprocal contrasting acting out, oriented on the one hand to controlling and judging teenager behavior in class as unruliness; on the other to deriding and rejecting the teacher-adult world-view, seen as being obsolete. If the local culture in question can evolve from the sterility of the acted out conflict, it will produce a lively, fruitful debate between adults and teenagers on the style and contents of learning. This debate will free learning from orderly repetitiveness on the one hand, and from reactive, unproductive improvisation on the other. We are describing, albeit in general terms, the function of fostering production, which is consistent with the goals, and which the local culture can assume in a specific organizational context.

We have also said that, to promote production, local culture must free itself of the emotional acting out of affective symbolization. This is a very important point, within the theoretical construct we are envisaging. The affective symbolization of the context can have two different destinies, in social relations experienced by the various symbolic areas, or if you like by the different cultural repertoires of the context itself. Collusive affective symbolization, in other words, can be *acted out* or *emotionally thought*. When it is acted out, it is difficult for collusive dynamics to place itself at the service of the production process. We must also add that the destiny of most collusive symbolizations is that of collusive acting out, of avoiding emotions from social relations.

In the model we are proposing, the acting out/emotional thought dichotomy depends on the level of polysemy retained by the collusive affective symbolization in the contextual relationship. The higher the degree of polysemy, the more likely it is for the collusion to be acted out; the more definite, precise and limited the collusive symbolization is in emotional thinking, objectified in objects consistent with the organization's goal of production, the more likely it is for the collusion not to be acted out but to be emotionally thought. It is the function of thought (which we call "emotional thought" insofar as it is organized in emotional dimensions and dynamics) that reduces the polysemy of collusive processes, and therefore of affective symbolizations. It is a type of thought that we, like Matte Blanco (1975), define as the establishment of "relations between" emotional-symbolic components; the establishing of relations, in fact, enables the objects symbolized to be at least partly removed from the polysemy of affective symbolization, and to be given an organization that underlies the experience of strangeness of the object, and therefore the need to construct a relationship of exchange with the object itself. Remember that polysemic symbolization of objects ties them to familistic emotional values, based only on the affective dynamics of friend/foe, with its infinite variations on the theme. The construction of relations between objects detaches these objects from familistic values and makes a decisive contribution to defining their extraneousness, an important potentiality for motivating the relationship of exchange between components in the context.

In our example of the school, the emotional thinking that establishes relations between objects makes it possible to free teachers and pupils reciprocally from emotional visions of a familistic kind: the teachers, like parents, intolerant of the new and unexpected, in the pupils' symbolization; but also the pupils like children to control and hold back in their potentially dangerous desire for innovation, in the teachers' symbolization.

THE PHASES OF COLLUSION

Carli & Paniccia (2002, 2003, 2005) proposed a series of empirically demonstrable phases in the construction of collusive symbolization in organizational contexts as well as in relations between the individual and the context.

1. *The phase of symbolization: this consists of the projection of affective elements belonging to one's bodily reality onto the objects of the context.* These are symbolic dynamics: inside/outside; tall/short; in front/behind. More generally, all these symbolic dynamics can be covered by the category: friend/foe. It is understandable that these collusive symbolizations, involving a high level of alarm in relation to the function of survival that they perform, both phylogenetically and ontogenetically, are very likely to be acted out in the collusive relationship.
2. *Symbolization concerns an affective-symbolic class that we call neo-emotions.*[7] These are symbolic processes concerned with relating to what is foreign; the function of the neo-emotions is to negate the extraneous and to transform it into a familiar object with which one can return to the primitive symbolizations mentioned in the previous phase. If this transformation takes place, then there is a high probability of collusive emotional acting out.

According to our proposal, the most primitive neo-emotion is *expecting*. Expecting is a neo-emotional modality that seeks to establish a relation where one wants to obtain something from the other person, but without entering a relationship of demanding, without negotiating a symmetrical transaction with the other person. The person who "expects" hypothesizes a relationship of power over the other person, taking it for granted that he will obtain what he wants. One who may expect is the sick person, because he is suffering and is therefore part of a collusive helping relationship, almost compulsory, on the part of the other person. The university student may 'expect' at a lecture, expressing his claim (to remain passive and uninvolved, but also possibly to reject the teaching he is being offered) with a detached, sceptical attitude.

One may respond to this expecting with another demand, for example that the patient recovers from his symptoms. The purpose of the one who expects is not productive but concerns the organization of collusive dynamics that ignore, at times successfully, the limitations of the context. For instance the one who expects can in turn become subject to expectations, thus being involved in a collusive relationship of reciprocal control.

The one who expects, on the other hand, may evoke a response that is not totally symmetrical. When faced with the rejection of the demand, there may emerge two different neo–emotions: *controlling* and *distrusting*. The first expresses an active reaction in the relationship of denying extraneousness, while the other involves a passive reaction. Controlling means acting so as to guide and direct the other person's behaviour, so as to make it predictable, in a relationship of conflict. This is a difficult emotional goal, often impossible because it can only evoke disturbing, symmetrical emotions in the other person. Distrusting means establishing a relationship in which one wants to show a friendly stance to one's friend, to reassure the distrustful person about one's real harmlessness: again an impossible task. Then again, controlling and distrusting can evoke collusive reactions in the other person but, like all neo-emotions, are not able to negate extraneousness. And here we see the reaction to controlling: *provoking* or *obliging*; and the reaction to distrusting: *complaining* or *worrying*. By provoking one tries to prevent the unpredictable variability of the other person's behaviour and of the emotions that such unpredictability can arouse, by laying down new rules of the game: these are personal rules that one wants to impose on the other person as if they were universally accepted rules. Obliging means acting out the fantasy of possessing the other person, by communicating in the relationship the feeling of having been defrauded and robbed, and therefore evoking guilt feelings. Complaining and worrying have a common meaning: calling into the relationship a third person endowed with power, so that the extraneous can be controlled. Figure 5.1 provides a graphic representation of what has just been said.

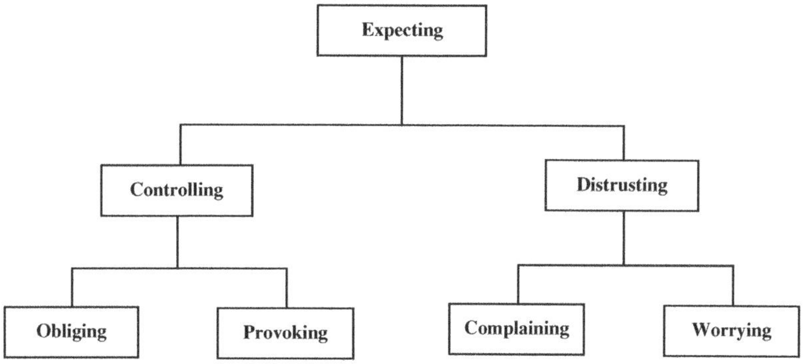

Figure 5.1. The Tree of the Neo-emotions

The neo-emotions are an adaptive resource of great importance: they enable relations to be structured ignoring the limits of the context. A "victim" who obliges can play his role of expecting, and can expect collusive responses at the bar just as in a board meeting. But this adaptive dynamic is not adequate for all situations; for example, it never responds to the need for growth.

The alternative to the neo-emotions is the *competence in convivence,* based on the knowledge of the stranger and on the productive use of this knowledge. How? It is the *history* of each of us, as well as the *context* we belong to, that characterizes us. These are the elements underlying the modality of the productive process, as well as its failures. It can be said, in the methodological perspective proposed here, that the development of every person, of every social group as well as organization, can be understood only in the history of these aspects. One must consider, on the other hand, that for the growth he or she can experience, each person is closely connected to others in the organizational context where he or she lives.

3. The third phase, in this path is marked by *the reduction of polysemy in relation to the symbolic objective nature of the productive process,* comes from the symbolic models underlying social relations. Think of the dichotomy between duties and goals, of that between the substitutive function and the integrative function in the organization (Carli & Paniccia, 1999), of the dichotomy between "given" and "construed" organization,[8] of the dichotomy between the social mandate and those commissioning interventions,[9] of that between user and client; in this case, too, the first dimensions mentioned are more likely to be affected by collusive acting out, the second have a lower probability.

The shift from highly polysemic symbolizations to symbolizations more oriented to the product and to the relationship with otherness is based on the emotional thinking that the components of the context are capable of developing about the symbolization itself. Emotionally thinking of the affective symbolization, on the part of a participant in the same context, on the other hand, is a function closely connected to the capacity to suspend collusive acting out in the contextual relationship. We therefore have a dichotomy in the affective symbolization process: on the one hand, there is the acting out of affective symbolizations, on the other, the emotional thinking about symbolizations, tending to organize the action according to the product. It should be pointed out that the first product is the knowledge of symbolic emotionality, as a crucial resource in the process of production anchored to the organizational goals. At this point an important clarification is needed. The choice between acting out and emotional thought is determined by the relation between the individual and the context; it is not an individual characteristic.

The Familist System

The place *par excellence* of emotional acting out is the familist system. We do not say "place" unintentionally. By saying this, in fact, we mean the relationship between individual and context. It is easy to see that the term derives from the family relationship.

In brief, familistic systems are the social and organizational processes that adopt the model of affective symbolization that is typical of the family. The family is a social system which, in the various historical periods, has played very different roles and has assumed different ways of being.[10] We can say that from the point of view of postindustrial culture, in the nuclear family there are symbolic-affective investments that may recall an institution based purely on the affective relationship, with no production goals. There is one exception, concerning a specific, idiosyncratic outcome: that of easing the young members, of the second generation, out of the original family system.

The absence, in the family we are talking about, of a differentiation of roles and functions involving productive objectives, implies relations that can be seen as establishing phantasmic acting out. The family social system seen in its relational reality, is characterized as we have said by the emotional acting out of reciprocal affective symbolizations. This can be linked, as we have said, to the specific relational modality characterizing the family system: Internally, there is no product; relations between the family members, therefore, are regulated only by affective symbolization, which does not serve its transformation based on thought and knowledge; as a result of what we have just said, there is the breakdown of the subdivision of roles based on the differentiation of competences; instead of the competent role we find the affirmation of the "given" role, based on gender differences (husband–wife; father–mother) or on generational differences (parents–children, in all the possible generational forms). Instead of the interaction organized around the difference of competent role, and aimed at the achievement of the product/objective, in the system of family relations a simpler dynamics is acted out, based on the need to possess the other person by expecting. The expectation appears to be the only organizer of family relations: one expects love, obedience, fidelity from the other person; every action based on expectation responds to a simple emotional "logic": "it's all for your own good!." Emotional acting out in the family is substantiated by expectation, such as the demand for emotional symbolizations in others, and therefore, the demand for others to act out, based purely on the "family" role played in the family system. The mother can expect to "be loved" by her children, as the "mother" ("after all I've done for you!"); children can expect to be gratified in their demands on their parents, as "children" ("I didn't ask to be born!"); the couple can expect "faithfulness" from each other, due to the mere fact that they are married and have shared family responsibility ...

In this system of relations based on expectations, there may be very violent symbolic acting out, which can be connected to the probable disappointment of the reciprocal expectations. When a demand is frustrated, one plunges into an anguished emotional state of "non existence," insofar as there is the loss of anchorage to the only possible identity in the productless system; hence, the violent aggressive acting out as a reaction to plunging into emotional "non existence." The only regulatory system "external" to expectations, and to the reciprocal control based on expecting, is the establishment of rules of the game that can be called "good manners." Since the production of "good manners" occurs at a higher level than that of expectations based on "given" roles, it is in fact the only possible product of the family social system.

Familist systems are social organisations, endowed with a product and a social function, which (for different reasons) lose the emotional symbolization of the product, and turn these symbolizations towards the internal relationship between people, roles, power systems: "as if" it were a social system with no product, comparable to the family. In analyzing familist systems the idea of power has to be introduced. We think there are two levels of power in organisations: *competent power*, based on the role that each person plays in the organizational context, in view of his/her competent contribution to the achievement of specific shared production objectives; and *power without competence*, which can be likened to the control present in family dynamics grounded on expectations based on the taken-for-granted role.

In the case of family and familist systems, collusion supports the system of relations based on expectation. Collusion in other words underlies the affective symbolizations of taken for granted roles, and justifies the emotional acting out that this collusion necessarily leads to, which can in fact be defined as expectation. It is also possible to analyze how failed expectation develops, going through the whole tree of neo-emotions, as it derives from the thwarting of expectation.

The alternative to the neo-emotions, as we have seen, is the competence in convivence, based on knowledge of the extraneous and on the productive use of the knowledge itself. We have thus reached the point of talking about systems that are able to develop emotional thinking about affective symbolizations; relational systems that use, and think about, affective symbolizations to know the emotional life of the organisation and to orient it towards an optimal functioning.

The organization, in this case, is constantly "constructed" by the thinking about affective symbolizations, and can therefore adapt to the demands of the broader social context. Emotional thinking is comparable to the two functions, assimilation and accommodation, which Jean Piaget (1964) considered to be at the basis of the individual's psychological life. Assimilating is, in short, reducing the unknown or the different, to the known; accommodating, on the other hand, is confronting and changing the known, on the basis of the unknown that one has known. Thinking of affective symbolizations, or if you like, knowing the local culture of a system one belongs to, means assimilating different cultural models to one's own, and accommodating one's own cultural model to the diversity of the "others," represented by the extraneous. The family system, closed and fixed in taken for granted roles, therefore changes in the social system open to dialog with the extraneous, in reciprocal processes of assimilation and accommodation which allow for the bridging of differences and interaction aimed at a productive objective.

Producing, literally "putting in front," means marking the dual relationship with the hoped for and constructed presence of a third person. Producing in other words means setting up the "growth" of the organizational system by planning and organizing competent dialog. If seen in this perspective, producing also means exploring the setting where the organization one belongs to is located; it means increasing the ties of exchange with other structures, potentially conflicting and threatening to the system one belongs to, if they are seen as closed alternatives of membership. There is no production without exchange. Nor is there exchange without production. But exchange and production are the results of thinking about affective symbolizations; without emotional thinking, there would only be an acting out rejecting or encompassing extraneousness, assimilation without accommodation, or accommodation without assimilation.

A CASE OF ANALYSIS OF THE DEMAND

In the terms stated above, we can now analyze the case of a mother worried about her depressed teenage daughter. The demand the mother addresses to the psychologist intends to reproduce an intervention system similar to her vision of the family: a psychologist-father, manipulated by the mother, intervening with the daughter so that the daughter will correspond to the behavioral models that the mother wants. She is a 45-year-old woman, separated from the man with whom she has had two children; the woman wanted a third pregnancy and she recalls that her purpose was to have a "daughter all to herself". She has never said clearly who the father was, she kept the child with her for all the years until the girl's adolescence, in an extremely intense fusional experience, where the mother's whole existence was devoted to her daughter, in the belief that there was also complete reciprocity on the girl's part. The relationship between the two has always been based on total frankness, trust in the other, without the slightest reserve. The daughter shared with the mother all her childhood and teenage friendships. Things started to go differently when the girl, now a 20-year-old, fell in love and had her first romantic relationship. According to the mother, she suffered a very strong conflict between the two desires: to talk to her about her love story or to hide the emotions she was feeling with the boy she was in love with. The mother repeatedly begged the daughter to keep these feelings to herself, granting her "permission" to have secrets that for the first time could characterize their relationship. It was in concomitance with these events that the daughter showed the first symptoms of "depression," as it was defined by her mother: she no longer wants to study or go out with friends; she stays at home doing nothing, often cries, has lost all interest in the music she loves; she is remote even with her mother, feeling a hostility towards her that she cannot explain. All this is recounted to the psychologist by the mother, who says she has a feeling of worried alarm at the worsening of her daughter's "symptomatology." The mother asks the psychologist to intervene with her daughter with psychotherapy; she also wants to work out with him the best way of getting the daughter to agree to psychotherapy, which the mother would like to see beginning as soon as possible. In the mother's vision, this decision to go to the psychologist, like her emotions towards her daughter, are comprehensible and justifiable: "What wouldn't a mother do for her daughter!." The woman is stunned and at first indignant when the psychologist suggests working on what she has said, so as to understand more clearly the emotions and attitudes that may have motivated a problematic reaction in the daughter, and that in any case are creating problems for the mother. She accepts the proposal to "think about her emotions" in the relationship with the psychologist: first of all, the fantasy that took her to the psychologist, though with the excuse of her daughter, and that allowed her to tell her whole, highly problematic, story. It is important to notice that:

1. If the psychologist accepted the mother's invitation to deal with the daughter, he would set up a sort of collusive family system, assuming the "parental" role, in a collusive relationship with the mother. This collusive system could later influence every possible intervention by the psychologist with the daughter and at the same time, would represent an unsurpassable obstacle to thinking about the mother's proposal;
2. if the psychologist establishes with the mother, the person who made the demand for psychological intervention, a relationship tending to think of the emotions acted out in the demand, he constructs a relationship that makes it possible to "think about" what the mother acts out; this is possible insofar as the collusion acted out in the demand does not find a response acted out collusively in the psychologist, but the construction of thinking about what has been collusively offered to him. The psychologist, by analyzing the demand, shifts from the level of acted out collusion, to the level of emotional thought on the collusive acting out.

The main aim of analysis of the demand is therefore to prevent the intervention from establishing a familist system (as defined above). This is important because in an intervention based on familist collusion, it is possible to interpret and analyze dreams and fantasies, "do psychotherapy"; but this may all be "fake" insofar as it is based on a collusive familist assumption, where each person plays his/her role as if s/he were in a taken-for-granted system, without any possible productive change. Certainly, the patient may be better, the psychotherapist may be satisfied with her work, those commissioning the psychotherapy may appreciate the progress made by the patient, but it all happens in a closed system, with no exchange and no product. A sort of rite, pre-scripted and predictable.

A note on this point: the mother's demand was motivated by the daughter's "feeling bad," by her rejecting the model of those who "feel good." The worried demand, in other words, is closely connected to the legitimation that a parent, a relative, a friend, a superior at work or at school, thinks they will achieve when they are concerned for someone else's state of mental health. It is the same legitimation envisaged by the person who asks for a psychotherapy intervention for himself, motivated by "feeling bad." This is in the perspective of attributing to psychotherapy the *restitutio ad integrum* of the person who feels bad. It is a very different situation when the intervention is requested by a person with the *desire to develop* in his work, studies, learning, or cultural growth. This is the case of the girl in the example we are discussing: some time after the mother came to the psychologist, the daughter *spontaneously* contacted another psychologist; not for "depression" but to get help in returning to her studies and social life, and therefore with clear developmental aims. Continuing with the example, the mother agreed to work on her phantasies of making her daughter go into psychotherapy. She therefore worked on the fantasies that had marked her whole relationship with her daughter from conception onwards; she explored her attempt to possess her daughter in a fusional relational system, where what clearly emerged was the value of compensation played out by the phantasy of possessing her daughter, as well as being possessed by her daughter. The aim of her work of analysis of the demand was not so much to separate herself from her daughter, which had in fact already happened, considering the daughter's adult age and the desire for independence that the daughter could not accept as a concession on the part of her understanding mother. The daughter was in fact claiming that independence as a right-duty of her adult state. The real aim of the work of analysis becomes, for the mother too, the pursuit of personal, professional and social development. The daughter had been a sort of tool for the legitimated gratification of the need to possess and of affirmation in a contextual culture that valorises the maternal role. It very quickly emerged that the woman had shifted onto motherhood, put off until the end of her daughter's adolescence, a need for self-affirmation that she had not dared to express in her professional work. One could say that the woman had been forced by her husband with her first two children, to give up her initial, promising professional activity in the field of interior decorating. Constrained by her husband: a constraint that she had accepted collusively, later developing a violent hostility towards the collusive system acted out. Her third pregnancy was a sort of revenge for the woman on her husband and the family and social culture she had collusively embraced. These familistic dimensions had forced her towards the "duty" of being a mother, as opposed to the desire for affirmation at work. A sort of revenge, played out in the same area of social constraint: "well, if I have to be a mother, I want to do it triumphantly, pushing every other person out of the relationship with my daughter, in a fantasy of exclusive possession." The work of analysis of the demand connected the woman's emotional involvement to the context of family and friends: an involvement that had led to her investing her new possessive motherhood with her need to succeed, confused with that of revenge and provocation, and had motivated her giving up professional success. Reporting the daughter's problem, in this analytical perspective, meant *also* hoping that the psychologist would notice her problem and her fusional relationship with her daughter. It was an implicit "demand," conveyed by the emotionality of the relationship in which the request was made to the psychologist, by her "manipulative" symbolisation of the psychologist, by the attempt to reproduce, with the psychologist, the relationship of control and power that the woman had established with her daughter and that she had systematically and regularly reproduced in relating to her friends and in her social relations in general.

The "boldness" of the demand can often be interpreted as the hope for a noncollusive reaction from the psychologist. One of the present authors recalls a phone call from a woman, who very anxiously asked for an appointment for her son. When asked the age of her son by the psychologist, the woman, suddenly calmer and almost smiling, said that he was 25 and that he consented to the appointment for psychotherapy. The psychologist politely told her that it was not enough to consent to start psychotherapy, but one had to be strongly motivated to work, something which could only be verified with the son. The woman, relieved, said she would get her son to call back. In this case, it is not possible, in a short telephone conversation, to analyze the mother's demand; it is however possible to postpone the fixing of an appointment and to leave space for the decision of who will ask for the appointment: the son if he wants to, or the mother, thus changing the point of view about the client that is more motivated and interested in meeting the psychologist.

NOTES

1. The term "collusion" comes from the Latin *cum ludere*, which means "to play together." Its etymology does not present the negative connotation that the modern term (both in English and Italian) has acquired.
2. It is useful to recall that the laboratory was constructed by psychologists conducting laboratory experiments: it is not a fact. The laboratory therefore is not only a limit to the experimentation but also a system of information that helps to understand the experimenter's culture.
3. For a more detailed examination of the analysis of the demand model (see Carli, 2006; Carli & Paniccia, 1981, 2003, 2005).
4. The term representation is linked, first, to S. Moscovici's theory of social representations (1961). We must remember that with the term social representations the Author refers to value system, ideas, and practices, that develop within and through social communication. Social representations are the elaboration of a social object by a community that allows his members to behave and to communicate in a comprehensible way. With regard to functions of social representation, we remember that they provide an order to the world, they help social communication and interaction, they demarcate and consolidate groups, and they make the unfamiliar familiar. As Grasso and Salvatore (1997) point out, social representations are not only a series of concepts, affirmations, explanations that grow out of daily interactions; they also express the way we acquire our knowledge. They are not only a series of opinions but they also act as value systems by which we construct and understand

our social reality. Social representations can be considered a set of meanings, often implicitly shared, on which social relationships insert. The development of the meaning of the term social representation, which we outline, conducts us to a second theoretical reference: Franco Fornari's theory of emotional code (1976). According to the author, the unconscious is conceived as emotional semiosis, which is a process of representation seen as attribution of meaning by emotional codes. The concept of collusion, which is at the base of the theory of the analysis of the demand to which the research refers, uses F. Fornari's emotional theory to categorize models of interaction between individual and social context. The term "representation" used in this work, mean collusive symbolization of the context.

5. We strongly emphasize this point. In much research, "data" is sought without an hypotheses about the models underlying the measuring tool and their meaning. The data is then "explained" on the basis of common attitudes, or of stereotypes present in the researcher's own culture. Such research is often pointless, and sometimes dangerous due to its claim to experimentally "prove" the experimenter's prejudices.
6. According to our proposal, "familism" is the extension of the model of affective symbolization that works within the family, to other social organizations. This model is characterized by the absence of reference to the productive aim of the social exchange and the assumption of the inner relationship as a unique criterion and value (see below, sub-paragraph "The familist system", p. 140ff).
7. By neo-emotion we mean emotional processes that do not belong to the individual, its intrapsychic world, akin to the emotions of anger, love, joy, fear, but always refer to the social relationship. We decided to call them neo-emotions because, although they are emotional processes among the best known, psychology rarely focused on them. This is because they are emotions that usually are not considered in the psychoanalytic and psychology literature because they do not belong to the individual.
8. By the expression "given organization" we mean an organization considered to exist independently of the procedure and the purposes of people working inside it. The experience is that of an organization separate from a specific historical, geographical, cultural context. Without time, space, or changes, the organization is perpetuated to infinity, always staying the same. Without relationships with the outside, all the emotional life is turned inside the organization, tied up with the rights and duties of its participants. In a given organization the professional function is anchored to obligations, not to purposes. The prevailing motivation, according to McClelland's model, is power and affiliation. A person that stays in a given organization feels reassured by the uncritical and foregone affiliation to the organization itself. In order to experience the organization as construed a third party has to enter: the customer of the organization. If the customer is at the top of the organization, the latter does not exist to perpetuate itself but its purpose is to earn its customer's satisfaction. In the construed organization participants have the feeling they contribute to its operation. Here, the prevalent motivation, still using McClelland's model, is achievement and not power and affiliation. For a discussion, see Carli and Paniccia (2002, pp. 124–130).

9. When the operation of an organization is anchored to the social mandate the procedure is built on aims that come from a socially shared system of values. Characteristic of the organization strongly oriented to the social mandate is the strong idealization of the organizational purpose. Organizational structures that work for commissioning, in turn, orient the practice to the knowledge of the specific needs of those who demand the intervention. The practice is innovative, varied, and oriented to the needs and constraints of the social context that makes the demand for intervention. For a discussion, see Carli and Paniccia (2002, pp. 134–143).
10. Suffice it to think of the family that is part of the clan or tribe, as it existed in the past, in western culture, and still exists in various countries today. Think of the extended family, where several generations lived in the same relational structure, with specific characterizations, whether patriarchal or matriarchal. Think of the nuclear family, characterized by the couple's relationship and limited to the presence of two generations, parents and children. Think, on the other hand, how the advent of the nuclear family created problems for the older nuclei, often with their return to the children's nuclear family; this offered family dynamics with very different features from the extended families of last century. We do not wish to stray into a field that is the domain of family sociology or cultural anthropology; this brief mention serves to get us thinking about the difficulties inherent in talking about the family without seeing the historical, cultural and structural depth of this ancient institution.

REFERENCES

Ainsworth, M. D. S., Blehar, M. C., Waters, E., & Wall, S. (1978). *Patterns of attachment: A psychological study of the strange situation.* Hillsdale, NJ: Erlbau.

Asch, S. E. (1955). *Social psychology*. New York: Prentice-Hall.

Achenbach, G. B. (2004). *La consulenza filosofica [Philosophic counseling]*. Milano: Apogeo.

Bion, W. R. (1961). *Experiences in Groups*. London: Tavistock.

Carli, R. (1987). L'analisi della domanda [Analysis of the demand]. *Rivista di Psicologia Clinica, 1*(1), 38–53.

Carli, R. (1992). L'analisi della domanda nell'intervento psicosociale [Analysis of demand in the psychosocial intervention]. *Il giornale degli psicologi, 1*, 13–20.

Carli, R. (1993). L'analisi della domanda collusiva [Analysis of collusive demand]. In R. Carli (Ed.), *L'analisi della domanda in psicologia clinica* (pp. 5–40). Milano: Giuffré.

Carli, R. (1994a). L'analisi della domanda [Analysis of the demand]. In G. P. Lombardo (Ed.). *Storia e modelli della formazione* (pp. 45–68). Milano: Franco Angeli.

Carli, R. (1994b). Psicoanalisi della collusione e conoscenza clinica [Psychoanalysis of collusion and clinial knowledge]. In G. P. Lombardo & M. Malagoli Togliatti (Eds.), *Epistemologia in psicologia clinica* (pp. 143–175). Torino: Bollati Boringhieri.

Carli, R. (1995). Analisi della domanda e integrazione individuo-contesto [Analysis of demand and individual-context integration]. In G. Trentini (Ed.), *Manuale del colloquio psicologico* (pp. 47–80). Torino, IT: Utet.

Carli, R. (1997). L'analisi della domanda rivisitata [The revised analysis of demand]. *Psicologia Clinica, 1*, 5–21.

Carli, R. (Ed.) (2004). *Culture giovanili: proposte per un intervento psicologico nella scuola [Juvenile cultures. Proposal for the psychological intervention in school]*. Milano: Franco Angeli.

Carli, R. (2006). Collusion and its experimental basis. *Rivista di Psicologia Clinica [On line Journal], 2–3*. Retrieved from http://www.rivistadipsicologiaclinica.it/english/number2/Carli.htm.

Carli, R., Guerra, G., Lancia, F., & Paniccia, R. M. (1984). L'intervento psicosociale nei servizi di igiene mentale: un'esperienza [Psychosocial intervention in mental health community centers. An experience]. *Psicologia Clinica, 3*(1), 75–96.

Carli., R., & Paniccia, R. M. (1981). *Psicosociologia delle organizzazioni e delle istituzioni [Psychosociology of organizations and institutions]*. Bologna, IT: Il Mulino.

Carli, R., & Paniccia, R. M. (1999). *Psicologia della formazione [Psychology of the education]*. Bologna, IT: Il Mulino.

Carli, R., & Paniccia, R. M. (2002). *L'Analisi Emozionale del Testo: Uno strumento psicologico per leggere testi e discorsi [The Emotional Textual Analysis. A tool for reading texts and discourses]*. Milano: Franco Angeli.

Carli., R., & Paniccia, R. M. (2003). *Analisi della domanda: Teoria e tecnica dell'intervento in psicologia clinica [Analysis of demand. Theory and technique of the intervention in clinical psychology]*. Bologna, IT: Il Mulino.

Carli., R., & Paniccia, R. M. (2005). *Casi clinici: Il resoconto in psicologia clinica [Clinical cases. The report in clinical psychology]*. Bologna, IT: Il Mulino.

Carli, R., Paniccia, R. M., & Lancia, F. (1988). *Il gruppo in psicologia clinica [The group in clinical psychology]*. Roma: Carocci.

Carli, R., & Salvatore, S. (2001). *L'immagine della Psicologia: Una ricerca sulla popolazione del Lazio [The image of psychology. A study on the population of Lazio]*. Roma: Kappa edizioni.

Festinger, L. (1957). A theory of cognitive dissonance. Evanston, IL: Row, Peterson.

Fornari, F. (1976). *Simbolo e codice [Simbol and code]*. Milano: Feltrinelli.

Galimberti, U. (2003, October 10). *Il successo della filosofia [The success of pshilosophy]* [Elettronic version]. Retrieved from http://www.repubblica.it/2003/i/sezioni/spettacoli_e_cultura/filosfi/filosfi/filosfi.html.

Grasso, M. (2006). Nails, fingernails and hammers: scattered notes on clinical psychology today. *Rivista di Psicologia Clinica [On line Journal], 1*. http://www.rivistadipsicologiaclinica.it/english/number1/Grasso.htm.

Grasso, M., & Salvatore S. (1997). *Pensiero e decisionalità [Thought and decision-making]*. Milano: Franco Angeli.

Grasso, M., & Stampa, P. (2011). Psychological normality, psychopathology and evidence-based psychotherapy: are we so sure "we're not in Kansas anymore"? In S. Salvatore & T. Zittoun (Eds.), *Cultural psychology and psychoanalysis. Pathways to synthesis* (pp. 225–278). Charlotte NC: Info Age Publishing.

Guerra, G., & Paniccia, R. M. (1987). Analizzare la domanda: un caso di intervento in un Servizio di Diagnosi e Cura [Analyzing the demand. A case of intervention in a Mental Health Center] . *Rivista di psicologia clinica, 1*(1), 54–64.

Lahav, R. (2004). *Comprendere la vita [Understanding life]*. Milano: Apogeo.

Mace, C. (2001). Formazione filosofica e filosofie di formazione in psicoterapia [High education in philosophy and the philosophies of high education in psychotherapy]. *Costellazioni, 6*, 37–55.

Matte Blanco, I. (1975). *The unconscious as infinite sets: An essay in bi-logic*. London: Gerald Duckworth & Company.

McClelland, D. C., Atkinson, J. W., Clark, R. A., & Lowell, E. L. (1953). Analysis of imaginative stories for motivational content. In D. C. McClelland, J. W. Atkinson, R. A. Clark & E. L. Lowell (Eds.), *The achievement motive. Century psychology series* (pp. 107–138). East Norwalk, CT: Appleton-Century-Crofts.

Moscovici, S. (1961). *La psychanalyse, son image, son public [Psychoanalysis, its image, its public]*. Paris: Presses Universitaires de France.

Paniccia, R. M., Giovagnoli, F., & Giuliano, S. (2008). For a clinical psychology of development: The competence in constructing contexts as the product of the intervention. *Rivista di Psicologia Clinica [On line Journal], 1*. Retrieved from http://www.rivistadipsicologiaclinica.it/english/number1_08/Paniccia_Giovagnoli_Giuliano.htm.

Piaget, J. (1964). *Six études de Psychologie [Six psychological studies]*. Genève: Gonthier.

Pollastri, N. (2005). *Il pensiero e la vita [Thought and life]*. Milano: Apogeo.

Ranchetti, M. (2003). Male: soggetto o aggettivo? [Evil: subjective or objective?] *Costellazioni, 7*, 53–62.

Salvatore, S. (2006). Models of knowledge and psychological action. *Rivista di Psicologia Clinica [On line Journal], 2–3*. Retrieved from http://www.rivistadipsicologiaclinica.it/english/number2/Salvatore.htm.

Salvatore, S., & Zittoun, T. (2011). Outlines of a psychoanalytically informed cultural psychology. In S. Salvatore & T. Zittoun (Eds.), *Cultural psychology and psychoanalysis. Pathways to synthesis* (pp. 3–46). Charlotte NC: Info Age Publishing.

Sini, C. (1993). I modi come cura [The modes as cure]. *Atque, 8*, 9–14.

Witkin, H. A. (1950). Individual differences in ease of perception of embedded figures. *Journal of Personality, 19*, 1–15.

CHAPTER 6

A GIRL LIKE A WILL-O'-THE WISP. LISTENING TO REPORTS OF CULTURAL EXPERIENCES AS A METHODOLOGICAL MEANS OF ACCESSING THE PRECONSCIOUS DYNAMICS OF SENSE MAKING

Tania Zittoun

Sociocultural research has to develop methods enabling to reveal thinking processes. One of the classical ways of accessing thinking has always been discourse: in effect, because one cannot have access to thinking "in the head," it concentrates on externalisations, and on what people can say about their thinking. One of the settings mostly often used to generate discourse is that of the research interview. Yet, this raises various issues, the main one being that discourse about the past is reconstructed in the here and now of the situation, and that therefore not much can be inferred about the past.

Cultural Psychology and Psychoanalysis: Pathways to Synthesis, pp. 151–179

In this chapter, drawing on psychoanalytical theory and method, I will outline a methodological strategy to overcome this limitation. It is based on two ideas: firstly, many externalisations studied by psychologists happen to be about contents to which people have deliberate, conscious access. However, psychoanalysis has made us aware of the fact that there is more to psychic life than this: the largest part of our psychic life is, according to this approach, made up of "preconscious" or "unconscious" processes, which are affective, embodied, and escape our control. The psychoanalytical therapeutic setting creates conditions for the verbal formulation of a stream of thoughts which enable patient and analyst to make hypotheses about such preconscious and unconscious processes. In that sense, psychoanalysis functions in perfect accord with current sociocultural psychology: externalisations are seen as material to work on, inferences are made about unseen processes, and eventually, the interactions in which the person is engaged, through internalisation, might also change the person him/herself, and hence his/her future externalisations. Secondly, the psychoanalytical setting is not the only one in which the person might be in touch with such preconscious thinking processes; cultural experiences also enable him/her to do so. As a sociocultural psychologist, I therefore offer an interview setting in which people are brought to discuss their cultural experiences, as a way of accessing some preconscious thinking processes.

THE THERAPEUTIC SETTING AND CULTURAL EXPERIENCES

How is it that the therapeutic setting enables psychoanalysts to make hypotheses about the unconscious of their patient? Features of the frames, as well as some theoretical tools, are used by them to reveal, make hypotheses about, and accompany the thinking processes of their patients. The reflection undertaken by psychoanalysts about the properties of a setting enabling such thinking processes offers a base to reflect about other frames for thinking.

Accessing Thinking in Therapy

The therapeutic setting creates a space where unconscious processes can be accessed, thanks to the explicit rules guiding communication, the actual frame of the exchange, the nature of the interpersonal relationship, triangulation of thinking, and the creation of a particular thinking space.

Psychoanalysis has been defined by Freud as a theory, a therapeutic setting, and as a research method. The rules of the psychoanalytic process have been set so as to take these three sides into account. One of the basic rules of the classical psychoanalytical process is for the patient to say whatever comes to his/her mind, that is, to "freely associate" (Freud, 1910/1961).[1] In Freud's first topological model, the psychic apparatus is a layered structure, where thoughts have to move through unconscious, preconscious and conscious processes, through a process of representational linking, that we can call semiotic elaboration. The move of thinking processes towards consciousness results from their progressive transformation into forms and contents which seem acceptable for the person in a given social situation. This acceptability depends both on values and norms internalised by the person (the superego) and on the person's capacity to stand the pain of some affects. The psychoanalytical setting creates conditions in which the person can freely associate, while suspending as much as possible the judgement she has on his/her discourse, that is, by lowering the control over what can be externalised. If this works, then the person might come to externalise much more than what he/she usually does; through this uninterrupted flow of externalisation, the psychoanalyst might also make hypotheses about parallel trajectories of thinking—precisely because the person's discourse is never purely free, but still avoids some themes or semantic fields, insists on others, chooses some words and some images rather than others, etc.

The safety of the frame appears as an important constituent of the therapeutic process, which can only take place in a space which is isolated from the outside world, where the therapeutic alliance guarantees confidentiality, and welcomes the person's thoughts, whatever they may be and however intolerable they might be in other settings. This is partly possibly thanks to the physical arrangement of the setting, i.e., a space or location in which one enters, at a regular time, and sits in a certain place in a certain position, in a room which creates a certain impression, inviting the person to a state of relative physical relaxation. It is also possible thanks to the institutional framing of the situation that is a guarantee of its quality. The therapist participates in the constitution of the frame: representing an institution, embodying expertise, he becomes a guardian of that frame (Grossen & Perret-Clermont, 1992; Viderman, 1982). A condition of the quality of the frame, Winnicott (1971/2001) mentions the ability of the "good enough" therapist to resist the attacks of the patient, to adjust to his or her needs, but without adhering too closely to them. This enables the patient to be sure that the therapist exists outside his or her own fantasy, as a person escaping his/her control.[2] Hence, the reiterative process of the session creates a specific frame in which the person might thus progressively reveal zones of his/her experience that otherwise escape his/her attention, and, through the mediation of the therapist, progressively elaborate these contents.

The therapeutic setting creates safe conditions enabling the person to enter in a state of relative relaxation, and therefore tend to lower the control over his/her discourse. In technical terms, the setting creates the conditions for a unique alliance of *primary* and *secondary* thinking processes (Green, 1973/1999). Primary processes are those that organise unconscious processes, while secondary processes characterise conscious thinking. In primary processes, thinking can be freely and independently linked following the principle of pleasure, and hence produces mechanisms of displacement, inversion and condensation, such as that seen in the dream-world or in slips of the tongue. In secondary processes, the train of thought is temporal, causal and logical—it obeys the principle of reality. In the therapeutic setting, primary processes are likely to be activated or to emerge thanks to the free association process; at the same time, the rules of the game require the person to intentionally address his/her discourse to another person. This discourse has to be organised into words and ordered into sentences, and hence, acquire characters of secondarity. The therapeutic setting hence creates a triangulation of thinking, where the person pursues two streams of thinking which mutually enable each other and generate a new type of discourse. Green proposes giving the name "tertiary" to the processes characterising this discourse, whereby primary and secondary processes can be articulated (Green, 1995, p. 152). Green's hypothesis is that such linking processes occur at the preconscious level (Green, 1992, p. 146). For example, reports of dreams made to an analyst are seen as a secondarisation of dreams, themselves occurring as primary processes (Freud, 1900/1953). Yet, in narrating a dream, a person can insist on certain points, repeat him/herself, or be self-contradictory, etc. Freud thus listened to the discourse of the dream, a secondary reconstitution of the dream experience in language, and through it, to the latent discourse—the "cloud" of experiences and perceptions that can be revealed by free associations and that are organised by primary processes. In that case, these two layers of discourse reveal something about the real dream, and about the thinking processes of the person which filtered that experience so as to let only some of its constituent coming to the fore.

Finally, this double anchorage of discourse in the therapeutic setting—a closed, delimitated, containing space—is also what enables Winnicott (1971/2001) to see the therapeutic process as occurring in a *transitional* space, that is, in a space where the question of whether what is being said is real or invented, belonging to the patient or to the shared situation, becomes irrelevant.

This setting thus creates conditions for unconscious processes to emerge, or be accessible through people's externalisations, to be reflected upon, and to be played with, in the interaction with another person. The setting therefore has the power to transform the person. Part of the transformative process occurs thanks to the semiotic elaboration of thoughts, the progressive distancing, unlinking and relinking of experience.

Such reading of the setting does not involve naïvely believing that some "truth" about the past life of the patient and hidden forces will emerge (see in this volume, Van der Veer, 2011; Cabell & Valsiner, 2011); rather, it supposes that in that very specific context, the person will attempt to produce a discourse, which might be impeded, or modified, by the person's apprehension of the nature of the setting itself. Movements of thinking might show through the discourse; these might be coloured and linked to traces of past events and situations; but of course all this is construed in the here and now.

Thinking in Cultural Experiences

In what other settings does our culture offer people an opportunity to have emotionally laden thinking processes made visible through a semiotic form, so as to give them a chance to reflect them?

Cultural experiences, such as watching a film, listening to tales, praying, contemplating an image, offer some of the features of the therapeutic setting. A cultural experience requires a jump into an *as-if* experience (Josephs, 1998), a form of imaginary thinking. Engaging in a cultural experience requires from the person a form of "surrender" to the flow of the experience (Benson, 2001; Dewey, 1934), which is only possible if the person feels safe enough (Winnicott, 1971/2001). Consequently, cultural experiences always require a framing of experience which separates them from the flow of daily life. This framing can be formal, such as the ritual introduction of a tale, or the habitual red velvet of the cinema lobby. It can also be informal, such as when a person simply changes his/her state of attention before "getting lost" in a book or in a painting (Nell, 1988).

Cultural experiences require two lines of thinking processes: an active, expert construction of the experience, partly drawing on the person's cultural literacy—such as that regarding the rules of the cinematographic game, knowledge of the basic genres of narration; and a less formal, perceptual, embodied emotional experience, by which the film, painting, or music resonates with one's sensibility, memories, and desires. This second line of processes consists in the creation of links between the form and content of the cultural experience and the person's traces of past experiences, thanks to perceptual resemblances, emotional similarities, and semantic proximities and so on, in other words, through the logic of primary processes.

Hence, as in the clinical setting, the frame offered by the cultural experience creates conditions for a certain state of relaxation, through which primary processes might take place relatively freely. The properties of cultural experiences have always interested psychoanalysts. Freud's interest for the arts is well known (see in this volume, Zittoun, 2011). Winnicott (1971/2001) suggested that any cultural experience requiring some form of suspension from reality—art, science, religion—take place in the area of transitional phenomena, in which the therapeutic process is also located. For Green, mythology offers an experience of strongly binding primary and secondary processes, thus promoting tertiary elaboration: in effect, their themes touch upon basic feelings and unconscious experience—the desire to kill or to love a parent, jealousy or despair (primary process-like experiences)—yet they organise them along some culturally set narrative canons (secondarity). Green (1992) suggests the possibility of seeing myths as collective transitional objects.

These authors, together with Vygotsky (1971), also came to consider the transformational power of myth and narratives. Because the person deploys some part of his/her internal life in the semiotic organisation of the cultural experience, the latter can guide a transformation of that experience (Valsiner, 2007; Vygotsky, 1971; Zittoun, 2006). Tisseron (2002, 2003) shows how much people's favourite book or song often precisely represents, or resonates, with part of their yet-unelaborated experience. Their fondness for a story might precisely be due to the fact that they recognise in it, under a semiotic from, some contents that reflect their inner, not yet accessible experience. People's strong connexion to a book which is then reread and reread might be seen a slow attempt to elaborate that experience more and more. It is a way of gnawing a bone, a slow process of digestion mediated by an external means (Zittoun, 2006). In other words, if the therapeutic setting enables semiotic elaboration through the words of the patient and the therapist, the cultural experience supports semiotic elaboration through its semiotic forms.

Hence, both the therapeutic setting and the cultural experience offer a safe space in which a transitional experience is possible. In the therapeutic setting, the transitional space first takes place in the intersubjective relationship before becoming an intrapsychological experience, while in the cultural experience, the transitional experience is mainly intrapsychological, even though it is created by the interaction between the person and a cultural element. In both cases, the flow of semiotic processes might change the linking of secondary processes and primary processes and their recombination. Both experiences might thus have a transformative effect for the person accepting the experience. Of course, one main component of the therapeutic setting seems missing in cultural experiences: the presence of the therapist. Actually, social relationships do occur through people's cultural experiences. On the one hand, it is very often another, emotionally significant person that has mediated a person's relationship to a type of cultural experience: a grandmother that read folktales, a best friend that introduced a rock band (Zittoun, 2006). On the other hand, people also very often either develop imaginary relationship to authors (composers, actors, artists, writers), or to characters (Zittoun, 2007)—processes often called identification (Bollas, 2003).

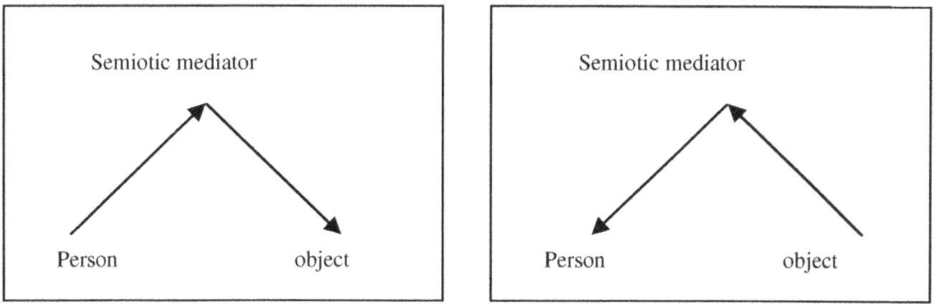

1.1 Sociocultural study of people's uses of a semiotic mediator

1. 2 Proposed inferential study of uses of semiotic mediator

Figure 6.1. Approaches to Semiotic Mediation

A person's preferred cultural element is doubly interesting for the sociocultural psychologist: on the one hand, it is in itself a potentially transformative mean; on the other hand, the cultural element chosen by a person precisely reveals something about the person's inner world, or at least, about current issues absorbing part of his/her preconscious attention.

Drawing on this, the present chapter is based on an inversion of the traditional sociocultural approach to cultural elements (see Fig. 6.1). Traditionally, sociocultural theory examines how people use cultural elements as tools to achieve some purpose (Zittoun, Gillespie, Cornish, & Psaltis, 2007). What interests the researcher is how the person learns to use the tool or the semiotic mediator, or how the tool or semiotic mediator expands the person's capacity to act on a mind or on an object. Here, I will examine how the person has acted with the use of the semiotic mediator, in order to make inferences about his/her thinking.

DESIGNING A RESEARCH PROCESS

Knowing of these two processes, I consider the research interview as a hybrid setting. Some of the features of the therapeutic setting are present: a safe space, institutionally located, and regulated by an expert, inviting some form of externalisation. However, the unique, short-term quality of the research setting, explicitly organised around a specific topic, is not likely to let much of the unconscious primary processes emerge. Therefore, in order to catalyze such emergence, I invited people to give some space to cultural experiences meaningful to them. Reporting upon these experiences, people were then invited to remobilise or invoke the resonances that cultural experiences had for them. With the mediation of these cultural elements, the interviewee is in a situation of having to call upon inner, sometimes preconscious experiences, and to organise them so as to address them to the interviewer. A form of tertiary process is hence created.

To summarise, what is sought, is part of a person's thinking processes. Yet, these processes are unattainable as such. Within a sociocultural framework, it is usually admitted that people internalise certain cultural elements, and that in doing so, they confer a personal sense to them, at times divergent from the shared social significance it might have (Vygotsky, 1934/1963). People then externalise various messages, which might be related to these elements, in different contexts, and for different purposes. In doing so, they both express (or conceal) something of the personal sense it has from them, and they might attempt to join or position themselves towards the shared meaning it has for others. The personal work of sense making, while invisible to the observer, can be induced somewhere "between" what is internalised and what is externalised—which are both observable.

This is highly consistent from what can be learned from the clinical literature. Indeed, we have seen that people are likely to engage in thinking about cultural elements which, for some reason, resonate, that is, easily create primary links with personal matters, preoccupations, affects and experiences. Hence, having people talk about these cultural elements is a way of gaining access to issues that people have in mind in a preconscious way.

Cues: Making Hypotheses About the Elaboration of Affective Processes

If discourse might be seen as revealing some aspects of the flow of inner experience, how can we go below the content of the discourse, so as to learn about the thinking processes? Given the parallel identified above, it might be useful to use some of the theoretical tools developed by psychoanalysts. Indeed, their theories enabled variations in the discourse to be captured, giving information about the degree to which the person has elaborated his/her experience. I propose to import these insights as methodological tools for sociocultural psychological work.

Thinking is largely the semiotic elaboration of affects (Freud, 1900/1953; Valsiner, 2007; see also in this volume Salvatore & Zittoun, 2011). Consequently, one important methodological need is to identify cues enabling us to infer how much the affective experience has been elaborated. In his study on affects, Green (1973/1999) identifies different typical types of discourse that can be heard in the clinical setting. The first type is characterised by the heaviness of its climate; silence is heavy, discourse is focused on the here and now; the tone of discourse is uniform, lacks melody; the analyst has the impression of being exposed to a compact substance. The second type is characterised by extremely quick and abundant representations; the patient has a lot to say, and creates links and associations. Green sees these two types as exemplifying, first, a discourse dominated by affect—where the affect is a defence against representations, while the second is exemplifying a discourse dominated by representations—where representations are a defence against affects. A third type of discourse is characterised by the centrality of the process of signifying—that is, the active process of linking separate experiences and affects to representation, and back. Hence, in the course of the session, an idea that comes to the mind of the person calls a dream back to memory, and as she re-experiences it, she embodies it—her hands and feet move, posture changes etc, and thus, affects are experienced; these, in turn, call for more representations, put into a narration, and so forth. Hence, in the third type of discourse identified by Green, language has a function of linking processes, and representations and affects exist in an equilibrated manner. Green distinguishes the modality of linking of affects from that of linking representations. If representations are linked by *concatenation*, that is, in terms of causes and effects, affects are linked by *diffusion*: like oil, they can expand and invade the whole psychic apparatus (Green, 2002, p. 178).

This distinction is not equivalent to that between primary and secondary processes. The dimension that connects primary to secondary processes is somehow orthogonal to the dimension that runs from embodied affect to representations. Hence, primary processes will engage affects and representations linked to some degree, and likewise for secondary processes. It is only in primary processes that the power of affects—their oil-like extension—is dominant, whereas they are limited and constrained in secondary processes. One might therefore say that processes of thirdness occur at two levels, or require a double branching: between affects and representations on the one hand, and between primary and secondary processes, on the other hand.

Methodological Implications

From these considerations, two methodological pointers emerge. Firstly, in terms of the identification of significant tasks or research objects, one might be willing to consider tasks that demand a substantial affective involvement, while offering people space in which representation or discourse is facilitated. The emotionally significant event considered here is the transition to parenthood,[3] which is likely to have emotional resonances, and requires some working through. Transition processes can be analysed following three lines of changes: processes of identity changes (e.g., from being an independent student to becoming a responsible father); processes of learning (e.g., how to deal with sleeping hours); and issues of sense making (e.g., what does it mean to have a child in my life?). Additionally, we have seen that tertiary processes as well as linking between affects and representations occur in specific situations of dialogue, or in specific interactions that people have with myths and other culturally generated transitional spaces. Here, we question people about the cultural elements that they considered and thought about while they were expecting a child.

Secondly, the psychoanalytical reflection of affects in discourse leads us to define significant cues when listening to interviewees. In order to access what is significant to them, what they can elaborate, or what they resist, attention can be paid to two types of elements:

1. The semantic contents of the discourse, not only in their discursive construction, but also, in the overall fabric of the discourse, in its repetition, contradictions, recurrences, silences, etc. In that sense, the discourse "under" the discourse can be listened to, that is, the traces of primary processes, or the effect of unbound affects at the representational or semantic level which can be propagated through the discourse.
2. The emotional quality of the discourse: rhythm, melody, or accents of the discourse are always revealing something of the balance between affects and representations. Green's typology gives us tools to identify these changing balances. In particular, beyond the general tone of a person's discourse in a given discursive context, the binding of affects and representations varies according to what is being talked about.

CAPTURING NAME CHOICE PROCEDURE TO REVEAL SENSE-MAKING IN TRANSITIONS

The clinical literature suggests that the transition to parenthood is an important moment of reelaboration of past experience and raises various questions which have deep unconscious prolongation. Authors note the importance of the changing relationship that the new mother might have to her parents, the closer contact she might have to her body, and her experiences of questions linked to sexuality and gender, but also to life and death (Bydlowski, 1997; Stern, Brunschweiler-Stern, & Freeland, 1998). Many of the feelings, memories, and echoes of these questions remain unconscious and preconscious; yet, authors also often mention the mother's particular receptivity to these contents, which seem to manifest themselves through dreams and daydreaming.[4]

In order to have access to people's process of making sense of their transition to parenthood, I questioned them about the procedures by which they had chosen first names for their children (Zittoun, 2004, 2005). The theoretical reasoning was the following: narrative and symbolic systems in traditional societies provided people not only with birth rituals, but also with naming principles. Names, which are public, always reveal something of the symbolic system to which they belong. Hence, in a modern society, first names might also indicate narratives and stories belonging to the parents' personal culture, which are mobilised in relationship to the birth of a child.

Forty semistructured reconstructive interviews were carried out with parents, alone or in couples, three or four months after the birth of a child, about the procedure of choosing a name (Zittoun, 2004, 2005). The parents, out of a group contacted in a French speaking Swiss town by way of their birth-announcements in the newspaper, came from different social classes and cultural backgrounds. Interviews included questions related to their choice procedure (names evoked but rejected, naming practices in use by their families), representations of the child, and the cultural elements mobilised through the name-choice procedure. Notes were taken during the interviews. The taped interviews have been fully transcribed and the corpus of transcriptions was submitted to four types of analysis. The first one was a content analysis documenting procedures of choices and negotiations of names ("what's in a name"). Case-analysis of each family constituted the second analysis; they enabled the trajectories of decision through couple negotiations and identity dynamics to be reconstructed. The third, quantitative analysis, was based on a systematic codification of the interviews on two dimensions. The first one, based on the clinical work of Ammaniti Ammaniti, Candelori, Pola, and Tambelli (1999)[5]—which can be seen as an operationalisation of Green's three types of discourses—classified the transcripts according to the balance between affective and cognitive dimensions of the discourse (by three independent coders); the second one identified the transgenerational transmission present in the interviews. Based on the idea that tradition offers resources to elaborate the newness offered by the transition to parenthood, the hypothesis tested was that discourses reflecting a transgenerational awareness were also more likely to have a cognitive-affective balance. Interviews without this transgenerational dimension, yet equivalently elaborated, appeared especially interesting, as they enabled us to explore which other symbolic resources were used by parents to elaborate such events. Consequently, the fourth analysis was a qualitative exploration of interviews corresponding to the hypothesis, or on the other hand, not predicted by the theory. It was an interpretative attempt to trace back processes of sense making in which the person had been engaged, and that might have been mediated by various cultural elements[6] (for an exhaustive presentation see Zittoun, 2005).

In the rest of this chapter, I will give an example of a case-study, which I have chosen because it mentions a wide variety of cultural elements and their uses. I will draw on the first, second, and fourth analyses mentioned above, and propose an analysis in four steps. First, I will examine explicit contents, showing how the interview starts, summarising the name choice procedure, and suggesting how it is linked to the process of becoming a parent. Secondly, I will identify significant cultural elements for the parents. Thirdly, I will make hypothesis about thinking processes through a closer look at "conflicting knots" of the discourse. Fourthly, I will consider the cultural elements as mediators, or as diffracting mirrors, to access to some of the person's preconscious thinking process.

BAPTIST AND THE WILL-O'-THE-WISP

Jean has been interviewed after the birth of her second son, Baptist, following Benjamin, 3 years older. According to the criteria defined by Ammaniti and colleagues (1999), this interview can be considered to be characterised by a relative balance between affective components and secondary elaboration. It is also an interview in which one finds a certain attention to transgenerational values and transmission. In that sense, this in an interview which is somehow "canonical," that is, that corresponds to the general expectations of the research project mentioned above.

First Turn[7]

Like all the interviewees, Jean had been expecting this interview—she had been contacted by means of a letter, and then by a phone call, explaining the purpose of the research and the definition of the situation—a young researcher interested in how people found first names for their children. Once I had arrived in her flat—in the living room, with the baby that would be breast-fed in my presence—the interview started rapidly, and after my reiteration of the question—"so, how did it happen for you, this choice of first name for your children?," Jean gave a first, long, relatively prepared answer. First turn answers are usually revealing something about what the person think is expected and her understanding of the situation. Yet, it has other informative qualities: firstly, it often repeats what the young mother usually answers to people who ask her about the origin of the first name; the answer is often quite stereotypical, and reveals some form of social representations about what is in a name (Moscovici, 2000). Secondly, this first turn also often informs about the emotional state of the interviewee: comparatively, some mothers' first turn about the same questions are very short, factual, while others are expanded, rich in emotions, and cover a good part of the interview. Thirdly, it often introduces the thematic threads which will have to be explored during the interview. Here, the first turn is quite interesting for this reason:

> **E** Let's start with the older one. He's called Benjamin, he's three years old, well, we just looked in a book of names, we tried to choose between names,

> and then I tried to make a list, and my husband too. And, well, we were unable to find a common name (laugh)—and well, we decided, we found—well, Benjamin was a smooth name, it wasn't heard too often, and I do quite like old first names, that's why we choose Benjamin. It's true that ... it sounds good. We have been looking with the surname, too, it's not so easy, we are called C., and my husband is a plumber, then if we had ... I liked William quite well but William it would have been WC, then WC for the plumber's son (laugh) it was (laugh) not so terrific, then now BC that's all right with the initials, too. Because it's true we have been thinking about all that stuff, because then later at school with the kids you know what happens, they won't do each other any favours. So, for Benjamin that's how it went, we kept the surprise until the end.

The first turn announces some of the traits of the procedure of choosing a name (each parent made a list and they tried to find a common name), and the resources used for it. Books were used to generate names, and various criteria were used as operator to restrain the choice: aesthetic (a smooth name), general harmony (it shall be fitting with the surname), frequency (not too often), identity related (belonging to a certain family), future consideration (what children will say at school). These criteria are among the commonly used. However, the first joke about plumbers is to be noted. It is the most connected here to transmission—what sort of son, what is the heritage in the family; and the theme will come back in the interview. After the first turn, Jean will expand on various aspects of this first turn, and consider various first names that have been considered for the two children.

Naming a Child: Insights into the Transition to Parenthood

A first analysis can remain close to the explicit content of the interview. It explores the name choice procedure, and highlights issues related to the transition to parenthood, especially, issues related to the affirmation of one's identity which comes to the fore as the parents have to decide "what sort of child" they will have.

Naming a child is choosing an explicit sign of belonging. Negotiations about names often turn to be identity negotiation between parents. These negotiation can be more or less conflictual, and parents find different strategies to resolve or repress the conflict—e.g., finding names which fit in two cultures, or out of them, or giving the space of the second name to the other parent's claims. In this case, Jean's husband wanted names that she found too common, too "Americanised"—Kilian, Kevin or Jonathan. The names she was interested in are more Christian, French names, which are related to her origins, that she defines as Breton and Christian. Her maternal grandfather is a "pure" Breton, and many relatives have such first names. However, she considers mainly Breton names for girls.

> **E** For a girl, the name we chose was Gwendolyn, because my mother is of Breton origin, I like Gwendolyn very much, kind of fairy-like, it was cute (…) **T** Is there a particular story about Gwendolyn? **E** Let's say it was ... In relation to what I had read in the fairy tales, she was running a bit ... I don't know if you know Brittany, there are some rather abrupt fields, where one can run, there are will-o'-the-wisps ... it's a bit strange at night.... There are all those stories with the standing stones ... then there was a little girl called Gwendolyn who took walks at night ... Well, I like the night very much, I adore going for walks at night (laughs), and I thought that it fitted well.... I had figured out a brown-haired little girl—because my husband has real brown hair—brown-haired, green eyes, who'd been running at night (laughs) sometimes one can have sort of images, when you're pregnant, that's true.... And even earlier.... That has always been the case, seeing such a little girl. I was sure that I would only have boys, anyway (laughs) I don't know how, but I just felt it.... I dreamed more about girls, but I've been feeling that I was going to have boys ...

We thus have a configuration in which two family lines merge, and the two parents' positions are slightly divergent. The young woman defines herself as French and Christian. The names chosen for boys refer to the Bible, the feminine one instead to Brittany. Actually, Jean has not been socialised to this Breton identity, it is more a root that she is actively reconstructing. This identity dimension is quasi-mythical, and the family seems to go back to the origins of history:

> **E** On my grandfather side there is a genealogical tree. They went far back, they went back to the times of the Mongols. The Mongols invaded Brittany ...

At some point the couple used a book on names to help their procedure, but it turned out to be too confusing:

> **E** We read [the book] "3000 thousand first names for boys and girls," but I *strongly advise* everybody *not* to look at these names. Because what happens for us, we were looking at the meaning of these names—and this is a pity.... Because so many names, it troubles the mind, it's frightening.

So they stopped consulting it. They then found Benjamin—and Jean explains that she listened to her body, asked the baby whether he liked it, and felt that he moved, which she interpreted as him liking it. We do not know exactly where the name come from, although Jean knows the biblical anchorage and the fact that it generally means the younger son, meaning that she reappropriates saying that Benjamin is the younger son of the family branch.

Jean and her husband do not follow any established naming rules; they also agree not to give second names, although they both have one. Jean explains that the reason for rejecting this tradition is that each of them had painful memories associated to their godfather (although the children do have godfathers).

Some identity and position differences between the partners have appeared during the first decision procedure. These are partly grounded in the more general trajectory of the young mother, and the previous transition she had experienced—that of being a migrant in Switzerland. Jean defines herself through her connection to France, but also through her status of "migrant" in Switzerland, which she experienced as difficult, while her husband is from a local Swiss family. She also places more importance on the real or imaginary memory of her family (she was typing the genealogic research undertaken by her grandfather), while her husband has more concrete links to his family, through large gatherings; and she attributes a high status to studies and literary culture, while her husband, a craftsman, does not. Hence, finding the name for Benjamin is also a task of conciliating these two stories, sets of values, and life experiences.

This conciliating task seems to have been difficult. Jean says that the couple had difficulties to find a name for their first son; in effect, "Benjamin" was defined rather late, at 8 months (first names are often thought about during the 4–5th months, or 8–9th). Jean also refused the help of the family in finding the name, and kept the decision secret until the end. Note that Jean also explains that, unlike her husband, she did not want to know the sex of the child—so she actually did not know it while the husband knew it.

For the second child, the couple seems more relaxed. No naming principles were chosen and the repertoires of possible names are relatively stable. Jean however refuses to use the name envisaged for a girl the first time for this second child:

> **E** For me it was like.... Not like a dead child, but another phase, it was another pregnancy ... Because in our bodies we have.... I don't know what you know about that, but we all have a masculine and a feminine side. So I thought, if I took this name from Benjamin, I would take away his feminine side ...

Jeans appears attentive to the imaginary child—the child growing and developing in her fantasy, that eventually meets the real child at birth (Ben Soussan, 1999). She observes her daydreams and fantasying. She reacts intuitively and chooses names that "flash" her. Hence the name Angeline:

> **T** Did Angeline come from somewhere? **E** No it came like this, I didn't find any meaning to it, I didn't look for it either as we discovered we would have a boy. I found that it was smooth, like an angel ... One evening I was thinking about names, I don't know, all at once I say, Oh, there is Angeline, I don't know, it's cute, it's smooth ... Well it must exist somewhere[8] ...

The parents this time know the sex of the child, a boy, and decide his name in an intuitive manner:

> **E** So for Baptist, I heard ... it's something else : we haven't looked in the book, I suddenly heard the name on television, well—I don't remember if it was in a movie, that name, Baptist, no actually it was Jean-Baptist that I heard. I said, Oh, Jean-Baptist it's too long, and my father's name is already Jean-Paul, and we found it too long to write down and everything, and my husband didn't like hyphenated names at all [in French: "composed"]. So I said, Ah, Baptist, I think that Baptist alone is possible, so we checked. Then we saw this little card, and the signification on the book I had, we found it nice. And since we are both believers, Baptist, he's the one who baptised Jesus, when one looks at it, and I found it good. Always a bit ... and connected to water, too, always plumbing, water, we like its contact. It rang a bell at once :

The procedure of choosing "Baptist" is presented as contrasting with that of choosing the older son's name; while the latter was rationally decided (list of preferences, identity negotiations) here the procedure is much more intuitive, in the sense that the mother was struck by a name heard while watching television. The first name "Jean-Baptist" (John Baptist, a common composition in French) rings a bell. Watching films or the television often put people is a state of relative relaxation, and preconscious thoughts are more likely to emerge. The criteria and identity claims of the first child are still present, and the name solves the equation by satisfying both Jean's demands (French, rare name) and her husband's (a plumber's son) thanks to its designation of a higher level category to which the two belong, Christianity. Yet, this is solved in a preconscious, or unconscious manner, through a very different logic of reasoning: the name appeared in a "flash," and the decision seems due to a free association based on images which I might reconstitute as following: Baptist, baptising Jesus in the river, the baptismal water, the running water, the pipes, the plumber.... Hence the name here solves the problem thanks to a primary process operation. Note that a large proportion of parents believe in the importance of a name given in a "flash,", and such names usually cancel the many contradictions and constraints people are dealing with. In the quotation, the report of this "flash" is followed by a sort of rationalisation, by which the name is linked to other surrounding facts: her father's name, from which she wants to differentiate, the length, and finally, a symbolic resource—a card about first names.

At this stage, we observe consistent semantic networks emerging from these chosen and possible names. Angeline can be connected to the angelic dimension of John the Baptist (see Fig. 6.2). It crosses another sacred, religious line—Benjamin, Baptist—to which another name mentioned also belongs, Blandine, referring to Saint-Blandine, a church in Jean's father's town;

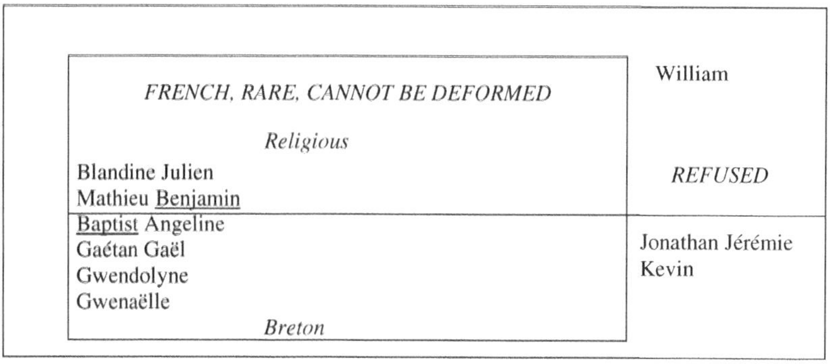

Figure 6.2. First Names Considered

the religious line comes from a spiritual—and perhaps desexualised—side with angels, baptismal purity; finally this sacred field finds a more pagan realisation—the will-o'-the wisp woman running at night, the importance of water and air (two of the basic elements of the old Breton tales). These networks are also characterised by phonological sets—the first names in B-, the endings in –ine; other names considered by Jean and refused for various reasons were Gaétan, Gaël, Gwendolyn, all Bretonic names starting with a G. Aesthetic preferences are the most difficult to analyse, as they directly touch upon embodied impressions and resonances.

Parents also have plans for their children. Jean intends to transmit her French identity, her religious identity, and the Breton origin that she is working at reconstructing. However, Jean did not hand down her maiden name. She wishes success in friendship to her children and at school. She also mentions the little books she is writing for the sons, about how the names were chosen, that is, with a story of their origin. Eventually, her husband will also hand down his business to his son. Finally, she also announces a desire to hand down her passion for reading historical books:

> **E** Oh, I like reading. And by the way for the kids, not for Baptist because he's a bit young (laughs) but I buy many books for Benjamin, well for his age, but I'll encourage him to read. I have never been forced to read, but I was encouraged, I was taught reading.

Relevant Cultural Experiences

Jean mentions many of the cultural elements that have been used during her transition to parenthood, or more generally, in her life. Mediating the name choice procedure were books of first names, books of tales, and the television.

For the first choice, none of these mediations were really relevant. Jean seemed to have felt that as invading and confusing. One might say that the infinity of possibilities revealed by books might just have reflected the couple's lack of direction at that point. It is by taking their distance from these books that the couple was able to find its way.

Another source of cultural experiences is television; although the name of Baptist came from there, Jean actually mentions television as a negative reference. In her view, television is propagating a loss of information which has rather negative influences on society, while more useful information is obviously missing:

> **E** If they showed less [violence] on the telly, there would be less in the streets. When you see those kids on the screen that can kill each other ... if they weren't shown how to do it, than they wouldn't do it ... I'm quite sure about this. The more you show the badness the more there will be badness. They don't show ... they hardly ever show something beautiful ... Some programmes are nice but it's still rare to see, Oh, well, a birth, or no, no, no one speaks about it, they always speak about, how many deaths this time ...

Hence, it seems that television is a potentially relevant medium for Jean, as she seems to believe in its power to influence people's actions, and to miss more important information, such as human birth.

Then, the most significant cultural experience for Jean is given by her reading of French history books:

> **E** And I do read a lot of historical things, yes. I am fond of history; it has always been my passion, so I read quite often. **T** About France? **E** Mainly about France, because let's say in my family we have got a lot of books that came from generation to generation, we hoard stuff (laughs). Here I don't have so many with me but since we have a chalet in France it's all there. (..) Now I am into the Kings of France ... I like it ... Maybe I find there ... I imagine as well, how it would be to be there ... **T** [And what do you imagine]? **E** I put myself in the shoes of one character, I imagine I was there ... I was there without being there ... To be like a dragonfly, that sees what is going on from high ... as I said I am into the kings of France ... **T** But what period? **E** Philippe le Bel. So if you know this period, it is not very joyful, this period. It was easy to get poisoned at that time ... (laughs). But there were already men living together, and it was not the end of the world. When you see nowadays the taboos around it, while it has existed for years, it's a pity. One should ... People could try to read more often, it wouldn't hurt them. You can't force—yet I believe that if people read more, they would be less narrow-minded about this which they believe they invented, while it has existed for years.

Jean evokes the origin of this interest: her mother read history, as well as her grandfather and great-great-aunt:

> **E** Many books come from my great-great-aunt. I loved, when she was alive—she died about ten years ago—I would go to her place, she would talk about the past ... she used to say ... for me it was great ... We were living almost next door, so on my way back to school, I would stop by, we would discuss [history]. She would give me books, she would say, Read this one, it's good, you'll see.

This great-great-aunt plays an important role in Jean's story; not only did she mediate her relationship to books, but probably also to Christian faith, as she used to go on pilgrimages to Jerusalem. If reading historical novels became important for Jean, then, it was with the guidance of this relative, who, in her way, became a "warden" of the specific cultural experience created there.

Jean also evokes Christian reading groups to which she used to belong, where people discussed biblical texts in the light of problems of actuality. Asked about similar links she could establish between historical texts and current events, she answered:

> **T** Do you think you still do the same kind of things, when you're reading history—connecting history with actual events? **E** It depends on the historical book. Because it's hard to find a coincidence with the Kings' story. But—there are things that, yes, I read them and I try to put them into practice. When I see how, at that time, the ... women were calmer with the children, how they used to live, they used to explain a lot of things to them, trying to understand, too, then it's true that I try to do it with.... Well, at least with the older, with Benjamin. By trying to see why he is like this, he did that, I try to be quite open. And it's true that I read in the book that they used to act like that. **T** In what period? **E** Eighteenth, beginning nineteenth century ...

Thus, not only are historical novels highly invested in by Jean, but they are also approached with more expert hermeneutic skills: her experience of reading biblical texts facilitates her entrance and exploration of novels, as well as her ability to create links between the space of fiction and real life. Hence, historical novels become a transitional space in which Jean projects herself, and plays *as-if* she was living at that time. In turn, she can bring back to her real life some semiotic means that enable her to guide her action with her children and to make sense to their conduct.

Finally Jean also comments on her "research" in more esoteric approaches to the person, which she has learned from her sister-in-law: chakras, care for the body, numerology and astrology. Here, she mentions how these techniques first enabled her to be more attentive to her intuitions and feelings, and to imagine the "life paths" for her children. Hence, these also become semiotic techniques used to open spaces to think about the future, and thus enable transitional experiences.

Conflicting Knots Arising

So far, the analysis has remained close to the content of the discourse: it has retraced the process of choosing names and, with it, some of the challenges of the transition to parenthood. In a second step, I have identified cultural elements significant for Jean, and especially, themes that she found particularly relevant. Now, in a third step, I propose to listen more carefully to what was said in the first part, to what remained implicit, and to what appeared as reflected, amplified or distorted through the magnifying glass offered by personally relevant cultural experiences. In other words, in this section, I use Jean's externalisation as a way of inferring some past and current thinking processes. This analysis leads me to identify a few transversal themes, or "conflicting" knots related to the transition to motherhood.

A first transversal theme is quite directly connected with the acts of becoming a mother, implying giving birth and taking care of a child. There are various cues that suggest that this might have been a sensitive issue: through her story and the cultural experiences she mentions, Jean seems to have felt relatively isolated when involved in her first pregnancy. As a "migrant," she cut her bonds to her family, and especially to the women that were close from her (mother, sisters, great-great-aunt, and friends). Studies in the migrant clinic show that the absence of this support might be difficult; gestures, rites, knowledge developed in the group which might help to deal with the newness, are then missing (Moro, 2001). In Jean's case, the difficulty appears at two levels. First, we saw that Jean refused to see the images of her first child and to know his sex; she also found it very difficult to think about the child, found attempts to help her do so very confusing (the family's help in choosing a name), and the name was chosen very late. This suggests that she had difficulties developing a representation of the child to come. Jean mentions how the help given by her sister in law, mediated by different esoteric techniques—numerology, discourses about chakras, developing awareness to one's body—precisely enabled her to initiate an imaginary dialogue with the child within her. This seems to have helped her to develop a representation of the child and to pick a first name for him. At the time, her situation made her feel very isolated. Above, Jean mentions that she would have preferred to see birth on television—in that context, we might think that she would happily have accepted this type of information when she needed it. She also mentions her loneliness with the children themselves. In that respect, her mention of the historical novels as sources of inspiration to guide her conduct with the children suggests, in the negative, that Jean seems to have lacked other, more relevant sources of support. Hence, Jean appears to have found herself very isolated when having to engage in the first care for her son, without the help of the women she knew; looking for other resources, she dismissed television, yet retained the historical novels in which she was already interested.

A second transversal theme is that of the trans-generational transmission. The young woman is the older of two sisters in a catholic French family, with a father from Alsace and a mother from Brittany, and grew up in central France, probably far from her grandparents. The father tried to find out information about the past of his family living in Alsace during the war. Apparently, the grandfather had to change his name so as not to be sent in Germany during WWII; the family line was lost because of some falsification of documents. The disappearance of this grandfather creates a doubt about the authenticity of the father's surname, and makes it impossible to identify more distant relatives. When the father wanted to find out more about this family, he was advised not to do so by people in Alsace. The forced secret surrounding the family history seems to have been experienced as shameful for the family. It is therefore better not to think about it. On the other side, the maternal grandfather from Brittany seemed to transmit more: he spoke about the family and its origin, and Jean transcribed her maternal grandfather's memories and research on his Breton roots.

This history is however a story of the mythical origins of the family, concretised in churches and places rather than in the living members of the family. Hence, even if this family line seems safer to emotionally invest, it is also somehow blurred into a "grand history." All together, from the two grandfathers—deceased before the birth of Baptist and Benjamin—there seems to be troubled family stories and blurred responsibilities, potentially generating shame (Tisseron, 1999). Jean's symbolic actions support this reading. On the one hand, she treats rather unequally the two family lines: the cultural space offered by Brittany is largely invested; Jean reads Breton tales, develops vivid fantasies in a Breton-like imaginary world, many of the first names considered by Jean are clearly Breton, and she seems to accept the "mythical" roots of this part of the family—while the Alsace family is hardly mentioned. Note that in doing so, she simply reproduces the symbolic interdiction promoted by her father. On the other hand, Jean is a passionate reader of historical novels of French Kings: as we will see below, these stories are mainly concerned with exploring issues of family transmission.

A third theme, which is harder to identify, is related to gender and sexuality. Jean's family comes from various places in France, and has lost touch with its regional anchorages. In contrast, the family developed a strong religious identity, which appears to offer more stability through time and space. It might be true that this religious commitment also makes it more difficult to discuss certain themes. In particular, Jean's enthusiasm for historical novels in which it is common for men to go with men, suggests that she discovered there a space in which questions related to gender and sexuality can be discussed—which, in turn, suggests that she did not find such a place in her family. Connected to this, Jean mentions that her father's brother died without having had children; consequently, her father who had three daughters saw the extinction of his surname. Jean and her sisters have rather masculine first names. As a child, Jean had decided never to marry, in order to carry on her father's name. Of course, by marrying her husband Jean had to renounce to this idea. In this line of consideration, Jean mentions that she refused to envisage children's first names that were sexually ambivalent.

Hence the three thematic knots emerging from the interview have to do with the main questions raised by the transition to parenthood and identified in the clinical literature: giving sense to the conception, the birth and the development of a child; trans-generational transmission; sexuality and gender conflicts.

Cultural Experiences as Symbolic Resources

The last step of the analysis is now to focus again upon the cultural experiences which have appeared particularly significant here. Jean mentions many of them: her Christian and biblical knowledge, and her practice of the bible reading group; her readings of French History; the written stories by the grandfather about the mythical past of Brittany; Breton tales she reads; esoteric research with her sister-in-law. In what follows, I will only focus my analysis of Jean's reading of French historical novels.

As we have seen, historical novels appear as transitional spaces in which Jean can think about questions related to family, as well as issues related to gender and sexuality. Interestingly, historical novels were very frequently mentioned as relevant cultural experiences during pregnancies by the women who were interviewed for this research, and especially the version written by Maurice Druon (1973). The main narrative structure is organised around issues of continuation and survival of the royal family through history—the figure of Philippe le Bel is an important character, faced with questions such as: how to save the name of the family, to be sure of the purity of the ascendants, to find an acceptable wife, and to be sure to have a symbolic and material heir? The figure of Philippe le Bel is also associated to war between families and between sexes, his main enemy being a woman who wants to recuperate the royal blood for her descendents. In a French dictionary of reference, le *Petit Robert des noms propres* (Rey, 2000), the note on Maurice Druon indicated that it belongs to a certain Romanesque tradition of the 19th century, "renewed by a certain obsessive fear of sex and death" (my translation). Hence these historical novels renew with a certain type of narrative in which the mixing of affects and representation is particularly strong (Green, 1973/1999). In that sense, it is likely to offer a reading experience which particularly works out the elaboration of affects. Also, the themes treated (family lines, loyalty and betrayal, gender conflicts) are likely to find echoes in people's personal experiences. Furthermore, as they particularly insist on the idea of historical time and transmission between generations, they are very close to questions typical for the transition to parenthood.

In the case of Jean, these stories have a double connexion to transmission, and historical inscription: on the one hand, they are about transmission and continuity; on the other, they are themselves the object of transmission in her family. These stories thus have a double function. First, as we have seen, the story seem to "offer words" for issues which seem hard for Jean to think about. The issues thus become fully and semiotically articulated. These representations take place in a specific frame of reference—the past history of France—that isolated them in a quasi-imaginary space. Losing oneself in the story is clearly an experience separate from one's daily life. In that sense, there is a safe containing space, enabling a cultural, transitional experience. Second, these issues and problems are not only represented, they are also part of full, complex narratives. The reader's emotional investment in a text can be seen as due to the fact that he projects some parts of herself into the text—we could say, she links some representational, affective contents to the semiotic structure. In doing so, these parts are "delegated" to the text, which then follow its own narrative logic. Hence, two characters which are enemies might enter into conflict and solve it, or one character might change and find new solutions to a problem. The idea is that the part of the reader's experience attached to the text—or represented through the semiotic means it offers—are in turn transformed by the narrative (Freud, 1908/1959; Vygotsky, 1971; Tisseron, 2003). Also, more generally, all the aspects of a fictional experience might find an anchorage in the person's experience. These descriptions find more perceptive actualisations in the reader—e.g., a description of the desert evokes memories and impressions of heat, dryness, loneliness, danger, whereas the description of a promenade under the trees along a riverside might evoke the feeling of coolness, smells of vegetation, the sound of the water, and with it, some form of calm and comfort. Just as the landscapes in which the narrative takes place might evolve through the story, so the reader's general emotional tone is also likely to evolve.

Altogether, the cultural experience enabled by a cultural element is likely to function like a symbolic resource (Zittoun, 2005, 2006). In Jean's case, historical novels are not only a mean to represent various contents. They are also quite likely a mean to transform the various affects and representations attached to the story. Firstly, as we have seen, the novel has its own evolving structure and narrative. As such, it is likely to play the role of a sort of "external thinking processor," supporting Jean's own elaboration of experience. Secondly, once in a semiotic form, these representations and affects can become objects of further reflection and externalisation; they can thus undergo further semiotic elaboration. Thirdly, Jean has developed some hermeneutic expertise through her participation in bible reading groups. These skills are guided attention procedures to identify common patterns between narratives and real life, and to elaborate various links between these two sets of meaning, representations or narratives (e.g., analogical, metaphorical thinking, and so on). She draws upon these skills when she is in need of specific skills to transfer from narrative to real life (e.g., using the mothering behaviour of late 18th century French mother to develop hers).

In Jean's case, the novels by Maurice Druon function as symbolic resources facilitating her transition to motherhood: they support identity processes—the reinforce her French identity, and scaffolds her elaboration of the idea of a transgenerational story; they enable her to develop concrete skills, such as mothering conduct; and they offer a transitional space for containing and elaborating complex issues related to family secrets, gender, transmission, violence, origins and death.

Finally, Jean's passion for historical novels has been legitimated by a significant person: the great-great-aunt that she used to visit on her way back from school. This relative guided her interest in these books, and mapped out her path as a reader. She is also the person with whom Jean started to discuss what she had read, her likes and dislikes and what it did to her. Hence, it seems that Jean actually developed this symbolic resource thanks to the active mediation of this great-great-aunt. It seems that Jean has understood the importance of this part of her experience, as she intends to transmit it to her sons. Hence, as there is a blurred and uncertain family story which renders intergenerational transmission very difficult, it seems that French History has itself become the mythical story which is transmitted through generations in the family.

CONCLUDING COMMENTS

Accessing thinking processes is one of the challenges of psychological research. Interviews are mostly at best considered as useful to get information about specific contents, about which a person intentionally expresses herself, the discourse being thus constructed as the interaction unfolds.

In this chapter, I proposed to draw on psychoanalytical insights to overcome these limitations. Especially, I consider that, although the discourse is a sequential reconstruction, there are traces and underlying currents in the discourse to which more attention can be paid. In doing so, hypotheses about preconscious thinking and elaboration in the making can be formulated.

Two main ideas were necessary to make such an analysis. Firstly, what legitimated the use of psychoanalytical analysis of the language of a patient in a clinical setting was my identification of some common features between a therapeutic setting, an interview setting, and more surprisingly, a cultural experience. To enable certain forms of thinking in which primary and secondary processes can be involved, a safe frame is required, where a transitional experience can take place, under a semiotic form connecting primary and secondary processes and thus transforming experience, and addressed to a real or imaginary person that guides or legitimates this processes. Secondly, because cultural experiences can offer a space in which people can engage in a process of semiotic elaboration of their experience, the externalisation they make about their experience usually suggests the issues which are currently the most relevant for them. In other words, as there are good reasons to believe that largely unconscious or preconscious issues with which a person is engaged find a semiotic elaboration in the cultural experiences reported by interviewees, a researcher can make hypothesis about an interviewee's preconscious thinking processes.

There are various ways in which the common semiotic grounding of sociocultural psychology and psychoanalytical thinking can be explored, as this volume suggests. Here I proposed one methodological exploration of this proximity, and I suggested that taking the developments of the two fields into account can only help us to explore human conduct beyond the immediately visible.

NOTES

1. However, such free associating flow of thinking and speech makes the person very vulnerable, given the fact that this discourse it always addressed to another person, to which the authority of the expert is conferred by the situation itself. It is partly to prevent analysts from abusing this power that the second rule is that of the abstinence of the analyst.
2. Of course, one important condition for the externalisation of rich discourse in this setting is the quality of the interpersonal relation between patient and analyst. It has been largely discussed under the name of transference (Freud, 1938/1964) —counter transference (Searles, 2005). Psychoanalysts considered that, because of the relative regression and lowering of control induced

by the setting—physical arrangement, trust, free association—the patient would recreate within her relationship with the therapist some of the emotional qualities of other relationships. In turn, the analyst might emotionally react to the attribution made by patient, which might find an echo in her own experience. These movements are analysed within the interaction; some trends of analysis are even essentially based on the analysis of these reciprocal movements. The setting thus creates a situation in which the analyst can be "used" by the patient to reincarnate the "others" of many of his past significant relationships; the externalisations generated by this process are used to make hypothesis about unconscious traces of present and past relationship which might be activated by the person in diverse settings.

3. It thus belongs to a series of studies about ruptures and transitions (see Zittoun 2006).
4. A second reason to be interested in this population lies in the fact that the transition to parenthood is one of the life changes which was traditionally heavily culturally mediated, by ritual practices, and narratives. Hence, the question of the origin of life is such a grounding mystery for all human groups, that all of them have developed, in parallel to the natural begetting, rituals of symbolic, second, cultural birth, in the realm of the human group. The question which interested me was thus, if it is true that collective modes of symbolisation of birth tend to vanish, yet if people's need to confer sense to their experience remain, what are then the modes of symbolisation of experience? In other words, in so-called traditional societies, people's individual modes of understanding are quite similar to the collective culture; in contrast, contemporary societies are characterised by a great distance between personal culture and collective culture, and by great individual variation. So what is it in people's individual culture, which has the function of conferring sense to this part of a person's experience?
5. Based on their clinical work, anchored in attachment theory, Ammaniti and colleagues (1999) defined a precise coding scheme to analyse mother's discourse. On this basis, they distinguish three types of representation in the discourse of women according to their openness to the new, the richness of their perceptions, traces of affective investments, consistency, differentiation etc. These three types of discourses are: (a) "balanced," where they are consistent, realistic and affectively invested; (b) "reduced/disinvested" when the discourse rationalises, excludes emotions, is abstract and disconnected from experience; and finally (c) "non integrated/ambivalent" when coexist different tendencies towards the child, and unsolved affective conflicts. These categories overlap with these proposed by Green: one might say that the first type of discourse gives the impression of an integration of representations and affects, that the second is characterised by defensive representations, and the third one, by the emergence of unbounded affects. Given this similarity—due to the psychoanalytical rooting of the two approaches—I used Ammaniti and colleagues (1999)'s coding scheme as a menas of operationalising Green's clinical insights in a research setting (Zittoun, 2005).

6. This fourth, interpretative analysis constructs and combines four layers of meaning:
    1. A reconstruction of the present transition period of the person, and of its relationship to his or her biographical lines (Bar-On, 1991; Riessman, 1993);
    2. A review of the cultural elements mentioned by the person, and a close examination of the most relevant books, songs, movies etc.; particular attention is given to the specific reports the person makes of the cultural elements. As I also have access to the cultural element, I can compare the shared meaning of the cultural element, to what the person reports; the second version, or the difference between the two versions, enables hypotheses to be made about the work of sense-making in which the person has engaged;
    3. An identification of the "conflicting knots' in the person's discourse, or of the less elaborated problems related to the transition to parenthood. When not explicitly mentioned as problems or difficulties, such "conflicting knots" are indicated by changes of emotional intensity in the discourse, by repetitions, contradictions, by cross-thematic semantic fields, by phonologic recurrences (Ammaniti et al., 1999; Freud, 1900/1953; Green, 1973/1999; Tisseron, 1998);
    4. A parallel reading of the personal story with its non-elaborated questions and in the cultural elements mentioned, both in their presentation by the person and in my own reading. This finally allows it to be seen whether and how these references could be seen as "symbolic resources" for indivduals (Zittoun, 2005).
7. Interviewed transcribed in French and translated by me. Transcription conventions: E = mother, T = interviewer; ... is interrupted sentence; (...) represents long sequences not reported; ::: indicates some long vowel; - marks a silence; [text in brackets] is added to facilitate the reading.
8. This took place before the large commercial success of Angelina Jolie.

REFERENCES

Ammaniti, M., Candelori, C., Pola, M., & Tambelli, R. (1999). *Maternité et grossesse [Maternity and pregnancy]*. Paris: Presses Universitaires de France.

Bar-On, D. (1991). *Legacy of silence: Encounters with children of the Third Reich* (2nd ed.). Cambridge, MA: Harvard University Press.

Ben Soussan, P. (1999). *Le bébé imaginaire [The imagined baby]*. Paris: Erès.

Benson, C. (2001). *The cultural psychology of self: Place, morality and art in human worlds*. London: Routledge.

Bollas, C. (2003). *Being a character: psychoanalysis and self experience*. New York: Routledge.

Bydlowski, M. (1997). *La dette de vie: Itineraire psychanalytique de la maternité [The debt of life: Psychoanalytic itinerary of pregnancy]*. Paris: Presses universitaires de France.

Cabell K., & Valsiner, J. (2011). Affective hypergeneralization: Learning from psychoanalysis. In S. Salvatore, & T. Zittoun (Eds.), *Cultural psychology and psychoanalysis. Pathways to synthesis* (pp. 87–113). Charlotte NC: Info Age Publishing.

Dewey, J. (1934). *Art as experience*. New York: Penguin.

Druon, M. (1973). *Les Rois maudits [The doomed kings]*. Paris: LGF-Livre de Poche.

Freud, S. (1953). The interpretation of dreams. In J. Strachey (Ed. and Trans.), *The standard edition of the complete psychological works of Sigmund Freud* (Vols. 4–5). London: The Hogarth Press and the Institute of Psycho-analysis. (Original work published 1900)

Freud, S. (1959). Creative writers and day-dreaming. In J. Strachey (Ed. and Trans.), *The standard edition of the complete psychological works of Sigmund Freud* (Vol. 9, pp. 141–153). London: Hogarth. (Original work published 1908)

Freud, S. (1961). Five lectures in psychoanalysis. In J. Strachey (Ed. and Trans.), *The standard edition of the complete psychological works of Sigmund Freud* (Vol. 11, pp. 1–56). London: The Hogarth Press and the Institute of Psycho-analysis. (Original work published 1910)

Freud, S. (1964). An outline of psychoanalysis. In J. Strachey (Ed. and Trans.), *The standard edition of the complete psychological works of Sigmund Freud* (Vol. 23, pp. 141–207). London: Hogarth. (Original work published 1938)

Green, A. (1992). *La déliaison. Psychanalyse, anthropologie et littérature [Unlinking. Psychoanalysis, anthropology and literature]*. Paris: Hachette.

Green, A. (1995). *Causalité psychique. Entre nature et culture [Psychic causality. Between nature and culture]*. Paris : Odile Jacob.

Green, A. (1999). *The fabric of affect in the psychoanalytic discourse*. (A. Sheridan, Tran.). London; Routledge (Original published work 1973).

Green, A. (2002). *La pensée clinique [Clinical thinking]*. Paris: Odile Jacob.

Grossen, M., & Perret-Clermont, A. (1992). *L'Espace thérapeutique [The therapeutic space]*. Lausanne: Delachaux & Niestle.

Josephs, I. E. (1998). Constructing one's self in the city of the silent: Dialogue, symbols, and the role of 'as-if' in self-development. *Human Development, 41*(3), 180–195.

Moro, M. (2001). *Parents en exil: Psychopathologie et migrations [Parents in exile. Psychopathology of immigration]*. Paris: Presses Universitaires de France.

Moscovici, S. (2000). What is in a name? In I. M. Chaib & B. Orfali (Eds.), *Social representations and communicative processes* (pp. 12–28). Jönköping, SW: Jönköping University Press. Retrieved from http://www.serge-moscovici.fr/biblioPS.html.

Nell, V. (1988). *Lost in a book: the psychology of reading for pleasure*. Yale, CT: Yale University Press.

Rey, A. (Ed.). (2000). *Le Petit Robert des noms propres [French dictionary]*. Paris: Le Robert.

Riessman, C. K. (1993). *Narrative analysis*. Thoudands Oaks, CA: Sage.

Salvatore, S., & Zittoun, T. (2011). Outlines of a psychoanalytically informed cultural psychology. In S. Salvatore & T. Zittoun (Eds.), *Cultural psychology and psychoanalysis. Pathways to Synthesis* (pp. 3–46). Charlotte, NC: Info Age Publishing.

Searles, H. (2005). *Le contre-transfert [Countertransference]*. Paris: Gallimard.

Stern, D. N., Brunschweiler-Stern, N., & Freeland, A. (1998). *Birth of a mother, the: How the experience of motherhood changes you forever*. New York: Basic Books.

Tisseron, S. (1998). *Y a-t-il un pilote dans l'image?[Is there a pilot in the image?]*. Paris: Aubier.

Tisseron, S. (1999). *Du bon usage de la honte [The proper use of shame]*. Paris: Ramsay.

Tisseron, S. (2002). *Les bienfaits des images [The benefits of images]*. Paris: Odile Jacob.

Tisseron, S. (2003). *Comment Hitchcock m'a sauvé la vie [How Hitchcock saved my life]*. Paris: Armand Colin.

Van der Veer, R. (2011). Tatyana on the couch: the vicissitudes of psychoanalysis in Russia. In S. Salvatore & T. Zittoun (Eds.), *Cultural psychology and psychoanalysis. Pathways to Synthesis* (pp. 49–65). Charlotte NC: Info Age Publishing.

Valsiner, J. (2007). *Culture in minds and societies: Foundations of cultural psychology*. New Delhi: Sage.

Viderman, S. (1982). *La construction de l'espace analytique [The construction of the analytic space]*. Paris: Gallimard.

Vygotsky, L. (1963). *Thought and Language* (Eugenia Hanfmann & Gertrude Vakar, eds. And trans.). Cambridge, MA & London: MIT press. (Original work published 1934).

Vygotsky, L. S. (1971). *The psychology of art*. Cambridge, MA & London: MIT press.

Winnicott, D. W. (2001). *Playing and reality*. Philadelphia/Sussex: Routledge (First published 1971 by Tavistock Publication Ltd).

Zittoun, T. (2004). Symbolic competencies for developmental transitions: The case of the choice of first names. *Culture Psychology, 10*(2), 131–161.

Zittoun, T. (2005). *Donner la vie, choisir un nom. Engendrements symboliques [Giving life, choosing a name. Symbolic begetting]*. Paris: L'Harmattan.

Zittoun, T. (2006). *Transitions. Development through symbolic resources*. Charlotte, NC: Information Age Publishing.

Zittoun, T. (2007). Symbolic resources and responsibility in transitions. *Young. Nordic Journal of Youth Research, 15*(2), 193–211.

Zittoun, T. (2011). Freud and cultural psychology. In S. Salvatore & T. Zittoun (Eds.), *Cultural psychology and psychoanalysis. Pathways to synthesis* (pp. 67–85). Charlotte, NC: Info Age Publishing.

Zittoun, T., Gillespie, A., Cornish, F., & Psaltis, C. (2007). The metaphor of the triangle in theories of human development. *Human Development, 50*, 208–229.

CHAPTER 7

THE DEVELOPMENT OF MEANING IN SOCIAL INTERACTION: EVIDENCE FROM EMPIRICAL RESEARCH ON PARENT–CHILD NARRATIVE CO-CONSTRUCTION

Nicolas Favez

NARRATIVES AND MEANING-MAKING

Telling narratives is a spontaneous social activity, which occurs as soon as the child enters into language. The first narratives are rudimentary as far as vocabulary and grammar are concerned, and they are built with a noncanonical structure (Peterson, & McCabe, 1983); even so, the core function of narratives may be fulfilled: to give meaning to lived events. Indeed, narratives are a powerful tool to organize social experiences. As Stern (1985) has pointed out, in infancy, affects, cognition and action are to a certain extent

Cultural Psychology and Psychoanalysis: Pathways to Synthesis, pp. 181–204

undifferentiated; the accession to narrative organization brings order and differentiation according to the narrative structure: events are organized around an agent, an action, an intention or motive, a goal, a scene, and they are interconnected with causal links and organized as antecedent and consequence. The construction of the narrative is thus a process of transformation, as it is not mirroring the "reality" but rather is a reconstruction of it according to the constraints of the narrative structure. Some authors have further argued that the narrative form is the basic unit of organization of the human intersubjective experience—that is, the perception of the social world is intrinsically narratively organized (Bruner, 1990; Stern, 1994). Furthermore, narratives allow lived events to be shared with significant others, even if they were not present at the time and place of the events.

Narratives provide a specific kind of knowledge about self and the social world. They allow an episodic knowledge (this particular event I have lived) and related to the self, they allow an autobiographical knowledge of who the individual is (by organizing self-defining memories—memories related to "who I am" in the social world). Thus, they participate in the definition of the child's identity. In this perspective, identity is defined as "the unity of a person's life as it is experienced and articulated in stories that express this experience" (Widdershoven, 1993, p.7). This knowledge refers to what Bruner (1986) has called "narrative knowledge" as opposed to "paradigmatic knowledge," that is scientific knowledge. Both these modes of knowledge establish causality between facts and events, but in two distinct manners. Paradigmatic knowledge aims to establish general rules of the world, based on deductive reasoning and on formal logic. Narrative knowledge aims to locate the experience according to a time frame and a space, and to establish connections between singular events. This mode is not based on logic, but on human motive and intentions—it gives meaning to the events in the social world.

One important aspect of meaning-making is what Ricoeur (1990) has called the "refiguration" process: narratives function as a laboratory which allows the individual to test experiences, to play with relationships between actors and actions, to test hypotheses. The individual can try several versions of the "reality" through different narratives. As an example of early "refiguration," Watson (1989) has described how monologues from the crib by a 2-year-old girl, Emily, are about daily routines (separation for the night and reunion the morning after) and how she plays in her narratives the negotiation with her father about bedtime, testing different scenarios about getting more time to play.

EARLY DEVELOPMENT OF NARRATIVES IN A SOCIAL CONTEXT

The first narratives are produced in the context of daily activities and routines; very early after the acquisition of language (as soon as 2.5–3 years), the child tells "emotional stories" to her relatives—that is, she shares the affects associated with lived events (Dunn, & Brown, 1991). These autobiographical narratives will progressively tend to be organized according to the classic structure described by Labov (1972) as development progress: orientation (specification of the time frame and the place of the story), complicating action (the first elements of the "plot"), high-point (the main event of the story), evaluation (the affects that the narrator associates to the event), resolution (how the plot is resolved) and coda (the announcement of the end of the story). This structure has been shown to be the "canonical" structure of autobiographical narratives made in a social interaction—be it in a group of peers or in the parent–child interaction (see Favez, 2000 for a review). In the first stage, narratives are context-dependent: the child talks about the here and now of an ongoing event; then, past references appear and the child begins to talk about events that happened when their adult speaker was not present (Fivush & Hammond, 1990; Nelson, 1992).

The first narratives are mainly co-constructions: the adult participates in the elaboration of the stories and helps the child to shape them in a coherent structure. The first co-constructions are asymmetrical in nature: the adult brings most of the "material" to the narratives; the child learns progressively in these dialogues how to tell story in a way that can be understood by others. Conversely, the narrative structure provided by the adult allows the child to give meaning to lived events and so influences the content of the child's autobiographical memory (Nelson & Fivush, 2004).

The two main dimensions of narrative co-construction that have been studied so far are the effects of narratives on learning and remembering on the one hand, and the narratives as shaping moral and cultural values on the other hand. Regarding learning, several studies in the field of cognitive psychology have shown that mother–child narrative co-constructions, also labeled "joint encoding," are related to later recall of an event by the child. The narrative context in which the child grows is related to the development of autobiographical memory; children with parents who encourage the narrative activity and help to elaborate stories are more efficient in recall tasks—as assessed by the number and the accuracy of memories of an event after a period of time: for example the birthday of a friend, or what happened during Summer holidays as the child reminds them 2 weeks later (Fivush & Haden, 1997; Haden, 2003; Leichtman, Wang & Pillemer, 2003). This effect is supposed to be active upstream of the recall task, when the child is telling the narrative for the first time and thus "encoding" memories, and at the time of the task itself: the support of the parent help the children to retrieve the events more efficiently (Nelson, 1996).

Research from the field of clinical psychology has on the other hand focused on narratives as the media of transmission of moral and cultural values, at two levels: on one hand, the ongoing activity of co-construction in itself conveys values (i.e., "how" to tell stories and to present oneself), on the other hand, cultural values are also transmitted by the parents at an explicit content level; parents may for example recount their own childhood experiences to compare with the story told by their child, or integrate their own beliefs in the co-construction, in order to give the moral of the story. Family stories are indeed not equivalent to family history (Fiese, Hooker, Kotary, Schwagler, & Rimmer, 1995): they give a window on how the family gives meaning to the intersubjective experience rather than being an account of the "real" experience itself. Narratives are co-constructed as a joint activity in the family; the family values (or not) the activity of telling a narrative, the kind of event that is narrated and the emotional tone given to it (Bruner, 1990; Stern, 1994). Moreover, research has shown that the content of family stories varies according to the developmental stage of the family: for example, during the child's first years, affiliation or the "sense of belonging" is a recurrent topic in spontaneous family narratives; as soon as the child reaches school age, the topic of achievement or academic success becomes predominant (Fiese et al., 1995).

One core component of autobiographical narratives is the affective evaluation of the experience, which is the narrative's motive (Labov, 1972). Families are not only talking about what happened, but also about how they feel about the event, what is the emotional meaning of what happened, and, what is more, they talk about what should have happened (Fiese et al., 1999). The affective content of narratives is sensitive to the quality of the relationship, as research on dyadic parent–child conversations has shown, in the area of attachment or in psychodynamic research about the development of self in childhood: a relationship which allows an open expression of emotions at a nonverbal level, or in the regulation of attachment needs, is associated with more elaborate narratives as far as affects are concerned; conversely, research has shown that preschoolers' narratives with coherent and detailed elaboration of affects are predictive of positive outcomes at the time of entry at school (Favez, 2003; Main & Weston, 1981; Oppenheim, Emde, & Warren, 1997).

Thus far, theory and research have shown that narratives are involved in the meaning-making process for the child at these two levels: first, autobiographical memory relies on the narrative structure. Second, co-constructing narratives is an activity of transmission and elaboration of social and family values. In both cases, the social interaction has an impact on narratives, either as facilitating the recall of an event—which will give more material "at hand" for the child to understand and interpret the world, or the sharing of emotions with significant others.

AIM OF THE CHAPTER

We present in this chapter two studies to illustrate these links between social interaction and narratives. The first study focuses on the "learning" level

(Favez, 2001, 2003); the second focuses on the "social-cultural" level (Favez, Abbet, & Frascarolo, 2006; Favez, Frascarolo, & Lavanchy, 2005). For each study, we give qualitative examples of narratives co-construction, and then we present results from quantitative analyses.

Study 1: Mother's Influence on Children Remembering

Population

46 mother–child dyads recruited in kindergartens. All children have French as their mother tongue. 21 boys and 25 girls. Mean age is 4 years 5 months (minimum 3 years 6 months, maximum 5 years 1 month). Socioeconomic status is middle-class to upper middle-class.

Procedure

The procedure includes two measurement points. At T1, the child, separated from her mother, is actively involved in a standard scenario, the Geneva Emotion-Eliciting Scenario (GEES), which involves different characters: a clown and a Queen of the Robots, played by women experimenters, and a large teddy bear (Favez et al., 1994). The central theme of the scenario is the separation of the clown from her friend the bear. The scenario is structured according to the labovian structure: (i) orientation (discovery of the characters), (ii) complicating action (playing together), (iii) high-point (the separation), (iv) resolution (comforting), and (v) coda (end of the story). Mothers are given instructions to ask their child to talk about what happened right after the scenario. At the end of the procedure, mothers are asked not to talk with the child about the scenario in the meantime between T1 and T2.

At T2, two weeks later, mother and child are received again to the lab and the same instruction is given to the mothers; there is no scenario, and no clue is given either to the mother or to the child about what happened at T1.

Coding

The dialogue between the mother and the child is transcribed verbatim and subdivided according to turn-taking. A microanalytical coding of the mother's discourse is done in order to determine the type of cooperation in maternal discourse in terms of speech acts, according to four dimensions: insistence, clarification, elaboration, emotionality (for the details of the coding system, see Favez, 2001). The combination of the four dimensions yielded three categories of maternal cooperation (Favez, 2003):

- Active omission: mothers oriented towards the recall performance, asking a lot of wh-questions (insistence), correcting the child's language (clarification), but not encouraging the child to speak about the emotions associated to the story (emotionality) nor to test different versions of the possible links between events (elaboration).

- Emotional facilitation: mothers are oriented to a certain extent toward the recall performance, asking some wh-questions (insistence) and correcting the child's language (clarification), but at the same time promoting the expression of affects (emotionality) and the search of different meanings for the events (elaboration).
- Disengagement: mothers provide very low support for the child on all dimensions.

Children narratives are coded for thematic content. Each utterance is coded depending on which part of the scenario it refers to (orientation, complication, high-point, resolution, coda). Two other categories of references have been added: a category for utterances which refer to the features of the objects and of the characters of the scenario (e.g., colour of the clothes, size of the objects), and a category for all other utterances which are not directly related to the scenario (features of the experimental situation, e.g., description of the room, of the camera, or negotiation with the mother, e.g. "I don't want to tell the story," etc.). We have thus seven possible categories of references in the child's narrative: the five parts of the scenario and these two supplementary categories of "Objects and characters" and "Others" references.

Reliability

Two judges scored independently 20% of the transcripts. The first coder was the author of this paper; the second one was an undergraduate student, blind to the hypotheses of the research. The reliabilities were computed at two levels (Cohen's Kappa): (i) Concerning the categories of cooperation, the raters achieved a reliability of $K = .69$. *(ii) For the child narrative categories, their agreement was between* $K = .71$ *and* $K = .78$.

Case studies

We will contrast two cases belonging to two different categories of maternal cooperation style as observed at T1.

Case 1: 4.5-year-old girl with mother at T1

Child	*Mother*
	1. So you tell me … What have you seen
2. Eeh a clown. Then we threw it	
	3. Threw what?
4. Eeh a teddy bear then we threw it	
	5. Yes
6. And. and … then we did. We were. the clown was gone	
	7. Where is it gone?

Child	*Mother*
8. Euh because it has someone to meet	
	9. Mm mm
10. And then a Queen came to take the teddy bear because it has to go and the woman was so sad so we did a dance	
	11. To comfort her?
12. Yes	
	13. Hey that's great. Mm mm was it a good story?
14. Mm mm	
	15. Did you have fun?
16. Mm mm	
	17. I'm reall happy for you ... and ... hum the Teddy Bear was soft?
18. Mm mm	
	19. Was it nice?
20. Mm mm	
	21. and the clown?
22. Mm mm	
	23. How was it dressed?
24. Mpff I don't remember	
	25. You don't remember? ... He had a big red nose?
26. No	
	27. And the Teddy bear, what colour was it?
28. White	
29. =Mm	30. White wow that's great and did you see the Queen again. The Queen who came. How was she this Queen. Do you remember her?
31. =She had a crown and something on the eyes	
	32. Yes. Something more?
33. No	
	34. So that's OK
35. Eh mummy	
	36. Yes
37. We did the «pont d'avignon» dance	
	38. You danced «le pont d'Avignon»
39. Sur le pont d'Avignon.	
	40. Mm mm! Did you do well?
41. Mmmm	
	42. With whom have you danced
43. With the clown and the woman	
	44. Ok alright....

In this excerpt, the narrative is structured in three steps: the child first tells a very condensed and almost comprehensive abstract of the scenario (1–12). Then, the mother evaluates the story and asks the child for the emotion he felt (13–17). Then she takes over the narration and asks the child for more details (18–44). The mother is thus following a double agenda: on one hand listening to the story as a social-emotional event and sharing the emotion with her child, and on the other hand engaging the child in a recall performance to ensure that the story is complete. Maternal cooperation style belongs to the "emotional facilitator" category, high on the dimensions of elaboration and emotionality, and in the middle range for insistence and clarification.

Case 2: 4.8-year-old girl with mother at T2

Child	*Mother*
	1. Oh Sandra. You tell me what happened? OK?
2. He is gone	
	3. Sorry?
4. Gone	
	5. What gone?
6. He is gone the clown	
	7. Please sit down properly Sandra. What?
8. We did soap bubbles	
	9. You did soap bubbles? Is that all you did? What did you do?
10. We sang «le pont d'Avignon»	
	11. Please sit down properly. So what did you do
12. We had the Teddy Bear doing somersaults	
	13. Mmm did you do that with the Teddy Bear?
14. Yes	
	15. Did you do somersaults yourself?
16. No it was the Teddy Bear	
	17. The Teddy Bear. Was it happy?
18. Yes	
	19. And then?
20. The Teddy Bear is gone	
	21. By itself?
22. Yes the Queen came to take it	
	23. Who?
24. There is a Queen who came to take the Teddy bear	

Child	*Mother*
	25. A Queen?
26. Yes	
	27. What Queen?
28. With a mask	
	29. Yeah
30. The one you love on the TV	
	31. Oh well
32. Yeah with the mask	
	33. Mm did she come by herself?
34. Who?	
	35. The Queen
36. Yeah	
	37. Why did she take the teddy bear away?
38. Well because the Teddy Bear was leaving	
	39. You don't know why
40. Now I'm hungry	
	41. Yes yes. So you came alone?
42. Yes	
	43. Who?
44. The woman	
	45. Mmm Mathilda?
46. Yes	
	47. Her name is Mathilda, the woman with whom you built the castle
48. Yes Mathilda	
	49. Mathilda but tell me. Please sit down. You will have something to eat later. You can do an effort please. Hmmm you remember what I told you. Please sit down properly
50. We came with/Mathilda and me we stayed alone	

This excerpt shows a mother focused almost exclusively on her child's recall performance. Although the child mentions some events of the scenario which are likely to be emotionally loaded [the arrival of the Queen (24) or the leaving of the teddy bear (38)], mother's replies are aiming at getting more details rather than sharing the emotions associated with the events. Moreover, there are several instances of "extra"-scenario details, especially toward the end of the excerpt (44–50). This maternal cooperation style belongs to the "active omission" style, which refers to a cooperation high on the insistence dimension, in the middle range on clarification dimension, and low on emotionality and on elaboration. Quantitative analyses show that at T1 (for $N = 46$, see Table 7.1) the three maternal styles are related to children's narratives (see Favez, 2003, for the details); children of mothers with the "emotional facilitation" style mention the high-point significantly more than the other children and children of mothers with a "disengaged" style produce narratives significantly shorter than the narratives of the other children. At T2, 33 dyads of the original sample (15 boys and 18 girls) were received for the "recall" task. Data (see Table 7.2) show that the effect observed at T1 is almost the same two weeks later; the "disengaged" mothers have children who significantly talk less about the high-point than the children of mothers of the two other styles and narratives are significantly longer for children with mothers of the "emotional facilitation" style than for children of mothers of the two other styles.

Table 7.1. Anovas and Specific Contrasts Between Maternal Patterns at T1 and Children's Narrative Content at T1 ($N = 46$)

Technical comments: Children of mothers with the "emotional facilitation" style mention the high-point significantly more than the other children (ANOVA: $F(2,43) = 7.21, p < .01$). Children of mothers with a "disengaged" style produce narratives significantly shorter than the narratives of the other children (ANOVA: $F(2,43) = 7.49, p < .05$).

	Maternal patterns at T1							
	Active omission (a) (N = 22)		*Facilitation (b) (N = 14)*		*Disengagement (c) (N = 10)*			
Parts of the narratives at T1	*Mean*	*SD*	*Mean*	*SD*	*Mean*	*SD*	*F (2,43)*	*Bonferroni contrasts*
Orientation	4.6	4.2	4.4	3.8	2.1	2.8	1.84	
Complicating action	7.4	6.4	5.9	4.7	3.5	3.5	1.73	
High-point	2.5	2.4	5.0	3.6	1.1	1.3	7.21**	b>a,c
Resolution	5.7	4.3	6.6	3.8	5.1	3.6	0.88	
Coda	5.8	4.1	7.3	5.3	4.1	5.0	1.61	
Length of narratives								
(all parts together)	52.5	20.1	66.0	23.1	26.7	18.5	7.49**	a, b>c

Table 7.2. Anovas and Specific Contrasts Between Maternal Patterns at T1 and Children's Narrative Content At T2 (*N* = 33)

Technical comments: He "disengaged" mothers have children who significantly talk less about the high-point than the children of mothers of the two other styles (ANOVA: $F(2,30) = 4.47, p < .05$), and narratives are significantly longer for children with mothers of the "emotional facilitation" style than for children of mothers of the two other styles (ANOVA: $F(2,30) = 5.69, p < .01$).

	Maternal Patterns at T1							
	Active omission (a) (N = 15)		*Facilitation (b) (N = 9)*		*Disengagement (c) (N = 9)*			
Parts of the narratives at T2	*Mean*	*SD*	*Mean*	*SD*	*Mean*	*SD*	*F(2,30)*	*Bonferroni contrasts*
Orientation	2.5	2.0	3.0	3.1	3.4	3.9	0.32	
Complicating action	4.8	3.9	4.4	3.9	3.9	3.4	0.16	
High-point	2.9	2.6	5.2	3.2	1.8	1.2	4.47*	B > c
Resolution	4.8	4.6	4.7	1.6	4.7	1.6	0.70	
Coda	1.0	1.1	2.0	2.4	2.4	0.8	1.22	
Length of narratives (all parts together)	35.6	16.6	50.6	12.3	27.8	13.2	5.69**	b>a,c

Study 2: Family Co-Construction of A Semi-Fictitious Event

Sample

25 families participated in this study, which is a part of a larger longitudinal study on the transition to parenthood from pregnancy to age 5 (see Favez, Frascarolo, & Fivaz-Depeursinge, 2006, for details). Different recruiting techniques were used: articles in the local press, notices in gynecologists' waiting rooms, advertising in a regional internet site dedicated to family issues, and contacts through midwives in the ultrasound scan unit of the regional University hospital. All families were middle-class (Hollingshead's ISP). Among the children, there were 16 boys and 9 girls. The mean age is 4 years 9 months.

Procedure

The family takes part to a standardized situation, the narrative version of the Lausanne Trilogue Play (LTP; Fivaz-Depeursinge & Corboz-Warnery, 1999), which is designed to make the family adopt the different interactive configuration in a mother–father–child threesome: mother–child interacting in presence of the father, father–child interacting in presence of the mother and finally the three of them interacting together.

The instructions are as follows: the family has to tell a story, whose topic is the parents leaving for the week-end, leaving the child in the care of relatives. Six Duplo toys (four adults and two children) are at hand as a support for the narrative activity. The topic of separation has been chosen as it is emotionally loaded and ecologically sound for a 5-year -old child. The family is asked to tell the story in three parts, according to the three triadic configurations: first, one parent begins to tell the story with the child; then, the other parents takes over the story with the child; finally, they continue the story altogether. The duration of each part and transitions between parts is up to the family.

Instruments

Coding of the narratives: NES (Narrative Evaluation Scales; Abbet, & Favez, 2005). 22 five-point Likert scales designed to assess the narrative co-construction, according to three dimensions:

1. Interactive context (seven scales; $\alpha = .83$). This dimension refers to the negotiation about the collaborative activity of telling the narration: mainly who will take part, what the roles of the participants will be. The seven scales are: participation, co-parental coordination, child scaffolding, engagement in the task, rules definition, parental guidance, level of child–parent intersubjectivity.
2. Structure of the story (five scales; $\alpha = .69$). This dimension refers to the way the events of the story are put together. The five scales are: the high-point structure, clarification of own elements, meta-comments, chronological order of the events, narrative stance (I/we or he/she).
3. Content of the story (eight scales; $\alpha = .80$). This dimension refers to the content of the story, that is, which are the events and details that are mentioned in the story. The eight scales are: mention of the separation, mention of the reunion, resolution of the story, positive affects, negative affects, details of the characters and environment of the story, inner state of the characters, elements of actions.

Narrations are transcribed verbatim and subdivided according to turn-taking. Two judges scored independently 25% of the transcripts. The first coder was the author of this paper; the second one was a graduate student, blind to the hypotheses of the research. The reliability was judged to be acceptable (Cohen's Kappa = .68).

Case 3: 4.9-year-old boy with father

Father	*Child*
1. You have to tell me a story, you have to tell me story. So here is a little character here mh this is Bob so which one do we have to take (.) this one this is Bob OK. And then we have to find one for Daddy and one for Mummy	
	2. This one is Mummy
3. This is Mummy and Dad is	
	4. This one
5. This one is Daddy, OK. So Mummy and Daddy really love Bob. Give me a kiss alright? Well, they have to do something this week-end and they have decided decided. What?	
	6. (?)
7. What did they decide?	
	8. Going holidays
9. They have decided to go away for a holiday, but only for two days, ok. Only for Saturday and Sunday. So they have decided to be just the two of them, because they love each other a lot as well, eh, they wanted to leave Bob with someone. Who with?	
	10. Jimmy
11. This one is Jimmy? Oh we also need two adults because you cannot stay on your own	12. So this one
13. Who are they?	
	14. Mummy and Daddy
15. Oh no, mummy and daddy are here, not there	

The first part with father begins with the organization of the narrative play. The father and the child are "setting the stage," first by designating the characters of the story (1–5, 10–15), then by giving the main elements of the plot (second part of 5–9) which correspond to the "orientation" phase described by Labov (1972) in the narrative structure. The content of the story, as prompted by the instruction, is mentioned in a straightforward way, and affects are directly evoked (love, 5 and 9). The child is encouraged to be an active participant.

Case 3: 4.9-year-old boy with mother

Mother	*Child*
1. Ring ring hello ring ring	
	2. Euheuh
3. Anyone on the phone?	
	4. Yes yes this is Gigi *(the Grandma in charge of the children)*
5. Hello Gigi, this is mummy. I hope all's well with the children	
	6. Yes
7. What did you do this morning	
	8. We watched TV
9. What did you see?	
	10. Jerry
11. Tom and Jerry	
	12. Fifteen Tom and Jerry
13. Fifteen? But I've told your grandma about not watching too much TV, hmm, wee, and everything is OK?	
	14. Yes
15. Yes daddy and mummy are very happy, they're going to the theatre tonight ah they are really looking forward to this evening but they just wanted to hear about you, to know how you are doing	
	16. Bye bye

The mother takes over the story by continuing and elaborating the topic proposed by the father. The plot is in a further stage, corresponding to the "complication of the action" in Labov's structure: the parents are away, and they call their child by phone to hear how he is. Again, the child is an active participant and he even plays another character apart from his own (Gigi, the grandmother)—by the way, the mother makes a slight misattunement (13) by talking to the "child" and not to the "Grandma," but the child shifts quickly to this new role and the narrative can continue. Again, affects and relational topics are mentioned by the mother (15).

Case 3: 4.9-year-old boy with mother and father

Mother	*Father*	*Child*
	1. Hello boys, daddy and mummy are back home oh are you happy to see us?	
		2. Yes
3. Hey, give me a kiss		
	4. So you are happy to see us	
		5. Yes, we can say that
	6. What did you do during this long week-end?	
		7. So we are finally back home
	8. That's right. Victor, mummy and daddy	

Ending the story all together, mother, father and child play the reunion at the end of the week-end. There is a "high-point" (1) and a "resolution" in which affects are evoked (second part of 1–5). Even if this last section is very short, it contains all the elements which allow a narrative to be concluded.

As a general comment, we can see that the instructions have been respected in this case: father first began the story with the child, then the mother took over, and finally they all did a final "coda" to the story together. Moreover, there is a connecting thread throughout these three parts, whose themes are interconnected: (i) first with the father, the "orientation" of the story is provided, then (ii) with the mother the action is "complicated," and (iii) finally there is a high-point and a short resolution all together. This is one story, in three acts. This narrative is high on the three dimensions of context (the roles have been distributed and respected), of structure (high-point structure and the story is temporally organized) and of content (details are elaborated and several affects are mentioned).

Case 4—4.9-year-old boy with mother

Mother	*Child*
1. Do you want one doll, or do you want to play with both?	
	2. With both
3. Are they brothers?	
	4. No, they aren't friends
5. They aren't friends?	
	6. Tttrrrrrchchch
7. Which one is the oldest?	

(*Continued*)

Mother	*Child*
	8. This one is the oldest (*showing a third doll*)
9. No, of these two	
	10. Mhmh him prr prr
11. Him? What's his name?	
	12. Cracou
13. Cracou, and the other one?	
	14. Coucou
15. Coucou and Cracou? And this one, who is this?	16. Coucou coucou prr
17. Who is this?Your mother? Or?	18. Aou who who who who who who who yes
19. Whose mother is this?	
	20. Kaaaarl's
21. Oh you did change the name	22. This is him
	23. From him
24. OK, this is his mother, and this one is his father as he is wearing the same shirt	
	25. Yes
26. So they can be easily identified	
	27. Ah
28. How are we going to do this? Will you go with Grandma and Grandad for the week-end?	
	29. No

In this first part, the mother begins by "setting the stage" (1–19), but the child is not cooperative and some kind of confusion occurs as the child changes the name of the characters in the course of the discussion (20–21). He finally refuses the plot proposed by the mother (28–29). This first part then goes on and on as an endless negotiation about who will be each doll; mother and child fail to give a clear "orientation" to the story. Interestingly, regarding the establishment of the context of the narrative, the mother continues to ask the child who, in turn, increasingly shows oppositional behaviour; there is no meta-comment done by the mother, or any disciplinary attempt to make the child more compliant.

Case 4—4.9-year-old boy with father

Father	*Child*
1. Do you want to go to the mountain with your friends	
	2. (*the child shouts*)
3. Which one is Coucou?	
	4. Coucou
5. Coucou	
	6. Here Cracou
7. And Cracou	
	8. Cracou Cracou Cracou Cracou Cracou Cracou Cracou Cracou Cracou Cracou AAAH *Shouts*
9. So Arthur	
	10. What (?)
11. Let's try to tell a story	
	12. Well
13. With the grandmothers and grandfathers	14. Mummy he's bothering me he's bothering me now they are friends with each other
15. Ah alright ah finally ah finally they will go skiing together in the mountains	
	16. Yes. Well, no. Now we are at the end
17. Alright. So do you know what will happen?	
	18. No
19. Well, the grandparents and the parents. They've had enough, they'll go. They are gone	
	20. (*laugh*)
21. They don't want to. They are tired of being hit all the time (.) What will you do, you little ones (.) Do you want to go to the mountains by yourself?	

The father takes over, but as the story is not oriented, he has to bring a new element (1) and has to try again to designate the characters of the story, but the child is still not cooperating (3–8). No complication of the action is made possible, and the father tries one instance of showing authority (11) but the child quickly returns to his oppositional behaviour and the father ends by making a harsh comment talking about the characters of the story (21) and not about the child himself.

Case 4—4.9-year-old boy with mother and father

Mother	*Father*	*Child*
	1. We take the bus, you take the bus	
2. And grandma, do you leave her with daddy		
		3. Yes, but I'll get up on gran-dad's head a AOUCH it hurts stop this (?)
		4. What?
5. Is grandma coming along with us?		
		6. Mh no
7. She stays with Dad?		
		8. Yes
9. Alright		
		10. (*shouts*)
	11. What happened?	
		12. What?
	13. What happened?	
		14. He hurt himself
	15. And?	
16. He will not be able to ski		
		17. (*shouts*) There is nasty people here, and behind us (*shouts*)
18. I think we have to get rid of the TV		
	19. Yeah	

The last part is on par with the other parts: the parents try to get the child to tell something, and he constantly refuses to participate. Thus, there is no "high-point" or "resolution" to the story, which is not concluded. Affects were not mentioned, neither in the story itself, nor regarding the behaviour of the child, to the exception of a rather disillusioned comment from the mother about the TV (18).

As a general comment, we can see that this case is contrasted to the first one on each of the three dimensions of narrative co-construction. To a certain extent, instructions have been respected, at least for the three parts of the interaction (one parent and the child, the other parent and the child, and finally the three together). However, the parents were unable to get the child to cooperate, partly because they did not place their discipline attempts at the adequate level: they tried to dramatize it by making the characters of the story play the discipline, at a content level, instead of establishing the rules at a contextual level in the "real" parent–child

Table 7.3. Correlations between the narrative dimensions (N = 25)

	Interactive context	*Structure of the story*	*Content of the story*
Interactive context	–		
Structure of the story	.70***	–	
Content of the story	.77***	.79***	
Spearman Rho.			

relation. As a result, the story fails to unfold and the labovian structure is not present. This narrative is in the middle range on the dimension of context (the parts have been respected, but the roles were not distributed and the child did not participate), and low on the dimensions of structure (no story) and of content (a very few details and almost no affects mentioned).

Quantitative analyses show that there are correlations between the dimensions (Spearman rho's all significant at $p < .001$); at a group level, it is thus unlikely that a narrative could be developed (at a structure and at a content level) if the context is not appropriate (see Table 7.3).

DISCUSSION

The aim of this chapter was to illustrate the links between social interaction and narratives and to present variations in family storytelling and narrative co-construction. The first study, which aimed at assessing the influence of different maternal cooperative styles on remembering, has shown that a maternal style-oriented toward emotional elaboration and at the same time providing a linguistic support for the child is associated with a better remembering of a lived event immediately after the event and again two weeks later.

Whatever the dimensions considered or the label given to them, different maternal styles in narrative co-construction have been constantly identified by researchers; these styles have been shown to be stable across time and types of past event that are narrated. Styles associated with a richer emotional elaboration have been consistently associated with richer narratives in children (i.e., more elaborate and with more information reported), concurrently and over time (see Reese, & Farrant, 2003, for a review). One of the main recurrent distinctions between parental styles is along a broad dimension of "collaboration" (Bohanek, Marin, Fivush, & Duke, 2006): either the parent acknowledges the opinion of the child and validates the emotions the child is reporting and integrates the child's point of view in the co-construction to make a collaborative story, or the parent tells the whole story from her perspective only, correcting the child in order to make its point of view true to his own version, or even just wanting to get information from the child about "what happened" without trying to co-construct a story with him, which will at best result in parallel stories—one from the parent, one from the child. The impact of the mother's style is all the more confirmed by an intervention study of Peterson, Jesso, and McCabe (1999) in a socioeconomically disadvantaged population which has shown that enhancing the mothers' style by coaching them to elaborate and to spend time in narrative activity increased language ability and narrative capacity in their children, compared to a control group.

On a methodological note, the originality of the research presented in this chapter is the inclusion in the procedure of a lab event, the scenario, to which we can compare the narration in terms of "absolute" exhaustivity—whereas naturalistic studies which are closer to the child's everyday life on the other hand only allow a "relative" assessment of elaboration or exhaustivity: the narratives of children are compared with one another, with the researchers having no knowledge of the "real" referent events—for example the actual birthdays each child is referring to, while some of them could be more favourable to elicit narratives.

Several hypotheses have been made to explain the association between mother's styles and children's remembering: first, the child learns in the narrative conversation the linguistic skills which enable past experiences to be reported, which will in turn increase the way he can organize and encode memories of lived events. Secondly, emotionally oriented narratives include references to thoughts, beliefs, intentions—that is, mental state language—which provides an understanding of mental worlds to the children and helps them to organise events around motives. Third, the narrative structure in itself allow events to be organized in a meaningful way for the individual. Finally, maternal scaffolding not only enhances remembering in children, but also adds new knowledge to the events by adding for example hypotheses about possible causal links between events, allowing different perspectives about the same "reality" to be "tested," which will promote problem-solving skills (Haden, 2003).

The second study was designed to explore the different dimensions in the family co-construction of a narration. Our results have shown an important variability along the three dimensions of interactive context (referring to the way the family cooperate to build the story), of story structure (the extent to which the story is close to the canonical narrative standard, with a high-point structure and a linking thread between the different parts) and of content (the extent to which emotions and inner states are mentioned and elaborated in the story). One can hypothesize that these differences are representative of the "meaning system" of the families, which play the role of protective or risk factors for the individuals. When family meaning is coherent—as in narratives high on the structure and content dimensions of our study—family life is more successful in terms of individual's adjustment and mental health (Sameroff & Fiese, 1999). When family meaning is not coherent, with fragmented stories, or contradictions between the emotions expressed and the content of the stories, the child cannot build a congruent image of self and of "self-in-the-world" and lack of meaning-making is related to difficulties in understanding and predicting the world. To explain the process underlying this association, Bohanek, Marin, Fivush and Duke (2006) have pointed out that controlling patterns of parental communication—that is, parents who are not empathetic with children's emotions and who do not integrate children's contribution in the narrative co-construction—do not allow acknowledgement for children's opinions and perceptions. This will in turn lead the children to question themselves about their value and worth as effective agents in the world—"did my opinion count or do I have to strictly adopt my parents' point of view?." These situations of incoherence are close to the classical description of family "mythology" as depicted by Ferreira (1963) in the field of family therapy, which refers to situations in which family stories are in contradiction with family practices: for example, the myth is one of a family with a strong father who is in charge of all the important decisions, while in the therapeutic sessions it appears that the mother is the one with the most relational power.

On the other hand, coherent family rituals foster child adjustment and ensure self-congruence in individuals. Our study has shown that at a group level there is a strong association between practice and the content of the story: establishing a favourable context for storytelling is associated with a structured story and content embellished with references to numerous emotional or inner states. We still have to test the extent to which these differences in storytelling are related to children's outcomes, such as, for example, the development of a theory of the mind or social integration at school.

In conclusion, both studies have shown the interrelation between the interaction during the narrative activity and the content of the narration, either evaluated as a learning or memory task for the child in the first study, or as a family co-construction in the second study. It is worth noting that studies from different fields (cognitive psychology versus clinical-cultural psychology) have led to the same kind of results regarding the relational format of narrative interaction: parents oriented toward more elaborate narratives, with an emphasis placed on the emotional experience, have children that are more efficient on the different outcomes measured, be it recall performance, or elaboration and mention of affective topics. This convergence speaks to the soundness of this process of co-construction and meaning-making resulting from social interaction.

REFERENCES

Abbet, E., & Favez, N. (2005). *Narrative evaluation scales*. Unpublished coding manual. Center for Family Studies. IUP, Department of Psychiatry, University of Lausanne.

Bohanek, J., Marin, K., Fivush, R., & Duke, M. (2006). Family narrative interaction and children's sense of self. *Family Process, 45*(1), 39–54.

Bruner, J. S. (1986). *Actual minds, possible worlds*. Cambridge, MA: Harvard University Press.

Bruner, J. S. (1990). *Acts of meaning*. Cambridge, MA: Harvard University Press.

Dunn, J., & Brown, J. (1991). Relationships, talk about feelings, and the development of affect regulation in early childhood. In J. Garber, & K. A. Dodge (Eds.), *The development of emotion regulation and dysregulation* (pp. 208–242). Cambridge: Cambridge University Press.

Favez, N. (2000). Le développement des narrations autobiographiques chez le jeune enfant [The development of the autobiographical narrations in children]. *Devenir, 12*(4), 63–76.

Favez, N. (2001). La régulation par la mère des émotions narrées par les petits [The mother's regulation of the emotion in children's narratives]. *Enfance, 53*(4), 349–362.

Favez, N. (2003). Patterns of maternal affect regulation in the domain of the co-construction of preschooler's autobiographical narratives. In R. Emde, D. Wolf, & D. Oppenheim (Eds.), *Revealing the Inner Worlds of Young Children: The MacArthur Story Stem Battery and Parent–Child Narratives* (pp. 302–323). New-York: Oxford University Press.

Favez, N., Abbet, E., & Frascarolo, F. (2006). Preschoolers' family narratives of an emotional event: Interactive precursors during infancy and toddlerhood. In N. Favez (Chair), *From pregnancy to school: Narratives as an index of family functioning and child social development*. Paper presented at the 10th WAIMH Conference, July 10, 2006. Paris, France.

Favez, N., Frascarolo, F. & Fivaz-Depeursinge, E. (2006). Family alliance stability and change from pregnancy to toddlerhood and marital correlates. *Swiss Journal of Psychology, 65*(4), 213–220.

Favez, N., Frascarolo, F., & Lavanchy, C. (2005). From family play to family narratives. *The Signal, 12*(3–4), 1–7.

Favez, N., Gertsch Bettens, C., Heinze, X., Koch-Spinelli, M., Mühlebach, M.-C., Valles Almela, V., & Stern, D. N. (1994). Réalité historique et réalité narrative chez le jeune enfant: présentation d'une stratégie de recherche [Historical reality and narrative reality in children. Presentation of a strategy of research]. *Swiss Journal of Psychology, 53*(2), 98–103.

Ferreira, J. (1963) Family myth and homeostasis. *Archives of General Psychiatry, 9*, 457–463.

Fiese, B., Hooker, K., Kotary, L., Schwagler, J., & Rimmer, M. (1995). Family stories in the early stage of parenthood. *Journal of Marriage and the Family, 57*(3), 763–770.

Fiese, B. H., Sameroff, A. J., Grotevant, H. D., Wamboldt, F. S., Dickstein, S., & Lewis-Fravel, D. (Eds.) (1999). The stories that families tell: Narrative coherence, narrative interaction, and relationship beliefs. *Monographs of the Society for Research in Child Development, 64* (2, Serial No. 257).

Fivaz-Depeursinge, E., & Corboz-Warnery, A. (1999). *The primary triangle.* New York, NY: Basic Books.

Fivush, R., & Haden, C. (1997). Narrating and representing experience: Preschoolers' developing autobiographical recounts. In P. van den Broeki, P. Bauer, & T. Bourg (Eds.), *Developmental spans in event comprehension and representation: Bridging fictional and actual events* (pp. 169–198). Mahwah: Lawrence Erlbaum.

Fivush, R., & Hamond, N. (1990). Autobiographical memory across the preschool years: Toward reconceptualizing childhood amnesia. In R. Fivush, & J. Hudson (Eds.), *Knowing and remembering in young children* (pp. 223–248). Cambridge: Cambridge University Press.

Haden, C. (2003). Joint encoding and joint reminiscing: Implications for young children's understanding and remembering of personal experiences. In R. Fivush, & C. Haden (Eds.), *Autobiographical memory and the construction of a narrative self* (pp. 49–69). Mahwah, NJ: Lawrence Erlbaum.

Labov, W. (1972). *Language in the inner city.* Philadelphia, PA: University of Pennsylvania.

Leichtman, M., Wang, Q., & Pillemer, D. (2003). Cultural variations in interdependence and autobiographical memory: Lessons from Korea, China, India and the United States. In R. Fivush & C. Haden (Eds.), *Autobiographical memory and the construction of a narrative self* (pp. 73–97). Mahwah, NJ: Lawrence Erlbaum.

Main, M., & Weston, D. (1981). The quality of the toddler's relationship to mother and to father related to conflict behavior and the readiness to establish new relationships. *Child Development, 52*, 932–940.

Nelson, K. (1992). Emergence of autobiographical memory at age 4. *Human Development, 35*, 172–177.

Nelson, K. (1996). *Language in cognitive development: The emergence of the mediated mind.* New York: Cambridge University Press.

Nelson, K., & Fivush, R. (2004). The emergence of autobiographical memory: A social cultural developmental theory. *Psychological Review, 111*(2), 486–511.

Oppenheim, D., Emde, R., & Warren, S. (1997). Children's narrative representations of mothers: their development and associations with child and mother adaptation. *Child Development, 68*(1), 127–138.

Peterson, A., Jesso, B. & McCabe, A. (1999). Encouraging narratives in preschoolers: An intervention study. *Journal of Child Language, 26*, 49–67.

Peterson, C., & Mc Cabe, A. (1983). *Developmental psycholinguistic: three ways of looking at a child's narrative.* New York: Plenum Press.

Reese, E., & Farrant, K. (2003). Social origins of reminiscing. In R. Fivush, & C. Haden (Eds.), *Autobiographical memory and the construction of a narrative self* (pp. 29–48). Mahwah, NJ: Lawrence Erlbaum.

Ricoeur, P. (1990). *Soi-même comme un autre [Oneself as another].* Paris: Seuil.

Sameroff, A. J., & Fiese, B. H. (1999). Narrative connections in the family context: Summary and conclusions. In B. H. Fiese, A. J. Sameroff, H. D. Grotevant, F. S. Wamboldt, S. Dickstein, & D. Lewis-Fravel (Eds), The stories that families tell: Narrative coherence, narrative interaction, and relationship beliefs (pp. 105–123). *Monographs of the Society for Research in Child Development, 64* (2, Serial No. 257).

Stern, D. N. (1985). *The interpersonal world of the infant*. New York: Basic Books.

Stern, D. N. (1994). One way to build a clinically relevant baby. *Infant Mental Health Journal, 15*(1), 9–25.

Watson, R. (1989). Monologue, dialogue and regulation. In K. Nelson (Ed.), *Narratives from the crib* (pp. 263–283). Cambridge, MA: Harvard University Press.

Widdershoven, G. (1993). The story of life. In: R. Josselson, & A. Lieblich (Eds.), *The narrative study of lives* (1–20). London: Sage.

CHAPTER 8

NARRATION BETWEEN LOGOS AND PATHOS. THE ROLE OF STORY-TELLING IN CLINICAL PSYCHOLOGY

Maria Francesca Freda

Although narration has always been specific to psychological research and intervention, it is only in the last two decades that the narrative method has taken on an explicit, relevant identity, putting forward a conceptual and methodological alternative which, despite obvious differences, has appeared as a "turning point" in several areas of the discipline (Bruner, 1990; Geertz, 1983; Shafer, 1983). This turning point became apparent in the different fields of psychology around the 1980s, with the publication of some volumes which would later become fundamental for the discipline, assuming and proposing that people construct and communicate their experiences through story-telling[1]. To psychology, the narrative turn meant an important link with other disciplines such as anthropology, linguistics, hermeneutics, and semiotics. At the same time, interest in story-telling has generated meaningful exchanges between and among different areas of the disciplines sharing a common interest in understanding the processes that

Cultural Psychology and Psychoanalysis: Pathways to Synthesis, pp. 205–223

enable people to construct meanings around their lives and experiences and to construct an order where, instead, countless possible orders reign.

This paper stems from a socioconstructivist epistemological paradigm that empathises the categorial and semiotic value of the mind as well as the symbolic processes of reality construction which the actors of the social relation perform intersubjectively.

Based on this perspective, the paper explores the construct of narrative thought as the link between the conscious and unconscious, operative and affective functioning of the mind. Starting from this hypothesis, the paper investigates the construct of narration as a symbolic process—the output of narrative thought—placed midway between the affective symbolisations produced by the unconscious dimension of the mind and the operative categories produced by rational and scientific thought.

The analysis is carried out by working on the comparison/integration of models of cultural psychology and psychodynamics. The paper and its focus on the device of narration are based on the idea that a comparison between socioconstructivism and psychodynamics could translate into an increased understanding of the symbolic dynamics of meaning making and thus of the links that are established between subjectivity, cultural models and cultural practices and of the symbolic models which may aid their transformation. I also believe that, in carrying out this comparison, the contribution of semiotics—viewed as a new cross-disciplinary science of sense-making processes, which considers narration as one of the ways through which a sense is given to the world—can constitute a major broadening for psychology and in particular for the connection between meaning making processes and intervention in clinical psychological counselling.[2]

Traditionally, two of the main perspectives in contemporary psychology—cognitivism with its social and cultural evolutions, and psychodynamics—distinguish the functioning of the mind in accordance to a binary logic. From the perspective of Bruner (1986, 1990) the unfolding of the mind and its functions is based on opposition and on the possible integrations[3] of two logics—one being based on classification and division, which is peculiar to scientific and rational thought, the other on analogy and configuration, which is peculiar to narrative thought and discourse (Smorti, 1994). Following Freud's fundamental contribution, in the psychodynamic framework the unfolding of the mind and its functions relies on the opposition of conscious thought, which is *secondary*, and on an unconscious functioning, which is *primary* and is based on drives and emotions. This paper stems from the hypothesis whereby a single conception of the processes of meaning making is possible within a socioconstructivist paradigm and when a semiotic perspective of the mind and of psycho-social phenomena is adopted. It is a model for meaning making which comprises unconscious emotional processes, cultural processes (often implicit) and processes of rational thought, through a process which is at the same time hierarchical and circular (Freda, 2008a, 2008b; Salvatore, 2004). In this specific field culture and narration are not viewed only as an alternative configuration to the more differentiating processes of logical and scientific thought: culture and narration, instead, qualify as emerging functions mediating between the mind's conscious and unconscious mode of functioning (Freda, 2008a, 2008b). Narration stands midway between the two, and it is this very position that gives it a significant role both in research and in the interventions of clinical psychology. It is an exploration of the narrative process which is not in opposition with the notion of "narrative thought" theorised by Bruner (1986, 1990), but rather contains it and leads narrative thought towards further outcomes. These outcomes are born out of a definition of narrative thought which is not only based on its comparison with logical scientific thought, but also with the mind's unconscious way of functioning—a process whereby we may assume the existence, for narrative thought, of a midway space between these two dimensions of the mind. This space appears to be particularly relevant, as we shall see, to counselling, as a bridge in a clinical dialogue aiming at the recognition of meanings while setting the conditions for their transformation.

Numerous studies and research works have been carried out concerning the hypothesis of an emotional root for narrative processes starting, of course, from Freud's works (1914/1958, 1918/1955, 1937/1964), as well as later Anzieu (1977)—who sees the narrative style as a fundamental defensive function of the mind and plot as a transposition of unconscious fantasies—and by Bucci's current studies (Bucci, 1997)—which aim at finding hints of the nonverbal unconscious processing modules of the relational experience that work simultaneously with conscious experience. An in-depth analysis of all these interesting theoretical contributions is beyond the scope of this paper, which however does follow the traces of a link between narration and the unconscious, starting from a semiotic approach to psycho-social processes in which narration could be thought of as a symbolic process bridging the unconscious and conscious on the one hand and the individual and the context on the other.

I believe this hypothesis of narrative thought and narrative as the link between emotion and the operative, rational categorial processes of reality construction is of particular interest in its ties with a socioconstructivist paradigm (Freda, 2008a, 2008b).

KNOWLEDGE BETWEEN LOGOS AND PATHOS

The thesis I am going to discuss is a cautious attempt to move towards a single conception of meaning making processes (Freda, 2008b; Salvatore et al., 2003; Salvatore, 2004; Salvatore, Tebaldi & Potì, 2009) built on a *process and semiotics-based interpretation* of the mind, linked to the recognition of the *intersubjective nature* of meaning making through which people define the world, the self and the social relationship.

This thesis stems from several areas of study within psychology aiming at combining emotion and thought in the processes of knowledge construction and thus aiming at processing and re-connecting the separation between the affective and cognitive processes, which are traditionally viewed as acting for feeling, thinking and knowing respectively. It is a task that since the 1990s has been undertaken by researchers studying emotion both in the cognitive framework and in the clinical and psychodynamic ones—a task designed to identify cognitive dimensions in emotion and emotional dimensions in thought, thus integrating the role of emotions and cognitions into the process of knowledge construction.[4] In this perspective, emotion is not seen as an antagonist of thought, but rather its basis, a primitive process of knowledge and orientation to action which lays the foundations of the differentiating and organising function of thought.

Another consideration which justifies a single conception of signification processes is the more and more widespread general reference to the concept of the unconscious in the same areas of psychological sciences. In his theory of social representations, Moscovici ultimately ascribes to the unconscious a transversal role in knowledge processes as well as a major regulating function in social processes (Moscovici, 1993). While these ideas allow us to draw lines which cut across the different perspectives of knowledge processes, on the other hand, they should serve as a pretext for the distinctions without which no integration would ever be possible.

The evolution of a semiotic and intersubjective conception of mental processes—in the field of both cultural psychology and psychodynamics—enables us to cautiously explore their possible integration. We can refer to the works of Geertz (1983), the transformations in Bruner's thought (1990) and, in the psychodynamic domain, to the concept of bi-logic put forward by Matte Blanco (1975, 1988), to the unconscious as the central element of symbolisation proposed by Fornari (1976), and his idea of the fundamental role of the processes of affective symbolisation in the construction of reality (see also in this volume, Salvatore & Zittoun, 2011). Albeit from different perspectives, all these scholars share a wish to contribute to the complex relationship between emotions, subjective experience and construction of reality.

The construction of knowledge, and the possibilities of processing experience, growth and learning, are not due to the functioning of the rational, conscious part of the mind only. According to Matte Blanco, knowledge cannot be founded on the functioning of one logic, but it is bi-modal in its very essence. Matte Blanco's significant and still original contribution lies in his reinterpretation of the conscious–unconscious distinction in terms of logical differences in the mind's functioning modes which, despite being diametrically opposed, still coexist. The mind's conscious way of functioning is asymmetric and separative: each category is build in terms of similitudes and differences, the principle of noncontradiction is respected, and each relation is different from its opposite. The mind's unconscious way of functioning is symmetrical and generalising: each category is build in terms of an identity between the part and the whole, the principle of noncontradiction is not respected, relations are symmetrical, each relation is identical to its opposite, and the categories of space and time disappear. The symmetrical and generalising logic of the unconscious homogenises what the conscious logic differentiates and puts in relation (Salvatore & Zittoun, 2011). Even if the two ways of functioning of the mind are untranslatable into each other, the mind's processes are always characterised by their constant interweaving—and such processes can be distinguished from each other by their different degrees of symmetry and asymmetry.

Thought for Matte Blanco serves to translate-unfold the symmetrical-unconscious being into an asymmetrical-conscious being. This entails a simultaneous, continuous presence of both modes of interaction with the object and reality, in thinking and in any other knowledge process (Oneroso, 2004). Emotion, viewed as the "mother of thinking" (Matte Blanco, 1975), thus becomes the foundation of mental life and of the symbolising function, seen as a prepositional function establishing links and relations.

In this chapter, the epistemological reflection leads us to identify a line that separates and joins one way of experiencing and of feeling the experience and another way that tries to tell and represent it.

In view of the above, it can be underlined that while emotionality does not destroy the constructed links of rational thought, it differs from it in that it refers to its object as a single whole, generating confusion between inner and external reality, whereas intellective thought always refers to a part, and from that point of view it establishes relations.

According to Moscovici (1993), too, nonconscious thought processes are not due to a limit of the human mind, to an uncontrollable automatism, but are determined by the mind's referring to underlying systems of representation. As stated by Moscovici, we are not unaware of something by default—that is because we have limited introspection abilities—but rather by excess, because we cannot resist the tendency to project our common, implicit convictions onto the object of reality. Following this perspective, at the time of knowing it is not possible to "wipe the slate clean," that is excluding all subjective interpretations alongside the shared beliefs reified in the community. Based on this assumption, implicit knowledge and even prejudice cannot be seen in negative terms alone, but must be enhanced as starting points for the effort of interpreting reality. This is an effort of the mind, which can get to know the object in its otherness precisely because of its ability to recognise its categories—implicit, but above all emotional—and to become aware of them.

The idea I am outlining certainly does not mean identifying the implicit with the unconscious; however, exploring it can help to identify different levels of meaning making and the role that emotions, implicit processes and thought play in them. One may hypothesise a pathway that, starting from the mind's unconscious functioning, moves towards a differentiation of emotions and feelings, and then towards the differentiation of shared implicit thoughts, until we reach conscious and rational thoughts. Indeed, despite their differences, both implicit and unconscious processes underlie the possibility of knowing and recognising the environment on the one hand, and they underlie the processes of repetition and of fixedness of meanings, discourses and actions on the other (see also in this volume, Cabell & Valsiner, 2011).

In this sense, the symbolic process can be treated as mental mode of working that acts as a *trait d'union*, making it possible to plunge into the unconscious dimension of the mind without losing oneself in it.

This logic[5] helps us unfold the process of conscience construction as a process that, from the polysemy of the infinitising emotional experience, progresses towards differentiation and thus towards the possibilities of representation, of which linguistic representation is one of the most important.

Although we are imagining the signification process as a flow, it must be stressed that very different logics operate at the various levels and that, in moving from one level to the other, a gap is generated which can never be filled completely; and it is because of this gap that any translation of one level into another has some limits, is confronted with the *incommensurability* of the mind's modes of functioning and carries a share of *incomprehensibility* (Martini, 1998, 2005). In this sense, it is only at the level of the implicit and of the conscience that thoughts can take a narrative form. Yet, in the following paragraphs I will argue that this form is rooted in the mind's emotional and affective modes of functioning.

STORY-TELLING BETWEEN LOGOS AND PATHOS

> One day, Andrea, a child who had always looked normal to me, started arguing with a schoolmate during a game. Andrea confronted his schoolmate with great violence: he threw chairs and desks at him. This violence was expressed also in name-calling and swearwords. At the end of the argument Andrea took off all his clothes and stood there naked. I couldn't do anything, and was in great difficulty. It was only at the end that I managed to calm him down by getting close to him and talking to him in a soft voice. A few days later, talking

> to his mother, I understood: a difficult family situation came out; Andrea was suffering because his dad was in jail.[6]

The excerpt you have just read was a narration. Whether it was a nice one or not, an interesting or a boring one, it doesn't matter. However, there are no doubts it is a narration. What is a narration, then? The first possible answer can be found in the sequence of words opening the tale: *one day*. Not all stories start this way, of course, but it is as if they did: saying *one day* is fundamental, as it means to establish some *distance* from the experience, without which no story can be told. Telling means opening up a world to representation; real or made up things can be represented, but what really counts is that they are always represented, that is they are not before us like the text or the person who tells them (Jedlowski, 2000; Ricoeur, 1985). When we listen to a story we place ourselves in two parallel worlds at the same time—the physical world in which we listen to or read the story and the possible world in which the story unfolds and to which we are referred: the phrase *one day* is the formula that uncloses this parallel world.

The second function of the incipit *one day* is to define uniqueness. A narration always refers to an event which is connoted as particular and incidental. This feature inevitably marks a difference from scientific discourse, where the events and phenomena are dealt with in general terms.

In this respect, cultural psychology provides a number of interesting contributions which see narration as a daily event, a universal way of constructing and conveying meanings about human events. According to Bruner (1990), human beings organise their experience mainly in the form of tales, stories, myths, and "reasons to do or not to do". In this perspective, the individual gives sense to his or her own field of life representing his or her experience in a narrative form, telling socially shareable stories about it. Bruner (1990), following Burke's (1945) dramatic pentad, highlights some fundamental elements to delineate a canonical structure of the narrative text that distinguishes it from other kinds of texts: *agents, actions, scene, aim and instruments*. These elements are organised in a text that we can define as narrative if the agents have aims and act on the violation, whatever the causes, of an initial state, moving towards a final state.

As can be observed, not all individual's experiences are followed by a tale that tries to attach a meaning to them: the individual generally experiences the canonical meaning emerging during the experiences as being appropriate and satisfying. There are, however, cases in which some incongruities appear between an action and its goal or between an action and its context, which prevent an automatic access to the meaning of what has been experienced and open up to the construction of narrative texts. These second-level texts take on the formal structure of a story and their function is to construct a meaning of the experience.

The relationship between the story-teller and the story, between mind and text, always takes shape within relational and social practices. In other words, story-telling is a social process bound to a context, or better to two significant contextual references: (a) a context viewed as the cultural code giving rise to the single narrations, which is modified by the presence of these narrations (Sarbin, 1997); a narration may be innovative or even devastating with respect to cultural codes, but can never be independent from them; (b) a local context, viewed as the contingent cultural model of the relationship between the norm and the exception, closely linked to the specific social position of the narrator and of his or her listener; the reasons for telling originate from a search for sense once the canonical systems of meaning attribution have failed locally.

The link between narration and cognitive processes is evident in the very etymology of the word: the verb is believed to derive from *gnarare*, *gnarus*, from a root *gna* which means *to know, to make known*. The root *gnarus*, *He who knows in a particular way*, entails a reference to the process of knowledge acquisition, but also to a specific process of knowledge organisation (Bruner, 2002). The epistemic function of narration is not considered only as a way of representing or corresponding to existing meanings, but rather as a way of constructing and bringing original meanings to our attention (Bruner, 2002; Polkinghorne, 1988). Bruner talks about *narrative urgency* as the way that humans have to construct models on the world, to come to terms with unforeseen events and their consequences. Telling a story equals seeing the world as it is embodied in the story (Bruner, 2002). The story is a social process of meaning making because the narrator does not confine him/herself to interpreting some events, to providing an acceptable translation of these, but organises them in a configuration of sense, in a specific structure which is typical of narrative thought. In this respect, narration appears as a space in which, in specific situations, it is possible to overcome the boundaries of the familiar in favour of the unusual and the unknown.

Narration thus produces a particular type of text in which the relationship between sense and reference is never one-way: the narrative text is polysemous in itself; it aims at triggering and guiding a search for meanings within a spectrum of possible meanings. As sustained by Bruner (1986) narration is telling reality in the subjunctive mode. Due to its use of an evocative language which in no way leads to clear and univocal references, narration (and the narrative thought that supports it) can be interpreted and dealt with as the space between the factual and emotional dimensions of experience.

The concept of *referential opacity* (Bruner, 1986) points to a suspension of the value of the external reality, a condition of flexibility between links that is based on a contamination between the narrator's inner world and the outer world, opening up to another fundamental function of the narrative process which concerns the link between thought and emotions. If, as I have shown, cultural psychology interprets story-telling as a product of narrative thought considered in its opposition with logical-scientific thought, psychodynamics considers narration as a process of putting into words, as the organisation of an analogical meaning which is generated starting from an identity defined by the mind being unconscious and affective. Story-telling envisages a two-fold functioning of the mind—affective and operative; these two aspects of the mind do not work alongside one another, but as complementary components in the construction of the narrative text.

Having a function of conveyance, the story behaves as a figure of speech, namely allegory,[7] and thus produces an additional sense for the understanding of the experience. According to Matte Blanco (1988) allegory offers an additional sense because it is a figure through which a circle of progressive symmetrisations and generalisations is accomplished (Matte Blanco, 1988; Milanese, 1999).

The term allegory derives from Greek *allēgoria*, made up of *allos* meaning *other, different* and *agoèuein*, meaning *to speak*, hence to speak of something else. This *other* may be considered as something hidden which the text symbolically refers to, but it may equally be meant as to speak in a different way, to speak another code which goes through the declarative code, underlies it and contributes to giving rise to its transformations. Dealing with narration in allegorical and metaphorical terms thus means treating the story in symbolical terms, as a transportation and transition process between different ways of functioning of the mind.

In Matte Blanco's view, metaphor is an act of novelty which is at the same time the invention and discovery of emotional categories: in the metaphor thought goes through a symmetrical logic to which it confers an asymmetrical sense, and in this passage it takes on a responsibility of meaning. In accordance with Jakobson (1956/1971) the metaphor is a figure of speech that offers, on the level of text structure, the logic of the unconscious founded on shift and condensation. Similarly, Ricoeur (1985) describes figurative speech as one which leads us to think of something based on a principle of similarity: what is felt as identical at the level of the logic of the unconscious is transformed by metaphor into a similarity through an iconic mode of meaning.

The processes of narrative construction are very similar to those occurring in the rules for the transformation of dream: events which are simply juxtaposed in space are connected by a logical link and events occurring one after the other are connected by a link of consistency. *Narrative transformation* (Corrao, 1991) creates a version of experience which has no connection with the experienced events, but shows a few invariants with respect to them.

In order to understand the emotional dynamics and mental operations that underlie the construction of a narrative text,[8] the theory of thinking put forward by Bion (1962, 1963, 1965) and its development following the model of "transformations" borrowed from mathematics is illuminating (Barbieri, 2007).[9] According to Bion's theory of thinking the first mental activity in the relation with reality concerns the generation of proto-sensory and proto-emotional conditions; these conditions can be metabolised and transformed by a mind which, by exercising the *alpha function*, works in configurations of sense called emotional pictographs and/or alpha elements. In the very early stages of development, as well as later in analytical experience, this transformation process is carried out with the aid of another mind which, by constantly repeating this conjoined operation, does not only transform proto-mental chaos into meaningful configurations but it also transmits the method and thus conveys thoughts together with an apparatus to think them (Bion, 1962, 1963, 1965). Alpha elements are not yet fully formed thoughts, but are used in dreams, memories and in waking dream thinking, and make up the first step towards the formation of a thought. *Pictographs*, the first product of the alpha function, are meaningful emotional configurations (Bion, 1962) which can be arranged in sequences and give life to fragments of text that we may call narrative derivatives (Ferro, 1996, 1999, 2007). Each pictograph is then arranged in a sequence with others: this sequence is not unconscious in its very essence and can only be known based on how it takes shape in the narrative derivative. These are narrative segments, with variable internal consistency and of different size, which make the emotions preceding the alpha elements thinkable by giving them a verbal expression. When we refer to a longer narrative production, we are necessarily referring to a discourse production which has undergone an additional transformation, in which more conscious modes of functioning of the mind play a significant role. Barbieri (2007) suggests that the narrative text is a further transformation of the pictograph, entaing a further change of form both in terms of a greater cohesion and consistency and of greater consciousness. Of course, once it has been included in a text the narrative derivative is no longer a fragment and becomes part of a cohesive and consistent whole. While in its relationship with reality it acts as "content," in its relationship with emotions it acts as a "container." While, following Ferro, the pictograph-narrative derivative relationship is a poem–prose relationship, the relationship between narrative derivative and narrative text is a work of signification which functions in terms of a container–content relationship and in terms of a relationship between disaggregated, still potential emotional states and clearly defined, accomplished states of mind. The narrative process helps the emotional states to play in a configuration that contains them and gives them meaning. In this sense, narration is not only a product of the mind, a product of the transformation of emotions and of perceptions into thought; it is also an apparatus of the mind, a mode of thinking emotions and thoughts.

By working as a container the narrative process enables the emotional contents to come on the scene within a texture that contains them and helps to give them a sense.

This process gradually transforms the identity on which the original relationship with reality is founded into equivalences: a linking process that acts by analogies and constructs configurations with an inner consistency. The persistence of invariants makes recognition possible, even though the narrative elements can be subject to shifts in both time and space. In this sense, narration can be considered an experience-transforming process which can contain and develop other types of transformation: as a *rigid motion transformation,*[10] story-telling brings the narrator's past experiences, feelings and ideas of life into the story by means of equivalence processes, hence today's story-telling makes past experiences and narrations current again; as process of *projective transformation,*[11] story-telling treats the story as the container of a number of projections of the author (Barbieri, 2007), who fills the narrative space with a multitude of fragments of its own inner world which are often so well disguised as to be unrecognisable. Being a process of narrative transformation, story-telling contains experience, processes it and produces connections.

The term *transitional* may be borrowed from Winnicott (1953) to assume that narration constitutes an intermediate area of experience including both inner and outer reality, where the conscious codes working for a consistent, articulated and differentiating organisation of experience live side by side with unconscious codes aiming at an affective assimilation of experience.[12] Besides, the subject—the story-teller in our case—is embodied in an affective role and from this perspective s/he organises a two-way affective relationship with his/her task and his/her interlocutor. The story-teller is a subject interacting with an interlocutor and a task. In this perspective, the construction of a narrative text is a task whereby the story-teller symbolises him/herself and establishes a two-way affective relationship with his/her interlocutor through the text.

The role of narration in the social relationship thus becomes a discourse process for the construction of meanings by which people bring order to disorder, combine emotion and thought, construct the relation and exchange the sense of their experience.

LISTENING, UNDERSTANDING AND TRANSFORMING NARRATIONS

If we move away from the theories on the way the mind functions and towards the professional field of action of clinical psychologists, what I have so far said about the transitional function of narration opens up further possible outcomes. These outcomes are closely linked to some particular methodologies concerning the use of narration as a device in clinical counselling (Freda, 2008a, 2008b; Mc Leod, 2006).

In this field, the interest in the semiotic device of narration as constructing the meaning of experience can be extended to the comprehension of those processes which support a transformation of meanings and the construction of original resources of sense[13] in the clinical psychologist–client relationship (Freda, 2008b).

As early as 1955, Walter Benjamin stressed the practical purpose of narration, whereby every story has either an implicit or explicit useful implication; every story is a source of advice for both the narrator and the listener. By "advice" the author did not mean an exhaustive answer to a question, but a hint to continue the story which supports the narrator in drawing what s/he tells from his/her own experience and in transforming it into an experience to share with the listener.

This means questioning common sense in order to offer some freedom in the rigid, repetitive categorisation of the meaning of experience, to discuss the implicit bond that is generated in any narration between the interpretation of the norm and the interpretation of its violation and enable the teller to regain the categorical criteria supporting his/her own construction of experience. The clinical relationship does not limit itself to recognising a sense, but uses it to construct new worlds of sense which the client may inhabit (Martini, 1998).

Let us consider, for example, the relationship between a clinical psychologist engaged in an activity of counselling with a client who is, in turn, engaged in the management of a personal problematic situation: in this relationship it will be necessary to promote functions to accept narrations, to understand them and to transform meanings, first of all in terms of a greater awareness and then of a greater ability on the part of the client to generate meanings able to support the effectiveness of his/her actions; the possibility for someone to open up to advice consists in the extent to which s/he is able to let the situation speak up; in other words, in order for someone to receive advice s/he must be able to tell the story. Exactly because they are sense-making processes, narrations can be open, at the service of what is new and original as a creative process of pursuit of meaning or they can be closed, at the service of what is known, presenting themselves as stories already told, ready configurations of sense available for coping with the unknown and the unpredictable. In the latter situations story-telling can act as a sense-making process attempting to reestablish a frail *status quo* or one that is perceived as lost; it can come up as a process connecting sense-making and experience in a defensive way. Although it appears as a symbolic process that can support a signification of experience, story-telling alone cannot support reflective processes and promote innovative sense resources which may help the subject to define and pursue his/her goals. So, if narration constitutes an early transformation of experience, which places it in a configuration of meaning and sets up connections between its parts, a narrative device in a setting of intervention becomes a method of reflecting on the narrative experience, with the aim of recognising and thinking of those symbolic processes which underlie the construction of the text in the relationship with the psychologist. This is a place where narrative thinking can be explored as a sense-making process, integrating emotional and operative categories, but also its inappropriateness, its failures to construct sense resources that can be used to support an effective transformative intervention.

The action of the one who, in a dialogue, listens to narrations with the intention of accepting, understanding and promoting transformation, cannot be seen as a process of unveiling meanings, but rather as a participation in a process of co-construction of sense (Sarbin, 1997). The listener is the one who contributes to the text's meaning by interpreting what is written between the lines; in this sense, every text is an intersubjective construction which takes shape on the collaboration with an interlocutor.

To understand narrations and to transform them means exploring different hermeneutical frames by performing functions of *semiotic connection*. By *semiotic connection* I mean the processes for the construction of links which may support sense-making and re-sense-making processes as well as connect the text to the dimensions of the field that has generated it.

The process of *semiotic connection* moves between different levels and planes of discourse and brings the text-generating process down to the emotional, intersubjective, and cultural processes on which it is based (Freda, 2004, 2008a, 2008b).

When moving from one connecting function to another, we may proceed from a process of construction and analysis of the *meanings* of narration towards a process of analysis and construction of the *sense* of narrating. While the meaning of a narration can be traced in its semantic content and in the specific structure that the narrative plot gives to this content, sense—namely the sense of narration—is related to the value narrative meaning takes on in the specific contingency of the discourse exchange conveyed by narration (Freda, 2008a, 2008b; Salvatore, Tebaldi, & Potì, 2009). In other words, what is the sense of the action of narrating one particular story in the *hic et nunc* of a particular relationship? Sense is related to the relationship and may only be understood by assuming narration as the criterion for the construction of a discourse context, narration as a function addressing a relationship. The client through his narration contributes to the construction of a relationship where some answers from the psychologist become more probable than others. In the search for the sense of the narration everything that the client is narrating of his experience must be connected to what the client is asking in the present within the relationship with the psychologist. Hence there is no story-telling produced in the intervention that is unrelated to the narrator–listener relational context.

Adopting a narrative device in the setting of psychological counselling sets up a context in which it is possible to proceed through a *transitional theory of knowledge* (Corrao, 1990/1998) that lies in an area between inner objects and objects of reality. In the intervention process this area is maintained through the continuous unfolding of the narrative discourse and of its constant shifting between opening and closing phases of the meaning.

In the circuit involving emotion and construction of the narrative discourse the psychologist can intervene through processes of semiotic connection. To perform this processes of semiotic connection in the relation between the psychologist and its client means suspending the automatic acting out of affective symbolisation in the narrative discourse, so to enable an acceptance, a recognition of emotions and—starting from them—an exploration of the experience and the relationship.

The implementation of semiotic connection along the different lines and planes of the narrative text calls for a greater number of criteria to interpret experience and gradually supports the development of an awareness of sense. The transformative value of a narrative trail does not lie in the extent to which it responds to the characteristics of the past experience narrated or in its effectiveness in transforming the narrator's inner world into dynamic words. The transformative capacity of a narrative trail lies instead in the ability of the narrator–listener relation to process it and to start from it so as to keep transforming the sense of experience in narrative terms.

From Ferro's latest work (2007) I would like to borrow the interesting idea of clinical work seen as a shift between the exercise of negative abilities—the expression successfully coined by Bion (1962) to refer to the ability of lingering in doubt, the ability not to know and wait for a sense to develop gradually—and the exercise of an option, *the chosen fact* (Bion, 1962), which leads to the selection of one trail around which to construct a particular form whereby we will eventually make one choice and ignore all the other possibilities. Adopting a narrative device in the intervention setting promotes a constant shift between "*transformative narrations*," which the author considers as the process by which narration supports the processing of the meaning of experience, and "*narrative transformations*" (Corrao, 1991), seen as the work on narrations that makes their expansion and transformation possible. It is through this swinging between the organisation of a narration-induced sense and its opening towards original configurations that a narrative device promotes, first of all, the possibility of recognising and sharing in the actors' point of view and, secondly, a process transforming the sense of experience. Above all, however, it promotes the ability to think of the shared experience in a transformative manner by connecting and integrating processes of affective symbolisation with processes of operative symbolisation.

In conclusion, if we look at narrations as a transformation of experiences (Bion, 1965; Corrao, 1991) in its bi-logic connotation (Matte Blanco, 1975, 1988) then we may try to capture the emotional sense at the basis of its cultural and communicative value. The act of narrating is not only invention and discovery of something in the world, but also transformation of the emotional matrix of meaning in a thinkable and recognisable configuration of sense. To consider narration as an analogical process of transition between codes, as a bridge between *logos* and *pathos*, I think will open new horizons of research and clinical practice, because it lets us see unfolding on a continuum methods of interpretation of meanings and of texts that were previously treated as conflictual, thus closing a dialogue between different domains of psychology. A dialogue that this book wants to start anew.

NOTES

1. Among these publications were *Narrative Psychology: the storied nature of human* edited by Theodore Sarbin (1986) which developed the idea of narrative as an alternative root metaphor to psychology; *Acts of meaning* by Jerome Bruner (1990) in which he suggested that narrative represents a fundamental "way of Knowing." Around the same time, leading figures in the clinical and psychodynamic field began to explore ways in which narrative concepts might be applied within therapy (Corrao, 1991; Ferro, 1999; Luborsky & Christ-Christoph, 1990; Polkingorne, 1988, Schafer, 1983; Spence, 1982).
2. Intervention in clinical psychology is always a mainly relational process, performed in a context to address specific demands. Clinical work, through the coding and re-coding of the relationship, identifies methods of construction, functions, illusory, defensive and innovative aspects. Clinical work tries to give a meaning to the client's request to relate to the psychologist so as to understand its complexity and support its evolution. It's a relational process through which those who make the demand receive back the meaning of their interactions and behaviours (Carli & Paniccia, 2003; see also in this volume Carli & Giovagnoli, 2011).
3. Bruner in later works (2002) distanced himself from the rigid opposition and comparison of these two modes of thought.
4. In this framework, there are also some conceptions that give emotion the fundamental role of primary judgement (Solomon, 1980). In this respect, there is interesting research in support of idea of an emotional activation of cognition: in one of these works, Murphy and Zajonc (1993) use the

priming technique and show that the emotional processing of the stimulus precedes and informs cognitive processing: "preferences do no require inferences."

5. Matte Blanco's theory (1975) shows significant ties with Parmenides' and Zeno's thought and, as the author himself said, on the way to Heraclitus.
6. The story was told by a nursery school teacher during a counselling group aimed at working with children at risk.
7. Allegory is a metaphor extended to the text.
8. In this paper the word "text" is not used to refer to a piece of writing in the common sense but in a semiotic logic where the term "text" is used to refer to a unit of meaning which is expressive, restricted and structured.
9. Links between Bion's theoretical model and a hermeneutical and narratological vision have already been highlighted and developed in Italy, in interesting works by F. Corrao (1987/1998, 1991) and more recently by A. Ferro (1999, 2007), with special focus on the processes leading to the construction of the analysis room setting (Ferro, 1996), and by Arrigoni and Barbieri, who have studied the ties between text construction processes and the unconscious, in and out of the analysis room (Arrigoni & Barbieri 1998; Barbieri, 2007).
10. Rigid motion transformations, typical of a non psychotic functioning of the personality, imply a low deformation and a movement of ideas and sentiments from one sphere of application to another (Bion, 1965).
11. Projective transformations, typical of the most primitive part of the mind, are related to splitting and projective processes and imply an elevated level of confusion and deformation (Bion, 1965).
12. A significant reference to the study of tertiary processes in a psychodynamic perspective is constituted by Green's contributions (Green, 1973), whereby tertiary processes are processes which intervene in the relationship between primary and secondary processes, and Kaes's studies (Kaes, 1994), whereby myth, utopia and ideology result from the functioning of collective psychic systems that enable us to understand the functioning of organised groups and institutions.
13. A resource of sense can be defined as a new configuration of meaning, elaborated in a relationship, which in a specific moment enables the construction of a unifying coherence that takes the subjects away from chaos and opens up degree of freedom in the logic that dominates and directs their actions.

REFERENCES

Anzieu, D. (1977). Les traces du corps dans l'écriture: une ètude psychanalytique du style narratif. [Body's traces in the writing. A psychoanalytic study of the narrative style]. In D. Anzieu, & A Anzieu (Eds.), *Psychanalyse et language. Du corps à la parole* (pp. 23–34). Paris: Dunod.

Arrigoni, M. P., & Barbieri, G. L. (1998). *Narrazione e psicoanalisi. Un approccio semiologico. [Narration and psychoanalysis. A semiological approach]*. Milano: Raffaello Cortina Editore.

Barbieri, G. L. (2007). *Tra testo e inconscio. [Between text and unconscious]*. Milano: Franco Angeli.

Benjamin, W. (1955). *Schriften [Works]*. Frankfurt: Suhrkamp Verlag.

Bion, W. R. (1962). *Learning from experience*. London: William Heinemann.

Bion, W. R. (1963). *Elements of psychoanalysis*. London: William Heinemann.

Bion, W. R. (1965). *Trasformation*. London: William Heinemann.

Bruner, J. (1986). *Actual minds, possible worlds*. Cambridge, MA: Harvard University Press.

Bruner, J. (1990). *Acts of meaning*. Cambridge MA: Harvard University Press.

Bruner, J. (2002). *Making stories: law, literature, life*. Cambridge MA: Harvard University Press.

Bucci, W. (1997). *Psychoanalysis and cognitive science*. New York: Guilford Press.

Burke, K. (1945). *A grammar of motives*. Berkeley, CA: University of California.

Cabell K., & Valsiner, J. (2011). Affective hypergeneralization: Learning from psychoanalysis. In S. Salvatore, & T. Zittoun (Eds.), *Cultural psychology and psychoanalysis. Pathways to synthesis* (pp. 87–113). Charlotte NC: Info Age Publishing.

Carli, R. & Giovagnoli, F. (2011). A cultural approach to Clinical psychology. Psychoanalysis and analysis of the demand. In S. Salvatore, & T. Zittoun (Eds.), *Cultural psychology and psychoanalysis. Pathways to synthesis* (pp. 117–150). Charlotte NC: Info Age Publishing.

Carli, R., Paniccia, R. M. (2003). *L'analisi della domanda. [Analysis of Demand]*. Bologna: Il Mulino.

Corrao, F. (1991). Trasformazioni narrative. [Narrative transformations]. In M. Ammaniti, & D. N. Stern (Eds.), *Rappresentazioni e narrazioni* (pp. 43–52). Bari, ITA: Laterza.

Corrao, F. (1998). Il narrativo come categoria psicoanalitica [Narrative as psychoanalytic concept]. In F. Corrao, *Orme. Contributi alla Psicoanalisi. Volume primo* (pp. 180–189). Milano: Raffaello Cortina Editore. (First published 1987).

Corrao, F. (1998). Epinoesis [Apperception]. In F. Corrao, *Orme. Contributi alla Psicoanalisi. Volume primo* (pp. 216–223). Milano: Raffaello Cortina Editore. (First published 1990)

Ferro, A. (1996). *Nella stanza di analisi [In the analysis room]*. Milano: Raffaello Cortina Editore.

Ferro, A. (1999). *La psicoanalisi come letteratura e terapia [Psychoanalysis as literature and therapy]*. Milano: Raffaello Cortina Editore.

Ferro, A. (2007). *Evitare le emozioni, vivere le emozioni [To evade emotions, to live emotions]*. Milano: Raffaello Cortina Editore.

Fornari, F. (1976). *Simbolo e codice [Symbol and code]*. Milano: Feltrinelli.

Freda, M. F. (2004). Metodi narrativi e formazione professionale: connettere e contestualizzare [Narrative methods and professional training: To relate and contextualize]. In B. Ligorio (Ed.), *Psicologie e culture. Contesti, Identità ed Interventi* (pp. 263–287). Roma: Edizioni Carlo Amore.

Freda, M. F. (2008a). Understanding narrative role in depicting meaning and clinical intervention. In S. Salvatore, J. Valsiner, S. Strout Yagodzynski, & J. Clegg (Eds.), *YIS Yearbook of Ideografic Scienc* (pp. 81–94). Roma: Firera Publishing Group.

Freda, M. F. (2008b). *Narrazione e Intervento in Psicologia Clinica [Narration and Intervention in Clinical Psychology]*. Napoli, ITA: Liguori.

Freud, S. (1958). Remembering, repeating and working-through (further recommendations on the technique of psycho-analysis II). In J. Strachey (Ed. and Trans.), *The standard edition of the complete psychological works of Sigmund Freud* (Vol. 12, pp. 145–156). London: The Hogarth Press and the Institute of Psycho-analysis. (Original work published 1914).

Freud, S. (1955). From the history of an infantile neurosis. In J. Strachey (Ed. and Trans.), *The standard edition of the complete psychological works of Sigmund Freud* (Vol. 17, pp. 1–124). London: The Hogarth Press and the Institute of Psycho-analysis. (Original work published 1918[1914])

Freud, S. (1964). Constructions in analysis. In J. Strachey (Ed. and Trans.), *The standard edition of the complete psychological works of Sigmund Freud* (Vol. 23, pp. 255–270). London: The Hogarth Press and the Institute of Psycho-analysis. (Original work published 1937)

Geertz, C. (1983). *Local knowledge. Further essay in interpretative anthropology*. New York: Basic Book.

Green, A. (1973). *Le discours vivant [The living discourse]*. Paris: Presses Universitaires de France.

Jakobson, R. (1956/1971). Two aspects of language and two types of aphasic disturbances. In R. Jakobson, & M. Halle (Eds.) (1971), *Fundamentals of Language* (pp. 67–96). Den Haag & Paris: Mouton.

Jedlowski, P. (2000). *Storie comuni. La narrazione nella vita quotidiana [Common stories. Narration in everyday life]*. Pavia: Bruno Mondadori.

Kaes, R. (1994). *La parole et le lien. Processus associatifs dans less groupes [The word and the bond. Associative processes within the groups]*. Paris: Dunod.

Luborsky, L., & Christ-Christroph, P. (1990). *Understanding transference. The CCRT method*. New York: Basic Books.

Martini, G. (1998). *Ermeneutica e narrazione. Un percorso tra psichiatria e psicoanalisi [Hermeneutic and narration. A path between psychiatry and psychoanalysis]*. Torino: Bollati Boringhieri.

Martini, G. (2005). *La sfida dell'irrappresentabile. La prospettiva ermeneutica nella psicoanalisi clinica [The challenge of the unrepresentable. The hermeneutic perspective in clinical psychoanalysis]*. Milano: Franco Angeli.

Matte Blanco, I. (1975). *The unconscious as infinite sets. An essay in bi-logic*. London: Gerald Duckworth and Company.

Matte Blanco, I. (1988). *Thinking, feeling and being*. London: Routledge.

McLeod, J. (2006). Narrative thinking and the emergence of postpsychological therapies. *Narrative Inquiry, 16*(1), 201–210.

Milanese, C. (1999). Antinomie dell'originario [Antinomy of the primeval]. In P. Bria, & F. Oneroso (Eds.), *L'inconscio Antinomico* (pp. 44–53). Milano: Franco Angeli.

Moscovici S. (1993). The return of the unconscious. *Social research, 60,* 39–93.

Murphy, S., & Zajonc, R. B. (1993). Affect, cognition and awareness: Affective priming and optimal and suboptimal stimulus exposure. *Journal of Personality and Social Psychology, 64*, 723–739.

Oneroso, F. (2004). Sistema Bioniano e sistema Matte Blanchiano [The Bion's system and the Matte Blanco's system]. In F. Oneroso, A. Gorrese (Eds.), *Mente e Pensiero. Incontri con l'opera di Wilfred Bion* (pp. 5–44). Napoli, ITA: Liguori.

Polkinghorne, D. E. (1988). *Narrative knowing and human sciences.* Albany, NY: State University of New York Press.

Ricoeur, P. (1985). *Temps et recit. Tome III [Time and narrative. Volume III].* Paris: Editions du Seuil.

Salvatore, S. (2004). Inconscio e discorso. Inconscio come discorso [Unconscious and discourse. Unconscious as discourse]. In B. Ligorio (Ed.), *Psicologie e culture. Contesti, identità e interventi,* (pp. 125–155) Roma: Edizioni Carlo Amore.

Salvatore S., Freda M. F., Ligorio B., Iannaccone A., Rubino, F., Scotto di Carlo, M., ... Gentile, M. (2003). Socioconstructivism and theory of the unconscious. A gaze over a research horizon. *European Journal of School Psychology, 3*, 1, 9–41.

Salvatore, S., Tebaldi, C., & Poti, S. (2009). The discursive dynamic of sensemaking. In S. Salvatore, J. Valsiner, S. Strout, & J. Clegg (Eds.), *YIS: Yearbook of idiographic science 2008* (Vol. 1) (pp. 39–72). Rome: Firera Publishing Group.

Salvatore, S., & Zittoun, T. (2011). Outilines of a psychoanalytically informed cultural psychology. In S. Salvatore, & T. Zittoun (Eds.), *Cultural Psychology and Psychoanalysis. Pathways to Synthesis* (pp. 1–46). Charlotte NC: Info Age Publishing.

Sarbin, T. R. (1997). The poetics of identity. *Theory & Psychology, 7*, 67–82.

Sarbin, T. (Ed.) (1986). *Narrative psychology. The storied nature of human conduct.* New York NY: Praeger.

Shafer, R. (1983). *The analitic attitude*. New York, NY: Basic Books.

Smorti, A. (1994). *Il pensiero narrativo. [Narrative thought].* Firenze: Giunti.

Solomon, R. C. (1980). Emotions and choice (pp. 251–282). In A. O. Rorty (Ed.) *Explaining emotions*. Berkeley, CA: University of California Press.

Spence, D. P. (1982). *Narrative truth and historical truth: Meaning and interpretation in psychoanalysis*. New York: Norton.

Winnicott, D. W. (1953). Transitional objects and transitional phenomena. *International Journal of Psychoanalysis, 34*, 89–97.

CHAPTER 9

PSYCHOLOGICAL NORMALITY, PSYCHOPATHOLOGY AND EVIDENCE-BASED PSYCHOTHERAPY: ARE WE SO SURE *"WE'RE NOT IN KANSAS ANYMORE"*?[1*]

Massimo Grasso and Pietro Stampa

evidence—n. 1. the state of being evident *2.* something that makes another thing evident; sign
evident—adj. [< L. *e-*, from + *videre*, see] easy to see or perceive; clear
Webster's New World Dictionary

INTRODUCTION

An ideological illusion turns up periodically on the scene of the cultural debate, appearing every thirty to fifty years. The last time it took the semantic form of the "neutrality of science," today it is in the guise of its

Cultural Psychology and Psychoanalysis: Pathways to Synthesis, pp. 225–278

"a-theoretical" nature. The scientific-professional community is saturated with a sort of repulsion towards the components and products of nonimmediately quantifiable thought, in favour of an objectivising reductionism that vastly overrates technology, servomechanisms, shortcuts and schematisms. The prevailing tendency is to reduce every continuum and all complexity to simple, discrete elements that can be measured in a linear way. The role of subjectivity in models of representation of reality is drastically cut down—subjectivity becomes "noise," and in order to get rid of it more easily without being forced to recognise it, it is translated into numbers. One imagines observable "facts" beyond all interpretation. This is a remarkable turnaround: it is no longer god that is dead, but Nietzsche.[1]

The illusion changes its name, but it is still the same. A historian of ideas could reconstruct its route from the middle ages to our times: but such an operation of *Begriffgeschichte* is outside our domain and outside the spatial and conceptual limits of this paper—we will therefore confine ourselves to talking about it in terms of current interest, with an occasional flashback to the 1950s-1970s. And we will obviously confine ourselves to the domain of the research and professional practice of clinical psychology and psychotherapy, in which the pervasiveness of the illusion, as if by a "domino effect," brings a certain number of conceptual consequences that constitute a corresponding number of epistemological pitfalls, which give rise to further systematic distortions of reality in the representations of interpersonal relations, and of the mental life of the single subjects involved in the relationships themselves.

This illusion has been the focus of some of our recently published work (Grasso, & Stampa, 2005, 2006, 2007, 2008; Grasso, 2006a) in which we have tried to examine in depth some questions concerning the concepts of health and mental illness and their connection to the diagnostic and therapeutic practice in the psychological and psychiatric domain, issues that will in part recur in this paper.

Let us go over the central issue. Thinking about clinical work in psychology and in particular about the outcomes of the clinical psychology and psychotherapy intervention, and about the dynamics involved in these processes, has in recent years been gaining in importance. But within this thinking the aspect that has been dealt with the least is precisely the one that, more than all the others, could give it meaning: we are referring to its methodological framework.

What indicators do we choose to state that a person marked by emotional suffering, inner discord, poor integration in a network of interpersonal relations—a patient in psychotherapy, for instance— "is better" or even "cured"? Subjective rather than objective indicators? If they are objective or objectivable, can they be made ostensible simply and clearly without losing precious qualitative information?

We are not at all sure that clinical psychology and psychotherapy can tolerate (not "follow" or "respect": literally *tolerate*) the same rules of operation as the natural sciences and as the corresponding practices, led by biology, medicine, pharmaceutical chemistry. But we will also say something about economics and perhaps about symbolic anthropology, linguistics and cultural politics.

As we will try to explain below, we have often found ourselves dealing with positions that have given sustenance to our observations and arguments, at times very critical because of the simplifications and reductionisms they feed on. As in the well-known film The Wizard of Oz[2] we have had the feeling that we have run into many Dorothy Gales, who, having left the mediocre reality of the farm where they live—sepia-coloured in the film—and with their big eyes wide open upon seeing a world suddenly in colour, where everything is big and beautiful, marvellous and amazing, turn to their little dog and say, "*Toto, I've a feeling we're not in Kansas anymore*."

But are we, researchers and professionals in clinical psychology and psychiatry, really sure that we are not in Kansas anymore?

In other words, we felt that research in clinical psychology and psychotherapy has often been fed by facile enthusiasm and dubious excitement about seemingly simple, brilliant solutions to complex problems: but often they are not simple solutions but rather, in our view, simplistic expedients.[3] As in the film promotion, we seem to have heard now and then resounding slogans like "*Mighty Miracle Show of 1000 Delights*" or "*Gaiety! Glory! Glamour!*," just as the belief has been passed on to us by someone that we are unquestionably on the *Yellow Brick Road*, that is, on what we could call the "right"[4] road, with no possible doubts or second thoughts.

We know very well the risk we are running by adopting a critical position (and we will state at the outset that we do not enjoy it), in order to dampen the raptures of the many elated Dorothies encountered, to embrace the viewpoint of the *Wicked Witch of the West*, if only to avoid ending up being melted by a bucket of water on the kitchen floor: but also because, more substantially, our intention is not to smother the yearning for research and for the new and find ourselves trapped in inertia and immobility.[5] Our position is therefore not an easy one and we realise that: however, we do want to point out, if our eyes reveal it, like Andersen's boy ("*but he has nothing on at all*"[6]), the "emperor's possible nudity" and perhaps remember, and remind ourselves, that behind the magnificent wizard of Oz, there may at times be hiding a harmless old man from Omaha, Nebraska.

Before examining our criticisms (constructive, we feel) in detail, we will offer the readers three brief examples of current clinical attitudes.

THREE CLINICAL FRAGMENTS

(1) A patient—a well-educated 50-year-old woman—during a psychotherapy session recounts the following experience.

Her gynaecologist, whom she goes to once a year for routine checkups, after asking her about her emotional state and some aspects of her sex life, expresses the opinion that she is suffering from a mood disorder linked to the menopause, and prescribes an antidepressant.

In the next few days, the patient goes to a physician who has been treating her for a lingering bronchitis. The patient feels well, and says happily that she is cured and has therefore stopped taking the antibiotics. The doctor kindly chides her: it is up to him to say whether or not she is cured! The patient gets undressed, the doctor proceeds with the auscultation using his phonendoscope. He promptly hears that the bronchitis is still active despite the woman's sensation of wellbeing, so she must continue the treatment for a while.

The patient then mentions the gynaecologist's prescription, asking the doctor his opinion. In response, first she gets questions: do you feel sad?—are you drinking too much alcohol?—when you wake up does the day seem to be pressing down on you, loaded with toil and problems?—do you cry often?—do you wake up at night and have trouble falling asleep again?—are you easily irritated?—do you feel a "reduced sex drive"?—do you think of suicide?—,etc. The patient cooperates as well as she can, but she does not answer a lot of the questions with a clear Yes/No, but rather, with "perhaps," "sometimes," "it depends"…

At the end of this examination, the doctor informs the patient that there is depression, but it is not as serious as the gynaecologist thought: he therefore prescribes another "lighter" antidepressant.

The patient comments on the story thus far as follows: "You know doctor, I would not like to take these antidepressants, in part because psychotherapy has got me used to considering my emotions in a more complex and nuanced way than how they can be expressed in schematic questions and answers; and in part because—to tell you the truth—I didn't always answer the doctors truthfully … On certain more intimate subjects I have difficulty talking about myself: in psychotherapy too, at the beginning, it took months and tens of sessions before I found the courage to reveal some of my thoughts and moods.… In short, what was the basis for the two doctors diagnosing depression, serious or not? I didn't let on, but actually I was a little reticent! Depressed? Of course I'm depressed. I already knew that myself!."

(2) A man of about forty comes to a psychological consultation. He has a specialised legal training but works for a public corporation where he carries out routine secretarial work and job placements, which makes him feel deeply angry and humiliated. He presents a major free floating anxiety disorder, which tends to dwell obsessively on properception (he feels a sort of itch in the head; what can it be?—he feels a "weight" on his stomach: is it serious?...)

The patient describes his meeting with a psychiatrist to whom he had initially been referred by the family doctor.

The patient explains in detail (and with some agitation) the variety and intensity of the symptoms: the psychiatrist, who up to now has been listening in silence, gives him a short questionnaire "Not at all/A little/Quite a lot/A lot," with items like: I feel upset, I feel cheerful, I am worried about possible accidents, etc; the patient compiles it carefully.[7]

At this point, the psychiatrist asks him to lie down on the couch and puts electrodes on his fingers, then turns on a device that makes a sound of varying loudness while lights come on; the patient is invited to relax and follow the rhythm of these sensorial stimulations—in short, a biofeedback programme.

The treatment ends after a few minutes: the psychiatrist asks the patient to come back to the desk and asks "How do you feel now?" Reply: "Exactly the same as before." The patient is asked to complete the questionnaire again, and—why doubt it?—the result is identical to the previous time. The psychiatrist then explains that the efficacy of a therapy is measured over time, and offers the patient a "package" of 10 sessions, also telling him the cost (incidentally, quite high). The first session, the demonstration, is free: the patient will only pay for the consultation (an average fee).

The patient leaves the consultation room thinking the psychiatrist must be mad if he expects him to come back, and later—hoping to find a very different welcome—he goes to the psychologist recommended by common friends.

(3) This patient is about forty years old, with a low education level, and is affected by a major disorder in controlling her impulses: she is bulimic, smokes too much, spends too much on useless purchases. She has been in psychotherapy for a while, and one day she tells the psychologist about yet another attempt to give up smoking. After uselessly trying nicotine patches, ear clips, acupuncture, acupressure, pranotherapy, Bach flowers ... she has come to a doctor who practises hypnosis and "guarantees"—as is explained in a brochure scattered around the crowded waiting room—a positive outcome in 85% of the cases (she was told about him by a friend who actually gave up smoking after attending several sessions).

After the introductions and having acknowledged the request to "make her get over the smoking habit" (not to "be helped to give up smoking," notice that the agreement therefore envisages that the result will be completely the responsibility of the doctor) the patient was asked to sit on a chair in front of the desk, and the doctor started talking calmly and evenly. He told her that when he was at primary school he used to go around with another boy who however turned out to be the classic "bad company," a kind of Lucignolo for Pinocchio: so he (the doctor, who now seemed to be at least 70 years old) played truant, did not do his homework, etc. . He realised that this was not the way a good student behaved, though. And so what did he have to do one fine day? He had to stop seeing the bad boy etc.

The patient, at this point, feels sleepy, her eyes close and she can hardly follow the story. The doctor then tells her to "let herself go," to lean back on the chair and not to think of anything. Who knows why (actually, the psychologist listening to the story has an idea, but no matter), at this point, the patient suddenly feels alert and also a little suspicious.... The doctor does not seem to notice and continues talking in a monotone: now he evokes the image of black mud that slowly spreads through the room, reaching the patient's feet, starting to come up, there, it's already at her ankles ...

When the mud reaches her calf, the patient pulls herself up and says words to the effect: "Excuse me doctor, but now I'm completely awake and I'm also a little irritated!," expecting the doctor to reorganise the setting in some way, to calm her down, so the session can continue.

"Madam," replies the doctor sharply, "it is you who is too stiff, too defended. If you do this you will never stop smoking. In these conditions, I cannot do anything," and he interrupts their meeting brusquely (Who's next?...).

The fee for the session, which lasted half an hour: €180, 00. The patient left feeling so angry that she smoked two packets of cigarettes, one after another, that afternoon.

Some Observations

Notice that these short sketches (as they appear both in the sense that the term has in English not only in clinical language, but also in that of variety theatre) present complementary situations.

The first case: the doctor who received the woman after the prescription for antidepressants by the gynaecologist had a totally different attitude in assessing the physical state and the emotional state.

As for the bronchitis—from which the woman "felt" cured, the doctor had no hesitation in relying for the assessment on an objective conceptual and clinical-instrumental system, considering the patient to be an unreliable source; for the assessment of the emotional state, the patient's subjective feelings and experiences suddenly become such a valid source that they even allow the doctor to estimate the "seriousness" of the disorder, which moreover in the patient's mind is not represented in terms of a "pathology" (unlike the breathing problems due to the bronchitis), but in an existential dimension which she is familiar with thanks to the introspective capacity developed and valorised by psychotherapy, endowing her with interpretative categories and models.

Just let us make an incidental observation on a question we will return to later. The "naive" representation that the patient has of her psychopathology (cf. for example, Di Nuovo, 2000) has long become part of the data on which qualitative research in psychotherapy can be based: in spite of this, it is somewhat strange that—both in the anamnesis, and in the diagnosis, and in the assessment of the treatment outcome—what is relied on is the patient's capacity to provide reliable data about herself when she reports her mental life, while it is quite clear to all the doctors that the patient is unreliable when she reports her impressions of her physical state.

Second case: The psychiatrist has found—though with a method that would seem to be verging on the comical, if it were not for the patient's psychic suffering—that the "therapeutic" intervention has produced no change in the mental state of the patient, who reports subjective symptoms that perfectly overlap those he had before having the treatment. But since that treatment is envisaged as being successful in curing those symptoms, its failure, as shown by the patient's words, is not predictive of later therapeutic failure. In this case, therefore, the patient is not considered to be a source of reliable data about himself, because this data does not match what is foreseen by the protocol of treatment.

And on the third case: here too it would be laughable if it were not bordering on extortion. The hypnotist doctor may succeed or fail to induce subjects into a psychophysical state of trance: if he fails, it is their bad luck. Who knows, if he had not ordered the patient to relax (the patient was already more than relaxed, but perhaps he did not notice this), he would have been successful in his intention: but the patient reacted (she detests anyone giving her orders), and the spell was broken. The obligation was to provide the means, not the results: the session must be paid for all the same. (We will return to the ethical aspects of the matter later).

Is there a difference between the approach of the psychiatrist (how can we define it: hyper-behaviourist? quantophrenic?)[8] and that of the hypnotist doctor? The latter was openly lacking in and uninterested in tools of verification, the former used them for false ends: the result is the same—by one and by the other the relationship was not for one moment considered as a factor for knowledge or for treatment at any level. The patients thus found themselves reified, reduced to objects devoid of personality and conscience, while in case (1), as we have already seen, subjectivity was promoted as being irrelevant to single-source diagnostic and prognostic purposes (bronchitis) and perfectly adequate and congruent with information for the same purposes (depression).

TWO MORE CLINICAL FRAGMENTS

So far, we have seen examples in which the physician makes an improper use of the methodological models of his scientific-professional culture to deal with the patients' emotional problems. Let us now see what may happen when a psychologist "imports" these same models and uses them a-critically without being aware of the trap he is getting himself into, and of the malpractice that will inevitably follow sooner or later.

(4) A young woman, intelligent and dynamic, who for her work spends many hours a day at the computer in an open space work area (she works in advertising graphics), presents at the psychology consultation saying she is suffering from an anxiety disorder defined as "a-typical" firstly by the GP and then by a psychologist who had been treating her for over a year, and as "panic attacks" by another she later went to. Tired of not seeing any results, after several months the patient stopped the second psychotherapy, and finally went to a third psychologist recommended by a friend who had been his student at university.

Her "attacks" seem to have the following dynamics. Typically, the frame is the workplace; while she is calmly attending to her duties (she elaborates texts and images in colour), she happens to feel the emotive and neurovegetative symptoms of an alarm reaction, although the feeling of anxiety and dismay is totally without ideative contents: she feels everything is spinning around, she trembles, she feels she is suffocating, she feels weak; she feels as if she is about to faint, although she has never actually done so; some indefinable change in her state of consciousness seems however to be present, at times it might be a sort of very intense "empty" daydreaming ("I feel as if I'm dreaming, but I don't actually dream any particular thing.... I see flashes of a bright white light and I feel desperate, I anxiously wonder what is happening to me"), other times a real episode of depersonalisation-derealisation ("I feel outside myself, I see myself as if I were another person observing... it seems that everything around me is false, like a stage set or a surrealist painting").

Her colleagues rush to her, they crowd around, they get her to lie down, they bring her water or brandy—to tell the truth, reports the patient with a smile, this confusion makes things worse, but after a few minutes it is all over, and there are no important consequences apart from an intense emotional pain, headache and a sense of confusion that lasts all day. A basic anxiety never leaves her now: when will the next attack come?

But in this subject there is something that does not fit in with the diagnosis that comes with her: despite the constant irritability—connected to the sense of an imminent, sudden "panic attack," she says—, the exposition of the problem is lucid and clear, and on the whole her style of communication is consistent and reasonable, very receptive and reflective to the psychologist's questions and comments; her mood is up, and in the flow of conversation when she talks about her relationship in the couple and her cats, there sometimes appears a touch of authentic, measured cheerfulness. She likes her work very much, she is respected and has a good salary. In short, if it weren't for the "panic attacks," this person would feel reasonably satisfied with her life.

So towards the end of the session, after having learnt of two other elements, and that is that (1) the "attacks" started to appear when the office the patient works in was completely computerised (we are in the middle of the 1990s; before that, the work was done with paper, rulers and pens), and (2) the patient does not like watching television because it has always given her a slight disturbance (e.g., tinnitus, eye pain) and nausea, the psychologist suggests an EEG, to verify or exclude the possibility that the symptoms are produced by a slight epileptic focus, normally silent, but activated by the visual stimulation of the screen.

When the test reveals the presence of this focus, the patient begins, on the neurologist's advice, to take a low dosage of barbiturates and to take some precautions at work to limit her exposition to the flicker effect of the cathode tube: the "attacks" quickly disappear, and with them any residual trace of anticipatory and consequential anxiety. The patient did not ask for psychotherapy, and now years later, she leads a quiet life without any further abnormal phenomena in her nervous system or mental life.

(5) This case, too, concerns a young woman aged nearer to twenty-five than to thirty, the mother of a beautiful healthy growing child aged two, of whom she proudly shows the psychologist a photo.

Although the patient is a pretty woman—quite short, with delicate regular facial features, a well proportioned body—the difference is striking: the child is an explosion of physical strength and health, the mother is very thin, and looks decidedly anorexic: her face is hollow, her arms almost without muscles, as are her calves; she is obviously asthenic, with greyish colouring and dull skin.

And that is why she is there with the psychologist: her family members insisted so much (one of them is a friend of the psychologist's), that in the end she made up her mind, more to keep them happy than out of conviction. The patient eats very little and unwillingly; she likes only a few light foods, and she eats very little of them too; she sometimes vomits, and always feels nausea at the mere thought of food. She reports that her companion, her mother and her two (elder) sisters do not believe her totally, and they are all convinced that both her constant semi-fast and the vomiting are voluntary; the same attitude was shown by the "female doctors" (at least one was certainly a psychologist, the other is unknown) at the centre for eating disorders under contract with the *Mental Health Services*, where she was sent by her GP.

The patient actually presents many signs and symptoms of this kind of disorder, which began at high school out of the blue with an "intestinal influenza" with vomiting and diarrhoea, after which the symptoms began to be more and more intense and pervasive, until the present situation that has now been going on for years. And yet to the psychologist the patient seems sincere when she says that her lack of appetite is due to the violent discomfort that food arouses in her: as well as nausea, as soon as she starts to eat she immediately has a swelling of the stomach, a sense of epigastric heaviness and at times also bad headaches. The patient does not show any signs of self-coercion to abstain from eating, but rather an involuntary refusal, primarily physical, accompanied by a sensation of disgust and irritation for the consequences of eating; her underlying depressive state depends, in her view, on secondary factors: the constant though slight general malaise, the insistent pressure of her family to start eating adequately, the discord deriving from the repeated quarrels linked to this problem.

On the other hand, the patient is a friendly young woman, lively in interaction, she appears very responsible when she tells of her relationship with her son, of the difficulties encountered in looking for work (she has a degree in classical letters), and also when she gives her opinion on the people in her family, whose concern she understands but does not know how to deal with. She does not present any dismorphophobia of distortions in her experience of her body: she likes to be thin, but admits that she would be happier if she could gain a few kilos.

Regarding her experience at the centre for eating disorders she says she felt welcome, but not understood: there too she went on the insistence of one of her sisters (incidentally, a psychologist) and it had been enjoyable to talk about her problems with the "female doctors," but when it came to the point, she did not identify with the restitutions they offered, and even less with the strategies of behavioural therapy that made up the treatment protocol.

During several meetings the patient seems to be satisfied to have found a new interlocutor, and talks about herself and the family she comes from, towards which there is no lack of old (and "classical") reasons for conflict but the characteristic forms of entrapment are not found, nor are polemical dependency or chronic festering anger, which are so recurrent in the cases of eating disorders. The patient's mother is a very anxious woman as are her sisters, who in fact are the daughters of a previous marriage: moreover, also the mother's second marriage ended quickly, so the patient grew up away from her father, who has never taken any interest in her. The patient's companion, the father of the child, is a young man she sees as solid and reassuring; he too is a little anxious, but supportive and tolerant towards the eating problem; the two love each other and have a good sexual and affective relationship.

On one occasion, in the fifth or sixth meeting, the psychologist questions her with more precision about the medical tests she has had and discovers with astonishment that she has never been examined by a gastroenterologist, and nor has her GP—an old family friend, asked to look into the problem by the patient's mother—ever given any other diagnosis than that of an eating disorder to be treated in a specialised centre. To the psychologist, on the other hand, it does not seem that the patient has, or not *evidently*,[9] a disorder of this kind, and tends to a diagnostic hypothesis (a hypothesis because it is not his job to make this diagnosis) of malabsorption due to intolerance to substances contained in common foods. He therefore sends the patient to a specialist he trusts.

The medical diagnosis of celiac disorder (a form that was presumably initially asymptomatic, brought out of its latency by the viral infection in adolescence) put an end to the misunderstanding, and a suitable diet in the following months enabled the patient to gradually return to a satisfactory state of health, thus bringing the interminable family discussions about it to an end.

Some Observations

In cases (4) and (5), we therefore have two different kinds of behaviour from psychologists in response to the demand.

The psychologists the patients initially contacted—after a very hasty diagnosis by the GP—applied a psychopathological method of evaluation, without taking into the slightest account the conditions of the context: the demand was, as it were, taken literally and inserted in a system of nosographic classification, no intervention was offered in order to construct the "competent demand" (Carli, 1987[10])—a process without which the psychological consultation is reduced to aping the medical consultation, with results that are predictably unsuccessful.

The other psychologists consulted went on with their tests until they identified a set of symptomatological variables that were incongruous with the overall picture of the patient's system of affective symbolisations and of relations, as they were presented in actual professional interaction: and since these variables were of *evident* medical interest, and had not yet been adequately explored—while there was the doubt that there was a primary physical cause underlying the emotive reactions—the patients had to be sent back for specialist tests.

Here, therefore, the psychologists did not apply the methodological models of medicine to their own discipline: instead they analysed with the patients the structure of the demand for intervention, placing them in a position to separate the objective aspects of the disorder from those connected to the emotions, to identify the links between the two, reconstructing the history of the disorder in affective symbolisations shared—mainly unawares—with the social environment, in the patients' culture. In both the cases presented here, the request for psychological help was the last link in a chain of emotional acting out: constructing thought about them makes it possible to break this chain and formulate clinical hypotheses finally free from prejudice.

Psychology is not the trash-can of medicine; it is not necessarily true that everything that medicine does not explain must have a psychological "nature"—at times, simply, medicine does not have elaborate enough concepts available to understand the nature of a problem. Or the physician makes an error, and it may happen that the psychologist follows him a-critically, perfecting and at times making the error definitive and complete.

An episode of Nanni Moretti's film *Caro diario* (Moretti, 1993) springs to mind, in which the director is telling of his experience with a series of negligent, incompetent doctors, mostly dermatologists, who kept on prescribing skin treatments for an intense itch with no specific clinical signs, until a reference book reveals that it is a pathognomonic symptom of Hodgkin's lymphoma. The illness is then treated successfully with the standard chemotherapy treatment. Looking at this paradoxical situation one wonders: is it possible that nobody thought, first of all, that the itch—especially since there was no reddening, blisters or other *evidence* of immediate dermatological involvement—is above all a coenaesthetic sensation? Something therefore between the neurological and the psychological dimension, deserving *prior* testing in that direction. Forcing phenomena to fit into one's preestablished schemas is always the most antiscientific—and most harmful—behaviour a professional can adopt, whatever his disciplinary area. The fact that the professional is incompetent and/or negligent, and that his repertoire of technical knowledge is shamefully poor, is an aggravating circumstance, not the substance of the problem. The substance is that the source of error lies in the suspension of critical thought, and in the search for concrete confirmation (nosographic classification, diagnosis *ex iuvantibus*) with simplifying, decontextualising interpretations of complex problems that are comprehensible only within (and thanks to) an adequate contextualisation.

And has the patient got nothing to do with the construction of the error? Did he never notice that his own fame, his prestige as a director-author influenced the doctor's attitude, making him want to please? One of the dermatologists, presented as the top authority in the field, calls him "maestro" and greatly flatters his vanity.... In the Moretti case, as it is presented in the film, there would have been excellent material for a psychologist: not to "treat," but to interpret the model of doctor/patient collusion that made it impossible to think about the demand and the protracted inefficacy of the diagnoses and the treatments. This would be interpretation not of a pathological situation, but of a form of interaction between two or more subjects strongly characterised in each other's eyes in terms of excellence, which prevents them (or at least contributes to preventing them) from establishing a correct supply/demand dynamic of professional consultation. This "normal" situation needs to be understood in order to be solved.

At this point, it would be opportune to take a step back and examine a fundamental question: what is the background of presumed individual and collective "normality" where phenomena classed as "pathological" are positioned, in the common culture of psychologists and psychiatrists?

COMMENTS ON THE CONCEPT OF MENTAL HEALTH

A review a few years ago, done by G. E. Vaillant (2003) as the outcome of funding from the *National Institute of Mental Health*, for the prestigious *American Journal of Psychiatry*, considered six different empirical approaches to mental health, deserving particular attention, according to the author. These include the "positive psychology" approach and the opinions on mental health of its most representative exponent, M. E. P. Seligman (1991, 2002; Peterson & Seligman, 2004).

As Vaillant (2003) writes:

Seligman has served notice that positive psychology will follow Meyer's rules of conscientious and impartial study and constructive experimentation. Seligman's concept of learned optimism incorporates the empirical advances in cognitive psychology that have taken place over the past three decades.

> [...] positive psychology is the only model of mental health that suggests, even tentatively, how a GAF Scale[11] score of 75 might be raised to 90." (Vaillant, 2003; pp. 1376–1377)

In the positive psychology model, mental health is based, among other things, on the possibility of implementing some "strong points" namely *love, moderation, wisdom and knowledge, courage, justice* and *transcendence*. Particular importance is placed on *optimism*. As Vaillant also writes:

> In part, the importance of optimism to positive mental health depends on an explanatory style that asserts, "The good things that happen to me will last

> forever. They are pervasive, and they are my own doing. The bad things that happen to me occur by chance, are limited, and are unlikely to happen again." (ibidem, p. 1377)

This statement allows us also to underline:

1. the impermeability of this vision of the world to any critical reflection and therefore to any possible psychotherapy process;
2. and at the same time, the singular closeness of such a statement to a perspective that we will not hesitate, according to the canons of traditional psychopathological nomenclature, to call paranoid.

But again as regards mental health and optimism, in the same review of the most authoritative and documented conceptions of mental health, Vaillant finds in the conceptualisation of "mental health as subjective well-being," a model worth particular attention due to the influence it has had, that it still has, and the prospects it opens in terms of scientific research. Although the author regrets that historically the Europeans have been

> skeptical of American concern with *happiness*[12] (*ibidem*, p. 1380—italics added)

he underlines that the term (*happiness*) presents an ambiguous meaning that has caused a great deal of confusion in the past, which makes him prefer the term *subjective well-being*. But things have fortunately changed. He in fact points out that:

> Until recently, the scientific parameters of subjective well-being were as vague as those for objective mental health. A 1967 definition suggested that a happy person is "young, healthy, well-educated, well paid, extroverted, optimistic, worry free, religious and married with high self esteem, a good job, morals, and modest aspirations." (Wilson, 1967) (*ibidem*, p. 1380)

However, there is the qualification that in the last thirty years, research has shown that such a vague generalisation is only partly true. Among others, it was Seligman (2002) mentioned above, for instance, that stated which of these adjectives should be considered correct.

We now know that "young, healthy, well-educated, well paid, extroverted, optimistic, worry free" can no longer be seen as the correct qualifications of a happy person. The research, serious and documented (!), carried out in these years has shown that only "religious, married, with high self-esteem and a good job" can be retained.

And it is in this picture that, though with a logical leap that may seem questionable, attention is drawn to one particular research project on nuns. Happy and long-lived, in certain conditions.

This research, published in 2001 (Danner, Snowdon & Friesen, 2001), has a title that leaves no space for doubt: *Positive Emotions in Early Life and Longevity: Findings From the Nun Study*. One of the authors, D. A. Snowdon (2001), has also published a book on the same subject: *Aging with Grace*.[13]

The research shows that 180 twenty-year-old nuns were asked to write an autobiography of a couple of pages. Among those who expressed mainly positive emotions, only 24% died before the age of 80, while among those expressing less positive emotions, 54% died before the age of 80.[14] Vaillant claims that this study highlights what is probably the most convincing connection between subjective happiness and health. But—and here the logical leap becomes obvious—happiness or subjective well-being, whatever is said, is impossible to earn. Vaillant notes:

> Indeed, subjective well-being is highly heritable and relatively independent of demographic variables. (*ibidem*, p. 1380)

In fact, the author stresses,

> The subjective well-being of monozygous twins raised apart is more similar than that of heterozygous twins raised together (...). Among the partially heritable factors making significant contributions to a high level of subjective well-being are a low level of trait neuroticism, high level of trait extra-version, absence of alcoholism, and absence of major depression (*ibidem*, p. 1380).

The scepticism of which Vaillant accuses us, as Europeans, now grows in view of the confusion of levels contained in these statements and of the reification and simplification of complex concepts that they offer. The very concept of "positive" mental health is probably a simplification. It is a simplification that does not hold up above all in view of the implicit misunderstanding of the cultural variables involved. We must add that it may also be a dangerous simplification with very clear consequences on the broader sociopolitical level. Vaillant also writes:

> Recent major psychiatric textbooks reveal virtually no serious discussion of positive mental health. An electronic search of *Psychological Abstracts* since 1987 turned up 57, 800 articles on anxiety and 70, 856 on depression, but only 5, 701 mentioned life satisfaction and only 851 mentioned *joy* (*ibidem*, p. 1373; italics added).

In this direction, we believe it is impossible not to feel ill at ease in supporting the approach that sees, for instance, the selection process in the Mercury program of the '60s to choose the first seven American astronauts, as the prototype of research seeking a scientific definition of mental health:

> This study underscored both the importance and the commonsensical nature of mental health. The final seven astronauts not only enjoyed exemplary

> work records but were also competent at loving. All had come from *intact, happy*, small-town families. In their '30s, they all were married with children. Although venturesome test pilots, they had suffered unusually few accidents during their years as pilots or even earlier. They could tolerate both close interdependent association and extreme isolation. They trusted others and were uncomplaining under discomfort. Emotions, both negative and positive, were strongly experienced. Not introspective, the astronauts seldom dwelled on their inner emotions; but they could describe them when asked. They were aware of the feelings of others, and they avoided interpersonal difficulties (*ibidem*, p. 1376–1376; italics added).

But above all,

> their group score on the neuroticism scale of the Maudsley Personality Inventory has been described as the lowest of any group reported in the literature (*ibidem*, p. 1376).

as was pointed out by one of their selectors, Captain Perry (1965).

If such a description is to be considered, a valid example of what can be meant scientifically by mental health, what is the appreciable qualification or innovation compared to the pre-scientific models that saw mental health as being closely connected to morality, models that Vaillant says we must repudiate?

It seems to us, on the other hand, that these statements take, as their main reference point, objectives of social control more than "purely" scientific objectives, as they would have us believe.

This risk achieving a paradoxical result: if mental health is due for instance to the fact that one belongs to a "happy united family," everybody can feel entitled to one. What are the actual questions that Vaillant, from time to time, poses in his work? For example, questions like the following:

> The perspective of mental health as Utopia is one of the bogeymen of national health policy makers. They are afraid, without directly expressing it, that this perspective (...) will put a backbreaking burden on health insurance. Is helping people to become happier with themselves a process that any health insurance program should be expected to cover? Over time society will have to decide who should pay for positive mental health: the individual, the educational system, third-party payers, religious organisations, or a combination of all four. (*ibidem*, p. 1377)

There is an answer, which is reassuring for the politicians, but less so for a self-respecting scientific community as we mentioned above, and with ineffable grace, at the right moment it is whisked out of the magician's hat:

> The answer is that subjective well-being has more effect on the environment than the environment exerts on it (*ibidem*, p. 1380).

In other words, it is argued that subjective well-being is due more to top-down processes, that is, factors of temperament governing subjective well-being, than to bottom-up processes—like for example the satisfaction of the universal primary needs.

So there is an answer. And the circle is closed. But it should be pointed out that it is getting more and more difficult for this to happen.

There have appeared, also in the United States, articles critical of the concept of subjective well-being as an indicator or as a factor making up mental health. We feel closer, for instance, to the point of view expressed in a study by Shedler, Mayman and Manis printed in 1993 in *American Psychologist*. Starting from the aspect stressed in the subtitle, "The *Illusion* of Mental Health" (original italics), the authors assume that

> standard mental health scales appear unable to distinguish between genuine mental health and the facade or illusion of mental health created by psychological defences. (Shelder, Mayman & Manis, 1993; p. 1117)

The article presents the results of a series of research activities based on the comparison of the responses of a group of subjects to questionnaires for the self-evaluation of the state of mental health, and clinical evaluations carried out blind by the researchers on the same subjects. The scales used tend to converge with the clinical judgments—expressed on the basis of direct contact[15]—only when the scores indicate the presence of situations of distress, while they diverge in a statistically significant way in the opposite case:

> [...] scores on mental health scales are valid when they indicates distress but ambiguous when they indicate health. If it is true (and if our clinical evaluations are valid), then the relation between the self-report Neuroticism scores and the clinical evaluations should be clearly asymmetric. People who report distress should be judged distressed by the clinician, but people who report health might or might not be judged healthy. This asymmetric pattern was in fact observed (*ibidem*, p. 1121).

CONSIDERATIONS ON THE CONCEPT OF MENTAL DISORDER

While the definition of mental health is having a hard time, the complementary one of mental disorder does not seem to be enjoying a better fate.

Let us look at what was recently written by J. C. Wakefield (2004), a respected clinical psychologist and researcher of New York University, who, in some of his previous works (Wakefield, 1992, 1997, 1999) had proposed the concept of disorder as "harmful dysfunction." Although Wakefield (2005) disagrees with Vaillant "because of some conceptual confusion" and due to the fact that "unfortunately his article does not contain a conceptual analysis either of the six models taken individually or of the concept of health in general", he initially attacks that

> improbable mixture of antipsychiatrists, behaviourists, postmodernists and socioconstructivists [for whom] there is nothing like a mental disorder in the literal sense of "disorder," and that is, in the way the concept is used in medicine. They claim instead that diagnoses of mental disorder are simply value judgments about the socially constructed categories of a disapproved behaviour, judgments that enable medical power to be exercised for the purpose of social control, over conditions that actually do not constitute disorders (Wakefield, 2004, p. 439; translation from the Italian original).

But the remedy identified does not seem much better than the problem.[16]

The model taken by the author and which he calls "hybrid," which in the basic formulation tried to harmonise the bio-medical and the sociopolitical perspectives, swiftly runs aground on a vision that cannot but envisage human behaviour and mental processes as unvarying and detached from historical and social processes. The concept that derives, of disorder as "harmful dysfunction" fails to keep either of the viewpoints happy. In fact, the author writes:

> In this model, "harmful" is a value term referring to a state judged to be negative by sociocultural standards, and "dysfunction" is a scientific factual terms based on evolutionary biology that refers to the failure of an *inner mechanism* in carrying out one of its *natural functions*. (*ibidem*, p. 440; translation from the Italian original)

But, when he has to explain what is meant by "inner mechanism" and "natural function" he inevitably writes:

> I will use the expression "inner mechanism" as a general term to refer to physical structures and organs as well as to mental structures and aptitudes, such as motivational, cognitive, affective, and perceptive mechanisms. Some authors distinguish between "disorder," "disease" and "illness"; I will focus on the term "disorder," or on the broadest term which covers both traumatic wounds and diseases, and which is therefore close to the global medical concept of pathology.
>
> [...] An additional factual component is needed to distinguish disorders from the many other negative mental conditions that are not considered disorders, such as ignorance, lack of ability, lack of talent, limited intelligence, illiteracy, criminality, bad manners, stupidity and moral weakness (*ibidem*, pp. 440–443; translation from the Italian original).

Yet, again we are forced to point out, if nothing else, the confusion of levels of analysis: the concepts used are levelled out and lose their connotations and their differences. It is true that Wakefield's aim is not only to "vindicates psychiatry from the antipsychiatrists" by explaining hoe genuine mental disorders con exist," but also to provide "grounds from within psychiatry's own implicit assumptions for critiquing the *DSM* diagnostic criteria as often pathologising normal conditions" (*ibidem,* p. 461):[17] however, the arguments used seem to us to be particularly weak and intrinsically contradictory.

We will quote two extracts, as an example:

> It is evident,[18] from the historical and anthropological documentation, that values, norms and ideologies strongly influence people's idea of what natural functions are, especially when there is an inadequate understanding of "function" and "dysfunction" (as happens with many mental characteristics). But none of this implies that the semantic content of "natural function" is value-based. In the same way, if a person's religious values lead him/her to reject the idea that the earth rotates around the sun and to assert that the earth is less than 7000 years old, this does not mean that the concepts "rotate around the sun" or "less than 7000 years old" are value-laden concepts; they are purely descriptive concepts, true or false as may be, about the earth, independent of the values of each person, even though the beliefs of each person about their applicability to the Earth are strongly influenced, or even entirely determined, by values (*ibidem*, p. 444; translation from the Italian original).

But doesn't the posing of the question in terms of the "truth/falsity" of these statements already imply, in itself, that one is adopting a value-based perspective? And, depending on the contexts, doesn't it therefore mean drawing the inevitable conclusions from those same statements? For all there is the reference to the human and scientific experience of Galileo Galilei, which has continued to resound until very recently.[19]

And again, if

> we think that the prewar Confederate doctors were quite wrong in classifying runaway slaves as being affected by "Runaway Slave Disorder (*drapetomania*[20])." (*ibidem*, p. 452; translation from the Italian original)

the problem, in our view, is not so much to establish whether this diagnosis was accurate or not, but to ask what contextual conditions made it possible and, yet again, what consequences this diagnosis had on the context.

And then, is there so much difference between a slave "affected" by "runaway slave disorder" and a "normal" citizen who is a victim of the disaster that for instance a few years ago struck New Orleans, rightly, in our view, desperate about what happened and therefore evidently not happy, but as a result eligible for being identified as not same on the basis of the model of "mental health as subjective well-being"—which, we repeat, says that "subjective well-being" depends on factor of *temperament* largely inherited and essentially independent of the environment?

A-CONTEXTUAL PRAGMATISM

But from the confederate doctors and their questionable diagnostic criteria, let us try to approach our own times, in which we believe the criteria used are far clearer and more scientifically grounded. And let us keep talking about the relation between white and black Americans.

We will start for example from a recent article (Ward, 2005) that sets out to explore the subjective experience of psychological counselling on the part of African American clients.

We therefore discover that African American clients, perhaps because they are (constitutionally?) "suspicious" of scientific research and, even more, of researchers—as Pinn, Harden, and Blehar, (2002) show—engage in (what a surprise!) an activity of continuous evaluation of their interlocutor (whether it be therapist or counsellor) to decide whether or not to trust him. And this activity refers to three main aspects: the importance they attribute to their black identity, any involvement in legal proceedings, and the similarity of ideological viewpoints. This influences their perception of security in a therapy and the assessment of the effectiveness of the counsellor, determining (who would have thought it?) greater or lesser degrees of openness and self-disclosure. Needless to say, *self-disclosure* is organised along a continuum that goes from absence of openness, through superficial openness, selective openness and lastly total openness.

It is interesting to notice that this exposition of commonplaces comes from an author who tells us she herself is black. It is also interesting to look at an episode cited in the article, which Ward finds emblematic in connection with her interest in the issue dealt with in her scientific work.

The episode is the following: our author is going to work (a *Community Mental Health Centre*) and on the bus, she happens to sit next to a black woman who immediately strikes up a conversation and identifying her as a student (it is well known that blacks are born evaluators!), asks her what she does. Ward replies that she deals with psychology of counselling and her interlocutor asks if there is one area she is particularly interested in (here too, it is well known that blacks are not open and are suspicious; by the way, who is the counsellor and who is the client?) and she says she is specifically interested in cultural problems and counselling. At this, the black woman compliments her saying, "we need people to deal with this stuff," and she tells her an anecdote.

> Girl, let me tell you what happened to me recently. Sometimes I have mood swings you know. When the weather gets cold, I sometimes get depressed and unhappy, you know. Part of my unhappiness is related to being a Black woman living in a White city. Anyway, I decided to tell my doctor about my mood swings. He recommended counselling. At first, I did not want to go, because you know how us Black folks feel about counselling. Plus, I don't want anyone to think I am "crazy."[21]

> Well, I finally got the courage to go to counselling; I thought it might be helpful. During the first 30 min the counsellor tells me I need to see a psychiatrist for medication. What's wrong with that damn counsellor? He didn't even spend any time getting to know me; he immediately started talking about medication. I just needed someone to talk to, but instead he is talking about medication. Well, girl, I never went back to see him (Ward, 2005, p. 471).

The author quickly points out that unfortunately, this woman's perception of counselling and counsellors is very common among African Americans who go to mental health services, especially among women. In fact, the decision to break off the consultations after only one session is in line with what Wade and Bernstein (1991) discovered: the scientific community is grateful to these researchers, who have the merit of revealing that African American women's attitude to counselling and counsellors (who knows why it is the women's attitude: maybe due to the very well known and scientifically proven phenomenon known as "female intuition"?) develops right from the first session influencing (here too, who would have thought it!) their decision whether or not to continue the consultations.

After the pioneering (!) work by Wade and Bernstein, the author complains that information on the issue is only anecdotal and this makes it necessary to explore the problem in a theoretically based analysis: the results of this analysis have been briefly outlined above.

We are not in a position to know the reactions of the person who inspired the work, the black woman on the bus, but we can imagine them: not one word is said, in Ward's work, on what she was told almost as an introduction to the short anecdote told by her chance interlocutor: "*Part of my unhappiness is related to being a Black woman living in a White city*."

The depth of such statement which, however, refers to a stratified contextual dynamic in hundreds of years of *black and white Americans* living together (in which some influence, especially as regards the confidence in professional mental health figures, must surely have been exerted by diagnostic operations and we suppose by therapeutic operations of the drapetomania type mentioned above!), is completely ignored in favour of general statements like the one in the conclusion, in which the author claims, among other things, that

> the findings from this study emphasise the importance of hearing and honouring the voices of the clients we serve (Ward, 2005, p. 480).

As if this were not so obviously implicit that one does not need sophisticated empirical investigations to demonstrate it and perhaps to remind those, like the counsellor in the anecdote, who are implicitly stigmatised *only* because they are not up to the task. In this way, a relational problem which, as such, is deeply influenced by contextual dynamics, is reduced to a *simple* fact of technical skill/lack of skill. Yet again, the importance of listening to and respecting the voices of the clients we serve, does not *in itself* constitute a basis of the clinical action in psychology, but it is worth underlining it insofar as clients' perceptions of counselling determine to a large extent the effectiveness of therapy (Constantine, 2002; Paulson et al., 1999—cit. in Ward, 2005; p. 480). And as we can see, this statement, which is so obvious that it almost sounds offensive, is supported by its own little repertoire of quotations to the point.

In conclusion, therefore, from what we read above it seems that the problem of the blacks vis-à-vis the institutions responsible for counselling and psychotherapy are both that they do not feel listened to and that they feel they are treated as being "mad." On the other hand, however, it seems that the psychologists (remember the anecdote) do actually tend to behave in this way towards them. This vision of the problem seems to us to be naïve and reductive, because it does not take into account extremely important contextual variables concerning the relationship, as it has developed over time, between blacks and whites in America (but there may also be something to say about Asians, Latinos, Italians, etc.).

THE RETURN OF REDUCTIONISM: WHAT HAPPENED TO COMPLEXITY?

And there is also something about counselling and its relationship with clinical psychology. As one of the present authors (Grasso, 2006b) recently pointed out, we have been witnessing for various years the growing spread of *counselling* and of practices inspired by it, that go by various names, along with the resulting creation of training courses and, at least in Italy, requests for professional recognition, and so forth. All these however have gone on in parallel with a process of progressively detaching itself from its matrix in psychology and more specifically in clinical psychology. The process of such a purely psychological practice moving away from psychology reaches its apex with the recuperation, for example, of *philosphical counselling*, whose "birth-date" has been fixed by common agreement among the experts of the sector, about twenty-five years ago.

Philosophical consultation is a discipline, as one can read in the ample space devoted to it on the Web, that aims to provide help and orientation for individuals that are unable to deal alone with the problems that daily life presents. The task of the *counsellor* is to help people reflect on their professional and affective choices and on relational and emotional dynamics and the meaning that can be recognised in any states of anxiety and depression experienced. These were the words of the philosopher and

Jungian analyst Galimberti (2004) in the Italian newspaper *la Repubblica* when announcing its spread to Italy:

> Those who ask for a philosophical consultation are not "ill," they are simply looking for a meaning. And where can we find a meaning, or rather the meaning that, underground and ignored, runs through our life unbeknown to us, if not in the suggestions of sense that constitute philosophy and its history? So it was, that in 1981, the German philosopher Gerd Achenbach opened in Germany the first center for Philosophical consultation, which was followed by the creation of a Society for philosophical practice, which then went international, spreading to Holland, France, the United States and Israel. In 1999, in Italy, the "Association for Philosophic Counseling" was established, translating the books by Pierre Hadot, *Spiritual Exercises and Ancient Philosophy* and by Lou Marinoff, *Plato, not Prozac*! and *The Middle Way*, which brought the general public closer to the figure of the philosopher who deals with individuals without presenting himself as a "therapist." In 2003, the Education Faculty at the University of Catania organised the first Conference on philosophical practices, while the University of Venice offered its first course in a broader project on philosophical practices that also envisages a Masters in the subject. The main Torin hospital "Le Molinette" has a philosophical consultant working alongside the psychologist at staff consultations, while District 4 of the Municipality of Florence has instituted a public service of philosophical consultation as an extension of the social services it offers the citizens. (Translation from the Italian original)

And again:

> And those who refuse to surrender to dullness, because they still possess a certain self-awareness, who do they turn to when they encounter not this pain or that pain, which the psychotherapies crowd around, but the essence of pain that is the inability to find a meaning? Here, the psychotherapies are of no use because it is not "pathological," as some would have you believe, to ask oneself questions, subject one's ideas to verification, examine one's vision of the world to see to what extent it is narrow, stuffy, fossilised, rigid, forced, unsuited to dealing with the changes in one's life and the rapid, unexpected changes in the world. If not all pain is pathology, a better answer to this kind of suffering and distress can be given not by psychotherapy but by philosophy. (translation from the Italian original)

It seems clear that psychotherapy and with it clinical psychology, in a mirror image of the fears of the stigma of madness mentioned before, are fully assimilated to the idea of "disease," of healing from a "pathology" that finds its necessary foundation in a decidedly medical viewpoint: in this, one might say, it satisfies those clinical psychologists that warm up their watered down identity with the comforting warmth of the white coat. The result, however, is a progressive erosion of the cultural and professional presence in the domains of so-called "normality," with which it would be natural for psychological counselling to deal.

On this point, the title of one of the books cited by Galimberti seems emblematic: *Plato, not Prozac*! (Marinoff, 1999).[22] As we can see, the medical-psychiatric intervention in mental distress is juxtaposed to the *philosophical* intervention in existential problems.[23] And psychology? Clinical psychology? Its specificity? Paradoxically missing. The assimilation of clinical psychology exclusively to the practice of psychotherapy involves, we believe, this sort of drift.

It is the psychiatrist, then, who is expected to face up to the pathology, and it is the philosophical counsellor who is given the task of helping to understand the roots of the dissatisfaction with daily life, with affective relationships, with work: so the "philosophical counsellor" is expected to act as a psychologist, a clinical psychologist.

The reduction of clinical psychology to psychotherapy involves on the one hand justifying the equivalence from a theoretical and methodological viewpoint, of the different models of psychotherapy, and on the other it is leading, we think, to the affirmation of the dominance of some models and consequently verification methodologies; these are the ones that are most compatible with naïvely (or not naïvely) dichotomic approaches, encouraging the temptation in the other models to avoid debate and to give up the connection with their original underlying hypothesis in the name of an a-critical support for simplifications of the type mentioned, for fear of being ostracised from international publications, from funding for research, and from participation in conferences.

This is what is happening consistently not only in our country, but to psychodynamically-oriented therapeutic models, or to spell it out, to those with a psychoanalytical orientation.

Reducing complex concepts in order to *operationalise* them is a current issue. To illustrate this, let us look briefly at one of the most problematic and controversial aspects of the therapeutic relationship in a psychoanalytical framework: the dynamics of countertransference.

How can this be explained unless by using the arguments just put forward, for example, the creation of the *Countertransference Index* (CI) (Hayes, Ricker, & Ingram, 1997), a tool made up of a single item which, thanks to a Likert-type scale, indicates to what degree the therapist's behaviour in the session just completed was influenced by counter transference?[24]

Or, still on the same question, how can we consider the process that led to the construction and subsequent use of the *Inventory of Countertransference Behaviour* (ICB) (Gelso & Friedman, 2000), where the initial 32 items which were supposed to describe countertransference behaviour were evaluated by 11 psychologists judged to be experts in the area of countertransference (by whom? And above all, based on what?), who, using the usual Likert scale, where 1 indicated that the item did not describe any kind of countertransference behaviour and 5 indicated that the item was an excellent indicator, selected the 21 which were then used?

In these cases, are we not dealing with a massive process of simplification? And what can be said about the measurements obtained from such tools? Judging by the uses made of them, which can be found in the literature, there are two kinds of outcomes.

On the one hand, the *concretisation* of the concept under study: what is obtained with countertransference, in other words, is not understood as a probabilistic at best, if not random, evaluation of the behaviours linked to countertransference dynamics, but *is* countertransference to such a degree that one then goes so far as to claim for instance that countertransference itself—the exact theoretical outlines of which have been progressively lost as research goes on—*is* defined and constituted by eight dimensions, which perhaps represent only the result of a simple factorial analysis.[25] Without counting that—as regards this last example on the *ICB*—the clinicians involved in the study had a psychodynamic, eclectic (?), cognitive-behavioural training: but didn't the concept of countertransference originate and develop within the psychoanalytical tradition (Freud, 1937/1964; Heimann, 1950; Racker, 1968 and obviously many others)? How might it have been, if it was, conceptualised elsewhere? For example, in the eclectic perspective, naturally by evaluating the type of eclecticism involved?[26] Far from being a process of integration of the different approaches, all these, in fact, seem like a melting pot where every distinctive feature is lost in the name of an unspecified *empiria*. On the other hand, there is a more cautious attitude which, aware of the critical nature of some assumptions, claims the entire right/duty to offer evaluations and/or conceptions that may be rudimentary (because, it is said, there is nothing better) in view of a later, progressive refinement. The problem is that based on what we have seen, it is often not a matter of inaccurate measurements, which can later be perfected, but simply a case of *non*-measurement. With the not infrequent result of starting from point A and of arriving, through a series of steps, at a point B that has little or nothing in common with the initial situation (Horvath, 2005b).

It makes one want to remark: but what happened to *complexity*? Is there anyone who remembers it?

How can we interpret all these? We seem to be looking at a sort of naive empiricism, descended directly from an obsolete *paradigm of simplification*. In this perspective, the world is complete unto itself, governed by linear mechanisms in which one can identify clear-cut categories of cause and effect. It is a paradigm, in other words, in which reality is assumed to be characterised by the order, stability and regularity of phenomena. If this were not so, it would not in fact be logical to try to identify precise connections between disorderly, unstable phenomena. The processes of isolation, separation and quantification required by the traditional experimental method are logically admissible only in a paradigm in which reality is described as a regular organic set, in which objects have their own characteristics, independent both of the observer and of the context in which they are found: in this case scientific knowledge is based on direct observations of reality—or on an *empirical* basis "free from any prejudice"—from which one starts, in order to reach the formulation of general principles that can explain the facts observed (Grasso, Cordella, & Pennella, 2003).

But is it not true that the contribution of epistemology, specifically within psychology and, in particular, clinical psychology (cf. for example, Lombardo, & Malagoli Togliatti, 1995) has produced an enormous amount of material for thought? Do we need to recall that it has been established that the interaction between the phenomenon, the observer and the tools used in the process of knowledge-getting is not only inevitable but must also be considered the *object of knowledge?* That the concept of *cause* has been joined by that of *condition* and that, as well as linear causality, different processes such as *interdependence* and *probability* have been highlighted? And that the latter is no longer considered an expression of the inability to define the *certainty* of the links existing between the phenomena observed, but rather, a characteristic that constitutes reality?

It is widely known how greatly the role of empirical induction has been cut down to size over time. When the idea of a permanent reality independent of the observer collapses and the observer comes to be placed in a complex network of interdependence with the phenomenon observed, it becomes inevitable to declare that observation heavily depends on the theories—naturally in the broad sense—of the observer. In contrast to what was stated by the empirical epistemology underlying the paradigm of simplification, the scientific theories therefore seem to be elaborated not so much starting from sensitive data, but more from the beliefs that can be held about the phenomena one intends to study. Something else that has collapsed is the idea of a *cumulative* dimension of knowledge—typical first of the enlightenment and later of positivist culture—in which scientific development was pictured as a sort of summation, in favour of the idea of knowledge as a process that comes about by eliminating errors.

The concept of simplification has long been replaced by that of complexity and by the consequent *paradigm of complexity* (Benkirane, 2002), in which the object of scientific interest is recognised in the totality of its elements and in the interactions between these elements and the environment in which they are situated. There has been much discussion around this concepts in the last thirty years. Where has the dimension of complexity gone now? How can it be found in the studies we have quoted? What we are seeing seems, if you will excuse the term, to be a sort of simplification of the concept of complexity.

We believe in fact that it is possible to regard a system of elements definable according to the functions they serve, as "complex." These elements, however, are not simply "part" of the system—if they were, the system would be fragmentable and therefore by definition not "complex"—but they have their own ontology that depends on the context in which they are located. Outside the system, these elements have no meaning and the system itself, without these parts, loses its identity.

Another example of simplification and reductionism?

The interesting book by De Coro and Andreassi (2004), which offers a broad overview of the empirical research in psychotherapy, concerning the studies on the efficacy of childhood psychotherapy, cites the research of Casey and Berman (1985), which is seen by experts in the sector as a turning point in studies on the subject. Using the technique of *meta-analysis* the two researchers analysed 75 instances of research into childhood psychotherapies (patients aged from 3 to 15) carried out between 1952 and 1983, with the aim of providing an *empirical* answer to questions like: does psychotherapy work with children? They obtained for the first time a more than affirmative result with an effect-size of 0. 71. One wonders: with children? From 3 to 15 years of age? One wonders whether Casey and Berman have ever even *seen* an adolescent aged 15 and a child of 3, to be able to think of them as being similar. One also wonders whether the two researchers have ever read or heard for example about the research of Estes (1938), a student of Allport, which led to the hypothesis of a "*trained incapacity*" to evaluate people for those who had studied psychology in the 1930s.

Underlying all these there seem to be what we can call a sort of *fetishism* of quantification. Statistical analysis is transformed in these cases, from a tool into an actual objective of the work: the research is carried out so that there can be quantification, regardless of what is being quantified, or how. And yet, again, in ignorance of the complex systems one is dealing with. But there also seems to be the deliberate disregarding (not just mere ignorance) of how widely and authoritatively these questions were debated and elaborated in the past, to such an extent that at least some people have an unpleasant feeling of *déjà vu*. Some questions come up again in cycles, some conflicts tend to be reproduced, as if everything that has been said, done, and written has not led to the slightest dimension of integration, or at least has produced no memory at all.

On the matter of the atomisation of behavioural dimensions, at times indiscriminate, carried out in measurement procedures, of which we have given a few examples above, is it really necessary to remember Rapaport? In the 1950s, when referring to a debate underway at the time, about evaluation and measurement, Rapaport distinguished between "molar" and "molecular" behaviour, and with reference to gestaltist conceptions, argued:

> Those segments of behaviour which are wholes, in that they have a self-contained *meaning* but which they would lose if further subdivided, are units of behaviour. Gestalt psychology calls these molar behaviour units, in contrast to the molecular units obtained by subdivisions disregarding meaningfulness. (Rapaport, 1950/1967, p. 341)

Again, in 1950, he warned against the reification that consists of attributing to conceptual constructs used to express data obtained from testing, the value of relations that *really* operate in the psychic organisation of any individual.

The problem we are dealing with therefore seems to be, first , a cultural problem. It is within the psychological disciplines on the one hand, and on the other, it is amplified by the connotations that social contexts tend to progressively assume—that is, by the superficial values that are being pushed more and more, by the highlighting of a culture of appearances and sensationalism fostered by the invasiveness of the media very often devoid of content other than the amplification of the image itself, by the tendencies to simplification, generalisation, reductionism, and conformism mentioned above. These are, we believe, aspects of the context that must be acknowledged and faced.

In the light of these considerations, let us now look at a singular debate that took place in March 2006 in the pages of the journal *Psychotherapy Research*. The issue opens with the introduction by the editor Clara E. Hill who presents the readers with the topic, to which a special section will be devoted, in the following words:

> In the psychotherapy community, the issue of whether the effects of therapy are due to the treatment itself or to the therapist has been hotly debated (Hill, 2006, p. 143).

And further on:

> If it is the treatment that works, the implication is that we need to have carefully specified treatment manuals that detail exactly what any good therapist would do at different points in the treatment process. If, alternatively, it is the therapist who is the responsible for change, we need to focus on selecting good therapists and fostering their personal growth and development. Finally, if it is actually the clients who are the major contributors to therapeutic effectiveness, we must focus on developing better diagnostic tools and tailoring our treatments to different types of clients. Hence, understanding more about the sources of effects directly influences practice, training and research. (Hill, 2006, p. 143)

One obviously tends to think of the vexed question of the importance of so-called specific or a-specific factors in determining the effectiveness of a psychotherapy treatment, dressed up for the special occasion in its Sunday best. But apart from anything else, the approach to the question seems to suddenly cancel out any reference to the most salient aspects of theoretical thinking in psychology and in particularly in clinical psychology and psychotherapy: the dynamics of relating. Or perhaps it seems to unilaterally highlight the dimension of individual behaviour, at the expense of relational behaviour. But in this case what is being referred to is a sort of old-style behaviourism, almost totally impermeable to any contextual reference.

Clara E. Hill's introduction leads into two research articles that offer to cast light on the topic, working, and this is undoubtedly a unique opportunity, on the same set of data: the results of the National Institute of Mental Health's Treatment of Depression Collaborative Research Program. The psychotherapy models considered are *cognitive-behaviour therapy* (CBT) and *interpersonal therapy* (IPT). The patients considered are 119 assigned randomly (!) to 17 therapists, 60 to 9 IPT therapists and 59 to 8 to CBT therapists. The two studies (Elkin, Falconnier, Martinovich, & Mahoney, 2006; Kim, Wampold, & Bolt, 2006), reach (would you believe it?) conclusions that are diametrically opposed.

In fact, the contribution of Elkin, Falconnier, Martinovich and Mahoney (2006a) underlines:

> There was no indication of significant therapist effects in the current analyses despite the use of a more efficient model (because all available data may be included) and a conception of treatment progress that focuses on rates of change, adjusted for baseline expectations, instead of focusing on status at a somewhat arbitrary point (p. 151).

Kim, Wampold, & Bolt (2006), on the other hand, state:

> Several multilevel analyses if the NIMH TDCRP data revealed sizable therapist effects, ranging from 1% to 12% depending on the outcome variable and the model adopted. Overall, a simple mean of all the estimates was about 8%. [...] it seems clear that therapists were an important source of variability in these data. [...] the results suggest that, with regard to outcomes, therapists are more important than treatments. (p. 167)

It would be sensible to stop here, and, as we used to say as children, have a good look at our conscience. In depth, Instead, in a sort of scientific-methodological-statistical *cupio dissolvi*, the analysis of these results, not so much diverging as decidedly contrasting, is entrusted to scholars of merit, Soldz (2006) and Crits-Christoph and Gallop (2006), for them to comment on and find justifications for the two different conclusions. And, that is not all: there is still space for a rebuttal by the coordinators of the studies examined (Elkin, Falconnier, Martinovich, & Mahoney, 2006b; Wampold & Bolt, 2006). As a result, over a third of the journal is taken up with this question.

Here we do not want to examine in depth the arguments produced. It is enough to underline the artificiality of the whole debate, as is also noticed by Dazzi and De Coro (2007), although they do not reach the same conclusions as us:

The central issue is: how can the effect of the "therapist" variable be reduced in outcome research, to obtain sufficiently "controlled" studies that document the effects of psychotherapy on the patient? The various authors debate the possibility of constructing multilevel models to enable the many factors to be kept together, and at the end of the debate, it is underlined that the attempts to construct models of data analysis that reduce the therapist effect have no sense, since all the research shows the importance of the therapist for the outcomes of psychotherapy and, as soon as the effects of the therapist are made to disappear, "all the rest will disappear"! (Wampold & Bolt, 2006, p. 186).

We wonder: wasn't this the expected result? Wouldn't we immediately say that the idea of seeing if the therapist variable can be eliminated in psychotherapy, or else proving that it counts, is an absolutely rearguard idea in the overall thinking on psychotherapy? And yet this "debate" takes up almost half the journal, only to reach conclusions, or rather, nonconclusions that seem to us could have been largely anticipated without being burdened with the highly sophisticated structure found in the two research projects. It is therefore impossible to avoid being malicious and quoting a well-known Italian saying, *it's a sin to think the worst, but it hits the nail on the head.*[27] In other words, it comes naturally to think that interest in research, and the attempt to look for answers, through research, to many questions posed by psychotherapy practice, actually represent something strongly conditioned by a "market," firstly, that of research and its funding, but also that of the provision of psychotherapy and its fruition by the clients, which in the United States is so markedly subordinated to the expectations of the insurance companies. Don't try to tell us that the purpose is the best use of available resources: also implementing this kind of research involves a precise choice about how to use the taxpayers' money.[28]

Soldz (2006) warns:

> Models, being idealisations, are not true representations of reality. [...] Thus, there is no such thing as a correct model. (p. 175)

If a scholar like Soldz finds it necessary to clarify such a *basic* point, then it means that he is not talking so much about the methodological aspects of the research in question,[29] as about the whole cultural design and, if we can use the term, about the philosophy of science governing the research designs being examined. The question therefore shifts from the sense of the research projects proposed, to the quality of the referees that evaluate such works for publication, in short, to the quality of the journal hosting them and to its cultural policy; yet again, we underline that, *thinking the worst may be a sin, but it hits the nail on the head*.

In this perspective, a particular position in studies on the efficacy of psychotherapy treatments is occupied by the so-called EST (*Empirically Supported Treatments*), that spring from so-called *evidence-based practice*. It may be interesting to quote on this the critical positions expressed, for instance, by Westen and colleagues (Westen, Morrison, & Thompson-Brenner, 2004), who though identifying some fundamental aporias in this kind of research, do not in our opinion take their analysis to the extreme consequences. They state, in fact, that

> many of the assumptions underlying the methods used to test psychotherapies were themselves empirically untested, disconfirmed, or appropriate only for a range of treatments and disorders. (Westen, Morrison, & Thompson-Brenner, 2004, p. 632).

And also that

> Unqualified statements and dichotomous judgments about validity or invalidity in complex arenas are unlikely to be scientifically or clinically useful, and as a field we should attend more closely to the conditions under which certain empirical methods are useful in testing certain interventions for certain disorders. (*ibidem*, p. 632)

Such statements basically seem to disprove not only the results, but also the overall methodological design of much of the research work in psychotherapy. Now, the malicious question that springs to our lips is the following: since such research work rejects any dimension of complexity (though still invoked by Westen and collaborators!), many of its basic assumptions, as we have tried to show above, immediately prove to contain very little sense, so how can it be that for twenty or thirty years they have found space and dissemination in numerous (respected!) journals, they have enjoyed conspicuous funding, and have involved scholars and researchers in conferences and symposia in many parts of the world? Perhaps once a "gold-bearing" vein is discovered, it is necessary to exhaust it (perhaps while "holding your nose"),[30] before going on to exploit the next one? If the blind adoption of a perspective made up of simplification and reductionism guarantees a consistent "yield," and if it still guarantees it, must we expect that in the near future, an equally sizeable advantage may come from the belated and perhaps fictitious (is it exaggerated to say crafty?), conversion to a hasty, superficial vision of complexity? It is as if the important thing is managing to remain part of the "scene."[31]

We therefore step warily when Westen and colleagues argue that

> however, is that the time has come for a thoroughgoing assessment of the empirical status of not only the data but also the methods used to assign the appellations empirically supported or unsupported. (*ibidem*, p. 632)

And so? How can one justify a debate like the one we have referred to above? Recently Westen (2006/2007) has again returned to the issue, reiterating that

> At a time when to be marketable, a drug or a therapy must prove its efficacy in carefully controlled studies, also psychotherapy—considered a medical therapy—must be promoted on the market of rival therapies and before possible users with a pedigree of empirical proof as to its efficacy.
>
> *The need of experimentation on EST*
>
> The requirements of research and the kind of epistemology and therapeutic modelling referred to by the EST researchers place specific constraints on the studies aimed at elaborating and assessing treatments (Chambless & Ollendick, 2000; Kendall, Marrs-Garcia, Nath, & Shedlrick, 1999; Nathan, Stuart, & Dollan, 2000). Here are some of them:
>
> 1. Psychotherapy validation studies must exclude subjects that undermine the homogeneity of the experimental and control samples.
> 2. The treatments to assess must be short, or at any rate must have a preestablished duration, because the protocol must be the same in all cases and the clinical situation presented by the patients at the beginning, must at the end of the therapy and in the follow-up be just as assessable as all the other conditions.
> 3. The treatments must be aimed at the treatment of a single clinical disorder that can be diagnosed with the psychopathological guidelines accepted by the international community (Goldfried, 2000) and they must be specific to that illness. This is why from the EST validation samples those patients who present comorbidity should be eliminated and the state and possible changes presented by disorders different from those targeted should be ignored. (Wilson, 1998).
> 4. The treatments to assess must be manual-based and the degree of adherence to the protocol of the real practice of the professionals involved in the studies must be monitored.
>
> In short, the EST movement tries to elaborate brief psychotherapy treatments, manual- based and aimed at the treatment of specific disorders, and it assesses them by means of samples of homogeneous subjects treated (and/or assessed) in an identical way and for the same target pathology. (pp. 17–18).

But what kind of psychotherapy and what types of patients are we talking about? About "real" therapies and patients? In the picture we are offered, it seems a little ambivalent to state weakly and overdefensively that

> we are not advocating against evidence-based practice. (Westen, Morrison, & Thompson-Brenner, 2004, p. 632)

A good question would in fact be: but what do we mean by evidence? We have tried to give an answer.

NOT EVERY PROOF IS EVIDENCE, NOT EVERY EVIDENCE IS PROOF

In a recent article—which appeared in the same volume in which we ourselves published one of the pieces cited above (Grasso, & Stampa, 2007)—Mancini and Barcaccia (2007) warn researchers and professionals to translate the expression "evidence based" properly from the English: medicine or psychotherapy based on *scientific proofs*. After quoting a work by Ravaglia (2003) in which the author attacks the concept of "evidence" which he considers philosophically "clumsy," Mancini and Barcaccia write:

> It is hard to prove him wrong. If it were not for the fact that *evidence* means "proof," not "the state of being evident," so *evidence-based* psychotherapy is [...] simply a psychotherapy based on experimental proof of efficacy [...] Nothing to do with the ideological arrogance inherent to the concept of "evident fact." In the domain of science nothing is "self-evident." (p. 130; translation from the Italian original)[32]

There are no objections on the linguistic level: just a slight slap of the wrists for those naive dunces who may have thought of "evidence" in a judicial sense (the suspicion is evoked with elegant understatement by Del Corno & Lang, 2006, p. 59). There is however one small problem, which we would like to point out. Can one talk about "scientific evidence" in the same way in medicine and psychotherapy? Yes and no. "Yes," if we are thinking of an abstract experimental condition, which manages to annul the context—not an easy feat. It is not simple matter, for instance to study tolerance to frustration, or the anxiety state (see clinical sketch n. 2 reported above) or the evocative memory, independently from the emotional/institutional dimension in which the setting develops, from the relationship between the experimenter/observer/agent and the experimental subject—which depends on several factors: personality, institution and organisation of the setting, implicit ideology of the conceptual design of the research and many others—and independently from the connections existing deep in the subject between the processes of acquiring, storing and elaborating information, of attention and concentration. And then it depends on the subject's basic culture and abilities etc. And yet this "yes" seems to dissolve in a labyrinth of uncontrollable variables.

And on the other hand, "no," one cannot talk about "scientific evidence" in psychology in the same way as in the natural sciences that underlie the thinking and the practice of medicine. The physiology experiments, the results of which were contrasted to the first Freudian approach—the exploration of the unconscious using hypnosis—still tell us little or nothing about how human beings, including therapists and patients, interact with each other.

We have already dealt with this question in Grasso and Stampa (2006), arguing as follows:

> In medicine, the distinction between "normality" in the statistical sense and in the clinical sense is at the centre of a literature that is now consolidated and clear in its conceptual structure (...). Most people have certain disturbances, produced precisely by the human organism's capacity to adapt to environmental conditions and individual and collective lifestyles in constant development: despite this, such disturbances have to be diagnosed, treated, "managed," subjected to adequate preventive measures where possible and so forth.
>
> The attitude on the part of medicine is made possible by the logical chain of knowledge that unwinds like a real hierarchy of knowledge: physics → chemistry → biology → physiology → general pathology → special pathologies → semeiotics... each of these disciplinary areas is methodologically "supported" by the one before it in the list.
>
> Now, thanks to this conceptual "pyramid," it can be established what "ideal" functioning is—and hence "normal" in a certain subject and in certain conditions—of an internal organ; and the range of variability that probabilistically defines its possibility of continuing to perform its role in the organism; and (if possible) how to intervene to ensure that the functionality is within this range. If and when it exceeds the upper and lower limits, a pathology is called a defect or an excess: also the second case is a deficit because the point is that "normal" functionality has been compromised. (p. 109; translation from the Italian original)

It is impossible to apply the same epistemological picture to psychology. There is nothing, in mental life that can easily be ranked, ordered, studied and, even less, modified using a linear logical procedure like the one schematised above.

At this point, we would like to say a few words in favour of a model of psychotherapy actually based on what is obvious, instead of on presumed "evidence." Del Corno and Lang (2006), quoted above, write on this:

> But what can we define as "evident"? Without getting into a philosophical discussion that would lead us astray (and that perhaps should be done,

> sooner or later),[33] we have to acknowledge that the "evidence" sought by those who investigate the efficacy of a psychotherapy is not confined to the domain of what is measurable in the best RCT tradition.[34] There is a more blurry or *fuzzy* area that belongs to the patient's subjectivity (as well as to that of the psychotherapist) and to the relationship between them. (p. 59; translation from the Italian original)

Moreover, what can possibly be meant in the DSM-IV-TR, when it says, on "Criteria for substance-induced disturbances,"

> B. There is *evidence*[35] from the history, physical examination, or laboratory findings of either (1) or (2):
> (1) The symptoms developed during, or within a month of, Substance Intoxication or Withdrawal.
> (2) Medication use is etiologically related to the disturbance.
> C. The disturbance is not better accounted for by a disorder that is not substance induced [...]. (American Psychiatric Association, 2000, p. 7)

It really seems that also in the *DSM-IV-TR*, as the support to descriptive psychopathology, there is a reassertion of the contextual paradigm, which is medicine's oldest model of clinical reasoning, based on the evidence. This is not "self-evidence"—a privilege accorded by science only to Euclid's first four postulates (the unnaturalness of the fifth postulate being the foundation of non-Euclidian geometries)—but the evidence deriving from an appropriate use of the procedure called "abduction."

For many years, the working group connected to some of the Psychology chairs at the University of Rome "La Sapienza" and to the *Rivista di Psicologia Clinica* has supported the model of the contextual paradigm as the best suited to explanation and interpretation in clinical psychology. In the Editorial of one of the last issue of *Rivista di Psicologia Clinica*, R. Carli (2007) again reminded us that he has repeatedly devoted articles to the question over the last twenty years:

> Recently, with some colleagues interested in assessment in, I posed a question which at that time remained unanswered: *What are the factors that have made psychotherapy an activity sought after and followed by a great many people in most of the world, despite the lack of valid research that can definitively prove the efficacy of psychotherapy, in its results and its process?* I think Clinical Psychology can assume two very different attitudes to this question. On the one hand, there are those who are trying to operationalise clinical psychology procedure so as to make it a diagnostic and therapeutic action with its standards and its protocols, with the aim of returning to the mainstream of western medicine, organised within deductive and inductive epistemology. This means that abductive logic is completely ignored: the paradigm of clues founded and supported, as Carlo Ginsburg reminds us, by *physicians* like Arthur Conan Doyle (the creator of Sherlock Holmes), Giovanni Morelli (founder of attributionism in painting)

> and Sigmund Freud. On the other hand, there are those who wonder what "force" lies in the Clinical Psychology intervention and in psychotherapy, what evaluation of it has enabled it to develop even without the contribution of the empirical approach. Perhaps those who practise psychotherapy organise its testing [Author's note: In meetings with psychotherapist colleagues, I suggested a testing "criterion" for psychotherapy work: the fact that the patient keeps returning to the psychotherapist, session after session. This statement may seem naive and misleading to some. I think one should consider it. Perhaps we have not yet identified the symbolic reasons for this "patient return," session after session; on the other hand, if this fact is considered apart from obligations and duties, it has an amazing force which deserves to be understood] a part of the procedure itself, in the relationship and the symbolic process characterising it. If that is the area where the testing should be sought, then the objectivisation of the disorder, the insistence on substituting the "objective" disorder for the problem as an eminently relational phenomenon, are aspects that may lead away from the more worthwhile road. (p. 217–218)

Let us return to *evidence* in the sense of a modality of knowledge-getting incorporated in the contextual paradigm. It is well-known that during the twentieth century, the prevailing logic in scientific research—thanks to the theoretical work of the neo-positivists, the Vienna Circle, and Popper and Khun—veered progressively towards hypothetical-deductive models, in which the departure point of an experiment concerning a phenomenon is the previous research on the same class of phenomena and the corresponding theories of reference: after the formulation of the hypothesis, observation is used to verify it (in Popper, to falsify it).

As has been pointed out by many scholars, the limit of this method is psychological: see for instance, Gangemi (2002):

> [...] every researcher reads many books on research or theory, formulates a more or less credible, more or less important theory of his own, and then tends to seek data that confirms his theory. Normally, he does this by looking for the data in which it is easier to find confirmation instead of following Popper's lesson that theories must be put to the test by trying to find evidence against them, not in their favour. (p. 87; translation from the Italian original)

This problem arises all the more when the theories and hypotheses concern research fields in which the variables are highly complex and their observation involves a massive "intrusion": if Heisenberg's principle of indetermination works in particles physics, it is amplified as the scale of the phenomena grows until psychological, social and anthropological research in which the researcher may aspire to be "neutral" or "noninterfering," is made literally impossible.

Alternatively, inductive models are still present and being used in research: an example could be the *grounded theory* of Glaser and Strauss

(1967), in which the formulation of hypotheses comes after the collection of data in the field

> In discovering theory, one generates conceptual categories or their properties from evidence, then the evidence from which the category emerged is used to illustrate the concept. (p. 23):

Therefore, here too, *evidence* is again seen as something in the data that strikes the observer—we would add, reflecting the part played by the observer in the context that the data itself belongs to.

In the abductive model, first formulated by Ch. S. Peirce (Peirce, 1935/1966), the process of collecting the data, formulating and testing the hypothesis follows a path that enables adjustments to be made during the operation: the hypotheses are formulated, accepted or rejected, and reformulated depending on whether or not they satisfy a criterion of maximum plausibility as regards the phenomenon observed.

The contextual paradigm supporting abductive reasoning, as C. Ginzburg (1979, pp. 111–115) pointed out, suggested a clear break with the traditional scientific paradigm, but at the same time, accounted for an empirical way of proceeding that was at once rigorous and a source of reasonable certainties and that had always been typical of humanity, from hunting times among primitive men, through the writing of history, and the philological study of ancient languages, to the sedimentation of clinical experience in medicine:

Between the Galilean physicist professionally deaf to sounds and insensitive to tastes and smells, and his contemporary the physician who risked making diagnoses by placing his ear to rattling chests, sniffing faeces and tasting urine, the contrast could not be greater.

The data on which abductive reasoning is based are *empirical facts*: but it is the observer himself that confers this status on certain data. The view of Peirce (1935–1966) of the three different logical procedures is the following:

Deduction	Rule:	All the beans from this sack are white.
	Case:	These beans are from this sack.
	Result:	These beans are white.
Induction	Case:	These beans are from this sack.
	Result:	These beans are white.
	Rule:	All the beans from this sack are white. (until proven otherwise)
Abduction	Result:	These beans are white.
	Rule:	All the beans from this sack are white.
	Case:	These beans are from this sack (probably)

Since Peirce suggests it, let us go back to the time of Galileo Galilei.

A good example of an erroneous deductive reasoning is in the chain of inferences that lead a minor character of *Promessi sposi* (Manzoni, 1840/1988), don Ferrante, to conclude that the plague is an illusion:

> *In rerum natura*, he said, "there are only two species of things: substances and accidents; and if I prove that the contagion can be neither one nor the other, I will have proved that it does not exist, that it is a chimera. And here I am. Substances are either spiritual or material. That the contagion is a spiritual substance, is a wild claim that no-one would support; so it is no use talking about it. Material substances are either simple or composite. Now contagion is not simple substance; and this can be demonstrated in four words. It is not an airy substance; if it were, instead of passing from one body to another, it would fly straight to its sphere. It is not acqueous; because it would become wet, and be dried by the winds. It is not igneous; because it would burn. It is not earthen; because it would be visible. Nor is it a composite substance; because in any case it should be sensible to the eye and to the touch; and this contagion, who has seen it? Who has touched it? It remains to be seen whether it can be an accident. Worse than worse [...]".
>
> *His fretus*, that is, trusting in these argumentations, he took no precautions against the plague, he caught it, and went to bed to die, like a hero from Metastasio, blaming the stars. (Chapter XXXVII; translation from Italian original)

The theory of the four elements linked to the syllogistics of Aristotle (who in fact was a great, open-minded observer of nature) did not enable the erudite fool don Ferrante to make hypotheses on the physical nature of the illness, and the deductive procedure provided the logical demonstration of this. But equally wrong was the conclusion reached inductively by the people and by the Health Tribunal on the same question: since at the same time as the plague was spreading, along the roads sinister figures had been seen daubing the walls with an oily potion, it was inferred that there was a cause and effect relation between the two events, and by arbitrary generalisation, the myth of the "plague spreaders" was created. The result was a totally futile method of fighting the epidemic, hunting them, as also the good Renzo Tramaglino was to discover to his cost. Manzoni writes at the end of Chapter XXXII:

> The magistrates, weakened every day, and more and more bewildered and confused, used all, so to speak, the little determination in their powers, to search for these plague spreaders [...] The trials that resulted were certainly not the first of that kind: and neither can they be considered a rarity in the history of the law. So, not to mention ancient times, but just something of the times closer to the age we are dealing with, in Palermo, in 1526; in Geneva, in 1530, then in 1545, then again in 1574; in Casal Monferrato, in 1536; in Padova, in 1555; in Torino, in 1599, and again in that same year 1630,

> sometimes one person, sometimes many wretches, were tried and condemned to tortures, mostly atrocious, as being guilty of spreading the plague with powders or with unguents, or with *malle*, or with all these together. (translation from Italian original)

On the other hand, it is historically well-known that at least in the Republic of Venice, the authorities responsible for protecting the population from the plague had understood very well that the epidemic spread in a circular fashion starting from certain critical centres, and the best way to contain it was to set up around these centres a "health barrier"; this often coincided with the course of a river, along which it was easier to control movements and to forbid travellers to pass (Cipolla, 2007).

This seems to have been the result of an abduction:

1. *Result*: in the towns and along the thoroughfares leading out of *x*, *y*, and *z* cases of plague were found in the days following those when the plague appeared in *x*, *y*, and *z*.
2. *Rule*: in the days after the plague appeared in places *a*, *b*, and *c*, there were cases in places *x*, *y*, and *z* which are situated along the thoroughfares.
3. *Case*: the plague (though we do not know how) spreads to towns along the thoroughfares (probably).

It followed that it was wise to close the thoroughfares in order to stop the epidemic from spreading. Abduction, Peirce underlines continually, not unlike deduction and induction, is a way the mind work spontaneously, but it is distinguished by its eminently pragmatic character: it serves to take decisions in the presence of "dirty" and/or partial data, since we may never have at our disposal data that is complete and/or "pure" enough.

It is all too true that the problem of criteria that somehow guarantee the reliability of the interventions, psychological interventions in our case, goes further than the understandable concerns of insurance companies and primarily involves the interests and rights of the clients/patients. Klerman (1989) starting from the discussion of the "Osheroff case" defines this problem with the expression the "challenge of efficacy," and that is linked to themes of great importance, not only clinical but also ethical and juridical (Stampa, 1990).[36] To the "challenge" proposed by Klerman, Stone(1989) juxtaposed the importance for a *respectable minority* of the scientific–professional community to have the possibility to put into practice models of clinical evaluation and therapeutic intervention not subject to the reassuring conformism of the guidelines, standards and protocols of diagnosis-care.

It is an open question. We therefore claim the independent space of a *respectable minority*, who do not accept the principle of a clinical psychology *ancilla medicinae*, and as such forced to accept the ideological illusion of a biological paradigm incorrectly applied to mental life.

What seems to us all the more misleading and confusing is the attitude of these researchers and professionals who seek a mediation between incompatible requirements, in the name of a neutral "scientificness" which gets its paradigms from natural sciences and restores medicine—in whose domain the contextual paradigm[37] was created—to a system of impoverished "evidence" of relational aspects, in which the observer is here and the object is there, and if the observer himself is the subject of the clinical act (in psychotherapy anything else really is rather improbable.) the subjectivity is "objectified" through computation.

And such behaviour seems all the more paradoxical (yet again!) when it is found among psychoanalysts, who on subjectivity as a working tool have age-old references at their disposal, repeatedly discussed, reviewed, corrected, perfected ...

The problem of the "scientific" nature of psychoanalysis was posed right from the beginning, when the young Freud was accused by the Viennese doctors of playing around with a charlatan's methods, and several thousands of pages have been devoted to the issue during the twentieth century and in these early years of the third Millennium: we will not even try to sum up its general outlines here, but we want to quote a comment made by E. Roudinesco (1999) relevant to the more limited topic we are dealing with. While psychoanalysis was able to save itself from Nazism thanks to the massive emigration of European Freudians towards the American continent between 1930 and 1940, this happened at the cost of a radical transformation of its ideals, its practice and its theory. The extremely pragmatic American therapists eagerly appropriated Freudian ideas. However, they immediately tried to *measure* sexual energy, to *demonstrate* the efficacy of the treatments by multiplying the *statistics* and to investigate whether the concepts were applicable empirically to the concrete problems of individuals. We have already expressed ourselves (Grasso, & Stampa, 2007) on this aspect of homologation of mental health to social conformism—and the consequent homologation of the process of "healing" to the client/patient's gradual assent to standards of self-representation consistent with those proposed by the establishment (it is inevitable that this corresponds to the preparatory homologation of the therapist to the same standards ...)

As Roudinesco maintains, in these conditions, across the Atlantic, independently of the orientations, psychoanalysis became the tool for an adaptation of man to a utopia of happiness. It took hold far less due to its system of thought or to the philosophical questions it raised, than to its capacity to bring an immediate solution to the sexual morality of the liberal and puritan society. After catalysing the elaboration of the psychiatric gnoseology for thirty-odd years, psychoanalysis was finally rejected. Did not the psychotropes or other explanatory models of psychism, based on the *DSM-IV* and on new cerebral mythologies, perhaps provide faster therapeutic solutions than those famous "disorders"[38] that fixed the subject in a behavioural symptomatology? So, as the historian Nathan Hale (1971) so well underlines, the American anti-Freud partisans between 1970 and 1990 put forward brilliant assessments, tests and investigations: a whole experimental arsenal unsuited to explaining the reality of psychoanalytical practice and theory.[39]

CONCLUDING REMARKS

One last comment: Most scholars engaged in the wide-ranging debate over research methods in psychotherapy seem to think of the question of its very possibility in diametrically opposed terms, at opposite extremes: as if a finding, an encoding and a rigorous mathematical treatment of the data were the only alternative to the rhapsodic intuition of imaginative therapists dangerously given to caprice or to intellectual *divertissement* at the expense of the reproducibility of "guaranteed" results.

The question of placing this whole problem in a broader perspective deserves future study: our epoch is fraught with numerous ideological illusions, whose greatest common denominator seems to be the widespread fantasy of producing safety and well-being through the use of "techniques" based on simple, a-contextual or metacontextual ideas, of general value—"creative finance" that generates money from money, without going through goods; the "war on terror," carried out on the one hand with traditional weapons, on the other with police measures, almost as if Islamic fanaticism could be identified with a country, with an "other" similar to the perfidious SPECTRE of the James Bond films;[40] the proliferation and uncontrolled spread of information technologies beyond all extra-technological control, as if their development should automatically produce nothing but positive effects (Stampa, 2006); and we could go on at length (remember Prozac, the "happiness pill" for example? …)[41]

What is the inevitable path of an illusion? There is no doubt—it is *evidently*—the final disillusionment. And in this strategic vision, the contrast between intellectual *divertissement* versus rigidity seems to us all the more dangerous for the future of psychotherapy as a discipline oriented to favouring the growth and development of the individual, instead of being interested in finding deficits and/or shortcomings to reclaim; moreover, we think that this controversy is of more interest to academic groups and circles than to the real professional practice of those involved as therapists and as "patients" in the complex "work" of psychotherapy.

We hope, with the optimism of goodwill, that we can find points of contact and integration between the two viewpoints: although the pessimism of reason points—and we hope we are wrong—towards other perspectives.

NOTES

*. A previous version of this chapter has been published with the title "Are We Really So Sure "We're Not in Kansas Anymore"? Quantitative Methods and Research Epistemology in Psychotherapy: A Critical Perspective", on *Rivista di Psicologia Clinica* [On line Journal] 1/2008–. Retrieved from http://www.rivistadipsicologiaclinica. it/english/number1_08/Grasso_Stampa. Htm.

1. Dedicated to those readers who love references even for the jokes—respectively, *Thus Spoke Zarathustra. A Book for All and None*: "Once the sacrilege against God was the greatest sacrilege, but God died, and then all these desecrators died."(Nietzsche, 1883–1885/2006; p. 6 English translation); and Section 481 of the posthumous collection published under the title of *The Will to Power* (Nietzsche, 1901/1910).
2. Famous movie directed by Victor Fleming with screenplay by Noel Langley, Florence Ryerson, Edgar Allan Wolfe, USA 1939, starring the 17-year-old Judy Garland. The film was based on the book by L. Frank Baum who wrote numerous children's stories about Oz, the fantastic land that owes its name to the two letters identifying the bottom drawer of the writer's filing cabinet. The film refers specifically to the book *The Wonderful Wizard of Oz* (Baum, 1900).
3. Those who have worked with psychosociology of organisations will recall a management by objectives slogan of the 1960s–1970s: "For every complex problem there is an answer that is clear, simple and wrong" (H. L. Mencken quoted in Odiorne, 1979).
4. The traps that can be hidden on this golden road were dealt with by, among others, Stuart M. Kaminsky (1978) in his most enjoyable Murder on the *Yellow Brick Road*.
5. On the other hand, it is Dorothy herself who paradoxically, but only seemingly, quickly gives up the fleeting and unfounded elation of the dream and the escape—"*There's no place like home*"—, like the right minded, conformist America of the 1930s–1940s, and soon proves to be the most strenuous defender of traditional values, conformism and the return to "normality." And as we have already got onto this subject, it is worth recalling the comments on the world of Oz and its deep roots in the "foundation myths" of the culture of the United States, made by a thoughtful critic, Neil Earle, who in *The Wonderful Wizard of Oz in American Popular Culture: Uneasy in Eden* (1993), argues that the work contains a series of profoundly American themes: the Frontier, the importance of hard work, the possibility of getting what you want and making your dreams come true thanks to personal gifts like willpower, intelligence, courage, a good heart, and lastly individual liberty seen as an absolute value. To further extend our metaphor, all these qualities and these values put together perhaps make a good pioneer, but—so it seems to us—they are not enough (and some are superfluous) to make a good *scientist-practitioner* in the field of psychology–psychiatry–psychotherapy…
6. *Cfr. Emperor's New Suit,* in *The Complete Hans Christian Andersen Fairy Tales* (edited by Lily Owens) (1981), New York: Avenel Books. "*Men han har jo ikke noget paa,*" in the original Danish "*Keiserens nye Klæder,*" published on

7 April 1837 in the collection "*Eventyr, Fortalte for Børn. Første Samling. Tredie Hefte*"

7. Probably the X-2 form of the *State-Trait Anxiety Inventory* by Spielberger, Gorsuch, & Lushene (1970).
8. The expression is well-known as belonging to the Russian sociologist P. A. Sorokin (1956), whose work it would be interesting to reexamine on another occasion
9. The reader will understand this use of italics by reading on.
10. For the sake of brevity, we quote only the first reference in historical order to this expression, which then became commonly used in Italy in the over twenty years of literature on *Analysis of the Demand*.
11. This is a method for empirical evaluation of adaptation's conditions, used in the *DSM* (note added).
12. A note of some interest to the not American reader may be as follows. The "American interest" of which we speak here arises from the Declaration of Independence of 1776, which states that all men are equal and all have equal rights, including the "pursuit of happiness" that since then repeatedly marked both the pedagogical and psychological literature that the activity of the institutions and even the law of that country: countless decisions of American courts have been and are still based on this principle.
13. A work that is part of a line in the debate that though almost totally unknown (so far) in Italy, is very lively in the United States, at least since, under the presidency of G. W. Bush, evangelical fundamentalism has become more and more closely aligned with conservative political culture. The interference of religious thought in the scientific field (think of the renewed opposition to Darwin in school curricula, or the anti-abortion movement that has reached peaks of violence never seen before) is also active in the fields of psychology and psychiatry. In response to numerous studies seeking to prove the beneficial effects of prayer and attendance of places of worship on the physical and mental health, the prestigious *New England Journal of Medicine* published in 2000 an article by Sloan and colleagues (Sloan et al., 2000) underlining that "prescribing" these practices for patients is to be considered useless and ethically incorrect.
14. We must admit that we wondered how a longitudinal research covering at least 65 years could have been implemented and carried out. This equivocation is created by Vaillant's exposition. In actual fact, by checking the original text by Danner, Snowdon and Friesen (2001), we were able to see that the autobiographical notes studied were not standardised: the researchers had access to the archives of the congregation of the American School Sisters of Notre Dame and worked on dishomogeneous material that was created for internal use (for social control, to have a basis for future obituaries, etc.). For all the Notre Dame nuns there is a document of self-presentation, written on their entry into the convent: those of nuns born before 1917 were used in the research, using language indicators to extract the positive and negative emotions then correlated to the life-span. Apart from the method used for this extrapolation, why was the exact heuristic value of those documents not considered? Two of them are given below.

Sister 1 (low positive emotion)—"[...] My candidate year was spent in the Motherhouse, teaching Chemistry and Second Year Latin at Notre Dame Institute. With God's grace, I intend to do my best for our Order, for the spread of religion and for my personal santification."

Sister 2 (high positive emotion)—"God started my life off well by bestowing upon me a grace of inestimable value [...] The past year which I have spent as a candidate studying at Notre Dame College has been a very happy one. Now I look forward with eager joy to receiving the Holy Habit of Our Lady and to a life of union with Love Divine" (p. 806).

We therefore wish to point out our doubts about this research.

15. "Our faith in qualitative clinical methods follows the principle that human communication can cover multiple levels of meaning beyond the most external or manifest ones, and that these meanings emerge more readily when communication is not rigidly structured (cf. Weinberger & McClelland, 1990) and that another human being is the best (and perhaps still the only) "tool" to record these meanings" (Shedler, Mayman & Manis, 1993, p. 1118).
16. Wakefield's definition has in fact been identified by some as the expression of a "biological reductionism" that does not take into account the aspect of *complexity* (cfr. Hansell, & Damour, 2005). Besides this, also the indistinct nature of the concept of disorder has been underlined (cfr. Kirmayer & Young, 1999), as we are trying to argue here.
17. However, Hansell and Damour (2005) do not agree; in their textbook they stress, on the other hand, the substantial convergence between the operative definition of mental disorder given by *DSM-IV-TR*, which includes many vague expressions like "clinically significant" or "behavioral, psychological and biological dysfunction" and that of "harmful dysfunction," as the collapse and consequent damage of a evolutionary human mental function, proposed by Wakefield.
18. Notice the use of this expression here: and keep it in mind later in this article, when we will go on to examine the uses in the scientific domain of the word "evidence" and its derivates.
19. Think of the mediatic furor caused by the controversial presence of the Pope at the opening of the 2007/2008 academic year at the "Sapienza" University of Rome.
20. Literally, "mania of running away," in the sense of the unauthorised leaving of an obligatory place; "deserting": in Greek military language *drapètes* (from the verb *drapetèuo*, run away, escape) is a deserter (*our note*). One interesting thing: the rough and short-sighted Confederate doctors did not realise that the culture produced in this sort of epidemic was not confined to expressing suffering, faith and hope, but also contained precise and constantly updated sub-codes with precise instructions for the treatment of the "symptom." As G. C. Roncaglia (2006) recalls, as regards spirituals, Martin Luther King pointed out that this way of singing was also a way for the blacks to communicate among themselves without their masters understanding, even if they were present: "We used to sing of the "heaven" waiting for us," wrote the leader of the black civil rights movement, "[and] the word "heaven" for us

meant "Canada," which we hoped to be able to reach." The songs contained directions in code about "safe houses, refuges, resting places and shelters" in a long chain that from the deep South "permitted and supported the flight of slaves across the United States as far as the border with hospitable Canada."

21. It is interesting to notice, as Sanders Thompson, Bazile and Akbar (2004) underline, that in matters of mental health, African Americans seem to prefer to go to emergency outpatients services: these facilities are in fact preferred because it is possible to be examined regardless of the ability to pay and, equally important, one can avoid being stigmatised, strongly felt when one goes to a public service, since it is difficult for *others* to ascertain the type of services needed. There is almost the need to hide the psychic behind the reassuring "free", shared somatic fragility to be helped and cared for—common to blacks and whites, rich and poor.

22. It seems, moreover, that there are many other things that are better than prozac—begging the pardon of some people and of the drug companies—and that have far fewer side effects: it is worth recalling here that these also include psychotherapy. It also received attention in the non specialist press (*The Guardian, The Times, The Independent* reported it; cf. also Franceschini, 2008), a work carried out by the Department of Psychology of Hull University in Great Britain, in collaboration with United States and Canadian universities and Clinical Centers (cf. Kirsch, Deacon, Huedo-Medina, Scoboria, Moore & Johnson, 2008) which, after reviewing numerous studies on the subject, reaches the conclusion that there are no significant differences between the improvement obtained with a placebo and that obtained with so-called "second generation" antidepressants (referring to the most common drugs in the antidepressant spectrum, known as SSRI—*Selective Serotonin Reuptake Inhibitors*—Prozac, Efexor, Seroxat).

23. Surfing the net, one can make some interesting and strange discoveries. For instance one finds out that in Italy there are at least two important associations linked to *philosophical counseling* (and we are certainly neglecting others): one, with some psychological contamination at least in the title, the AIP (Italian Associated Psychophilosophers), the other SICOF (Italian Society of Philosophic Counseling), which has its own school, a journal, and even a professional register (?) with a list of members. One can also read, gleaning information from the CVs that are given by the most representative exponents, that some of them can boast a basic training with specialisations in psychiatry, and perhaps professional competences linked to hypnosis, sexology, and even electroconvulsive therapies, as is shown also by teaching and publications: *primum vivere*, one might say, as the old adage warned, *deinde philosophari*. Moreover, one may discover the recent establishment of the International Functional Neurology Society, which, with the aim of in-depth examination of issues like neuroethics and neurophilosophy, in Decemebr 2007 in Rome held its first conference entitled "Neurophilosophy: the early years and new directions."

We can even discover that there is a *Center Sophon* which has for some time been offering the service of *Philoso-phone* which intends to provide, over the phone, "a first-aid hot-line for ethical dilemmas and existential problems" (cf. www.geocities.com/centersophon/pc-sophon.html).

24. And what about what happens to the psychotherapist in relation to a certain patient, *outside* the therapeutic setting?

25. Specifically: *Overwhelmed/Disorganised, Helpless/Inadeguate, Positive, Special/Overinvolved, Sexualized, Disengaged, Parental/Protective, Mistreated/Criticized* (Cfr. Zittel, & Westen, 2003). More than just a comment should be devoted to the presence of the dimension defined as *positive*. This is because this definition seems to us to be clearly connected to the reductionist perspective underlying the whole operation: yet again the connotation of complexity that is inherent to the concept of countertransference is simplified into a basic positive/negative dichotomy. One might then ask, positive or negative for whom, for what, and above all, in what sense? One might answer that obviously, positive and negative are to be seen in relation to the progress of the treatment underway: as if *positive* countertransference, to use the term proposed, were not already in itself a complication for a psychotherapist, but as if it were simply, as seems to be implied, *non-countertransference*, a non obstacle. In short, countertransference, in this perspective, may be there, and in this case, if it is not connoted negatively, it is nonexistent: is the positive pole equated to normality and the negative one to pathology? It would actually seem so, with the not negligible result, in our view, that normality is seen at the same time, as an absence of response to the relationship offered by the other, in a word, as an absence of relationship.

26. Might countertransference be, in the term used today, a *pan-theoretical concept?* This little formula is used for example for the therapeutic alliance (Horvath, 2005a). It seems to us to be a shortcut to avoid arming oneself with the conceptual rather than empirical tools to account for and make sense of what happens in the relational dynamics of psychotherapy.

27. *By the by*, life senator Giulio Andreotti, indestructible icon of the Italian political scene since the postwar period, who is credited by the *vox populi* with being the author (!) of the saying, has several times ceded the honour to an unnamed cardinal of the Vatican Secretariat of State.

28. We are advised, for instance, that the work cited by Crits-Christoph and Gallop (2006), "was funded in part by National Institute on Drug Abuse Grants R01-DA018935 and R21-DA016002" (p. 180). Our curiosity is whetted: what is the connection between drug abuse and therapist influence in psychotherapy, from the point of view of research funding? Don't they seem, at first sight, different issues and therefore with different sources of financial resources? Perhaps part of the explanation can be found in the simultaneous presence in the same journal, but in a different section, of an article on drugs and counseling written by the same authors (Cfr. Barber, Gallop, Crits-Christoph, Frank, Thase, Weiss, & Connolly Gibbons, 2006)?

29. Although, also at this level, Soldz feels the need to point out several things that seem to us not unimportant. In fact, they seem so important that they cast doubt on much (all?) of the research dealing with these issues: "it is important to keep in mind that the TDCRP data set, although one of the

larger psychotherapy data sets, is quite small for sustaining the analyses reported here" (p. 175).

30. *By the by* 2, this other widespread totally Italian commonplace was claimed by the well-known journalist Indro Montanelli concerning his vote for the Christian Democrats in the turbulent 1970s, when the Communist Party seemed to be about to gain the relative majority in Parliament.
31. On this point, an in-depth study should be made of the importance for psychologists and psychiatrists of publishing in journals with a high impact factor (IF), to which it is not easy to gain access if the experimental design of the work presented does not respond to the standard research criteria in the natural sciences field. Although this should not have much importance (in fact it has "zero") from the point of view of clients/patients, it has a very great deal for the professionals and researchers whose access to prestigious positions in Universities and Health Services, public and private funding, etc, depends on the IF. In Italy, too, some doctors have temporary contracts with Scientific Research Institutes (IRCCS) with payment directly proportional to the IF. We will examine this issue on another occasion.
32. The short-circuit "evidence = self-evidence" here seems to be highly significant of the pressure to eliminate subjectivity from science in general. It did not come into Mancini and Barcaccia's heads that a real fact could be "evident" *for somebody that enters a relationship with that fact*, rather than evident "in itself"? There are also some who, when faced with the same fact, do not find it obvious: it is the classic gag of Holmes & Watson, of Poirot & Hastings, or other detective couples when faced with the clues to a crime. We deal with the question a little later in this chapter.
33. We agree: and let us eliminate the "perhaps," and replace "sooner or later" with "soon." We in our humble way are already trying (our note).
34. The reference is obviously to the Randomised Clinical Trials model, in which the patients are assigned randomly to different groups with different kinds of treatment, in (theoretically) controlled conditions (our note).
35. Our italics.
36. The case concerns legal proceedings taken by a Dr. Osheroff, against the clinic of Chestnut Lodge, in which a psychotherapy approach had been tried with the depressive phase of his bipolar disorder. In the first weeks, the clinical picture worsened considerably compared to the situation on admission and the patient was admitted to another clinic, obtaining a rapid remission of the symptoms (we do not know the length of time) thanks to the application of a standard protocol of therapy with antidepressants and electroshock. Chestnut Lodge decided to settle out of court and paid Dr. Osheroff a substantial sum as reimbursement. The affair (from 1983) gave rise to a heated debate between supporters of experimenting with innovative approaches to mental disorders and supporters of the need to provide patients with prior, reasonable guarantees of positive results in terms of remission of symptomatology.
37. On this, see a book, which has aroused interest and curiosity in some sectors of our country's medical world: *Evidence-Based Medicine in Sherlock Holmes'*

Footsteps by Jorgen Nordenstrom (2006), in which the author—who works at the Karolinska teaching hospital in Stockholm—proposes an application of the abductive procedure for the collection of clinical information and the monitoring of treatments.

38. Significant, though not developed by the author, is this reference to the *disorders* that psychopathology tends to deal with descriptively and "objectively": the term itself evokes the break with a previous order, and the resulting confusion and malaise (due to the prefix *dys-* which from Ancient Greek we translate with a pejorative of the term it is linked to; in Rocci dictionary, Rocci, 1974, *ad vocem*, "indicates opposition, contrariness, doubt, difficulty, uncertainty, pain"). The breakdown of this order in mental life is therefore an existential event or condition, which appears *before* the psychopathology intervenes to describe, classify, and impose gnoseographic "discipline."
39. Any radicalization of this approach had already been opposed in the 1980s by M. Edelson (see above all 1984) with a research program that rejected the objections made by Grünbaum (1977a, 1977b, 1978, 1979) and tried to incorporate the "symptom-context" method of Luborsky (1967, 1973) and the bootstrap strategy of Glymour (1974, 1980): however, his efforts seem to have had little effect on the more recent debate.
40. SPECTRE appears in many 007 films, but in only one Jan Fleming novel, *Thunderball* (1961); here is a definition provided (anonymously) by the best documented of the websites devoted to the legendary character of espionage literature: "The word SPECTRE stands for Special Executor for Counter-Intelligence, Terrorism, Revenge and Extortion. The powerful and ruthless criminal organisation is dedicated to gaining wealth and power though criminal schemes that involve extortion, instigation of major wars to gain power and acts of revenge. Throughout several missions, Bond has been dedicated to the destruction of SPECTRE and its leader, Ernst Stavro Blofeld" (cfr. http://www.mi6.co.uk/sections/villains/spectre.php3).
41. Here, for the sake of brevity, we refer only to the work of Kirsch, and colleagues (2008) on the efficacy of antidepressant drugs, already cited in endnote 22.

REFERENCES

American Psychiatric Association (2000). *Diagnostic and statistical manual of mental disorders* (4th ed. Text revised). Washington, DC: Author.

Barber, J. P., Gallop R., Crits-Christoph, P., Frank, A., Thase, M. E., Weiss, R. D., & Connolly Gibbons, M. B. (2006). The role of therapist adherence, therapist competence, and alliance in predicting outcome of individual drug counseling: results from the National Institute Drug Abuse Collaborative Cocaine Treatment Study. *Psychotherapy Research, 16,* 229–240.

Baum, L. F. (1900). *The wonderful wizard of Oz*, Chicago, IL: G.M.Hill.

Benkirane, R. (2002). *La complexité, vertiges ou promesses: 18 histoire de sciences [The complexity: vertigo or promise. 18 stories of science].* Paris: Editions Le Pommier.

Carli, R. (1987). L'analisi della domanda [Analysis of the demand]. *Rivista di Psicologia Clinica, 1*(1), 38–53.

Carli, R (2007). Editorial. *Rivista di Psicologia Clinica [On line Journal], 3*. Retrived from http://www.rivistadipsicologiaclinica.it/english/number3_07/Editorial.htm.

Casey, R. J., & Berman, J. (1985). The outcome of psychotherapy with children. *Psychological Bulletin, 98*, 388–400.

Chambless, D., & Ollendick, T. (2000). Empirically supported psychological interventions: Controversies and evidence. *Annual Review of Psychology, 52*, 685–716.

Cipolla, C. M. (2007). *Contro un nemico invisibile. Epidemie e strutture sanitarie nell'Italia del Rinascimento [Against an invisible enemy. Epidemics and sanitary structures in the Italian Renaissance]*. Bologna, ITA: Il Mulino.

Crits-Christoph, P., & Gallop, R. (2006). Therapist effects in the National Institute of Mental Health Treatment of Depression Collaborative Research Program and Other Psychotherapy Studies. *Psychotherapy Research, 16*, 178–181.

Danner, D. D., Snowdon, D. A., & Friesen, W. V. (2001). Positive emotions in early life and longevity: findings from the nun study. *Journal of Personality and Social Psychology, 80*, 804–813.

Dazzi, N., & De Coro, A. (2007). Psychotherapy and empirical research: two irreconcilable terms or the blueprint for a new paradigm in clinical psychology? *Rivista di Psicologia Clinica [On line Journal]*. 1. Retrived from http://www.rivistadipsicologiaclinica.it/english/number1_07/editorial.htm.

De Coro, A., & Andreassi, S. (2004). *La ricerca empirica in psicoterapia [Empirical research in psychotherapy]* Roma: Carocci.

Del Corno, F., & Lang, M. (2006). Empirically Supported Treatments vs Empirically Supported Relationships. N. Dazzi, V. Lingiardi, & A. Colli (Eds.), *La ricerca in psicoterapia. Modelli e strumenti* (pp. 49–64). Milano: Raffaello Cortina Editore.

Di Nuovo, S. (2000). Strumenti qualitativi per la ricerca sulla psicoterapia; intervista sul cambiamento terapeutico di R. Elliott [Qualitative tools for the psychotherapy research. The Eliot's interview on the therapetic change]. *Laboratorio di ricerca*, 2–3. Retrieved from http://www.isuri.net/Dinuovo2000.Html.

Earle, N. (1993). *The wonderful wizard of Oz in American popular culture: Uneasy in Eden*. New York, NY: The Edwin Mellen Press.

Edelson, M. (1984). *Hypothesis and evidence in psychoanalysis*. Chicago, IL: University of Chicago Press.

Elkin, I., Falconnier, L., Martinovich, Z., & Mahoney, C. (2006a). Therapist effects in the NIMH treatment of depression collaborative research program. *Psychotherapy Research, 16*, 144–160.

Elkin, I., Falconnier, L., Martinovich, Z., & Mahoney, C. (2006b). Rejoinder to commentaries by Stephen Soldz and Paul Crits-Christoph on therapist effects. *Psychotherapy Research, 16*, 182–183.

Estes, S. G. (1938). Judging personality from expression behavior. *Journal of Abnormal and Social Psychology, 33*, 217–236.

Fleming, J. (1961). *Thunderball*. London: Viking.

Franceschini, E. (2008) (February 27). Addio Prozac & C. Gli scienziati: Farmaci inutili [Goodbye Prozac & Co. Scientists: useless drugs]. *la Repubblica*.

Freud, S. (1964). Constructions in analysis. In J. Strachey (Ed. and Trans.), *The standard edition of the complete psychological works of Sigmund Freud* (Vol. 23, pp. 255–270). London: The Hogarth Press and the Institute of Psycho-analysis. (Original work published 1937).

Galimberti, U. (2004) (December 15). Se un filosofo ti prende in cura [If a philosopher takes care of you]. *la Repubblica*.

Gangemi, G. (2002). *La costruzione sociale della logica. Tra concetti di relazione e concetti di attributi [The social construction of the logics. Between concepts of relationships and concepts of attributes]*. Milano: Giuffré.

Gelso, C. J., & Friedman, S. M. (2000). The development of the inventory of countertransference behavior. *Journal of Clinical Psychology, 56,* 1221–1235.

Ginzburg C. (1979). Spie. Radici di un paradigma indiziario [Spies The root of the clues-based knowledge paradigm] (pp. 59–106). In A. Gargani (Ed.), *Crisi della ragione*, Torino, ITA: Einaudi.

Glaser B. G., & Strauss A. L. (1967). *The discovery of grounded theory: Strategies for qualitative research*. Chicago, IL: Aldine.

Glymour, C. (1974). Freud, Kepler, and the clinical evidence. In Wolheim, R. (Ed.), *Freud. A collection of critical essays* (pp. 285–304), Garden City, NY: Anchor Book.

Glymour, C. (1980). *Theory and evidence*. Princeton: Princeton University Press.

Goldfried, M. (2000). Consensus in psychotherapy research and practice: Where have all the findings gone? *Psychotherapy Research, 10,* 1–16.

Grasso, M. (2006a). Modelli di salute e patologia mentale: implicazioni per la ricerca in psicoterapia [Models of health and mental pathology: Implications for the psychotherapy research]. *Trasformazioni, 2,* 52–73.

Grasso M. (2006b). Nails, (Finger) nails and hammers: Scattered notes on clinical psychology. *Rivista di Psicologia Clinica [On line Journal],* 1. Retrieved from http://www.rivistadipsicologiaclinica.it/english/number1/Grasso.htm.

Grasso, M., & Stampa, P. (2005, September). *Correzione di deficit vs promozione di sviluppo in psicoterapia: implicazioni per la valutazione e per la ricerca clinica [Correction of deficit* vs *promotion of development in psychotherapy: implications for the clinical assessment and reseach]* Paper presented at the V National Conference of the Society for Psychotherapy Research—Italian Group. San Benedetto del Tronto (ITA).

Grasso, M., & Stampa, P. (2006). Chi ha slegato Roger Rabbit? Diagnosi psichiatrica e modelli di salute mentale: osservazioni su alcune criticità metodologiche per la ricerca in psicoterapia [Who Un-framed Roger Rabbit?—Psychiatric diagnosis and models of mental health: Observations on some methodological issues in psychotherapy research]. *Rivista di Psicologia Clinica [On line Journal],* 1. Retrieved from http://www.rivistadipsicologiaclinica.it/italiano/numero1/Stampa_Grasso.htm.

Grasso, M., & Stampa, P. (2007). Diagnosi psichiatrica e modelli di salute mentale: osservazioni su alcune criticità metodologiche per la ricerca in psicoterapia [Psychiatric diagnosis and models of mental health: Observations on some methodological issues in psychotherapy research]. In G. Nicolò, & S. Salvatore (Ed.), *La ricerca sui risultati e sul processo in psicoterapia* (pp. 109–128), Roma: Edizioni Carlo Amore.

Grasso, M., & Stampa, P. (2008) . . . Are we really so sure "We're not in Kansas anymore"? Quantitative methods and research epistemology in psychotherapy: A critical perspective. *Rivista di Psicologia Clinica [On line Journal]. Teoria e metodi dell'intervento*, 1. Retrieved from http://www.rivistadipsicologiaclinica.it/english/number1_08/Grasso_Stampa.htm.

Grasso, M., Cordella, B., & Pennella A. R. (2003). *L'intervento in psicologia clinica. Fondamenti teorici [Intervention in clinical psychology. Theoretical foundations]* Roma: Carocci.

Grünbaum, A. (1977a). How scientific is psychoanalysis? In R. Stern, L. S. Horowitz, & J. Lynes (Eds.), *Science and psychotherapy* (Vol. I, 2nd ed.) (pp. 219–254). New York: Haven Publishing Corp.

Grünbaum, A. (1977b). Is psychoanalysis a pseudo-science? Karl Popper versus Sigmund Freud, (I). *Zeitschrift für philosophische Forschung, 31*, 333–353.

Grünbaum, A. (1978). Is psychoanalysis a pseudo-science? *(II). Zeitschrift für philosophische Forschung*, 32, 49–69.

Grünbaum, A. (1979). Is Freudian psychoanalytic theory pseudo-scientific by Karl Popper's criterion of demarcation? *American Philosophical Quarterly, 16*, 131–141.

Hale, N. G. (1971). *Freud and the Americans*. New York-Oxford: Oxford University Press.

Hansell, J., & Damour, L. (2005). *Abnormal psychology*. New York: John Wiley & Sons.

Hayes J. A., Ricker, J. R., & Ingram, K. M. (1997). Countertransference behavior and management in brief counseling: A field study. *Psychotherapy Research*, 7, 145–153.

Heimann, P. (1950). On counter-transference. *International Journal of Psycho-Analysis, 31*, 81–84.

Hill, C. E. (2006). Introduction to special section on therapist effects. *Psychotherapy Research, 16*, 143.

Horvath, A. O. (2005a). The therapeutic relationship: Research and theory. *Psychotherapy Research, 15*, 3–7.

Horvath, A. O. (2005b) (September). *L'integrazione dei trattamenti e la ricerca* settembre. Paper presented at the V National Conference of the Society for Psychotherapy Research—Italian Group. San Benedetto del Tronto (ITA).

Kaminsky, S. M. (1978). *Murder on the Yellow Brick Road*. New York: St Martin's Press.

Kendall, P. C., Marrs-Garcia, A., Nath, S. R., Sheldrick, R. C. (1999). Normative comparisons for the evaluation of clinical significance. *Journal of Consulting and Clinical Psychology*, 67, 285–299.

Kim, D., Wampold, B. E., & Bolt, D. M. (2006). Therapist effects in psychotherapy: A random effects modeling of the NIMH TDCRP Data. *Psychotherapy Research, 16*, 161–172.

Kirmayer, L. J., & Young, A. (1999). Culture and context in the evolutionary concept of mental disorder. *Journal of Abnormal Psychology, 108*, 446–452.

Kirsch, I., Deacon, B. J., Huedo-Medina, T. B., Scoboria, A., Moore, T. J., & Johnson, B. T. (2008). Initial severity and antidepressant benefits: A meta-analysis of data submitted to the Food and Drug Administration. *PLoS Medicine*, 2. Retrieved from http://www.plosmedicine.org/article/info:doi/10.1371/journal.pmed.0050045.

Klerman, G. L. (1989). Psychotherapy on trial? Osheroff vs. chesnut lodge. *The Harvard Medical School Mental Health Letter*, 4.

Lombardo, G. P., & Malagoli Togliatti, M. (1995). *Epistemologia in psicologia clinica [Epistemology in clinical psychology]* Torino, ITA: Bollati Boringhieri.

Luborsky, L. (1967). Momentary forgetting during psychotherapy and psychoanalysis. *Psychological Issues*, 5(2–3), 175–217.

Luborsky, L. (1973). Forgetting and remembering (momentary forgetting) during psychotherapy: A new sample. *Psychological Issues, 8*(2), 29–55.

Mancini, F., & Barcaccia, B. (2007). Psicoterapia "*cum grano salis*" [Psychotherapy cautiously]. In G. Nicolò, & S. Salvatore (a cura di), *La ricerca sui risultati e sul processo in psicoterapia* (pp. 129–133).Roma: Edizioni Carlo Amore.

Marinoff, L (1999). *Plato, not prozac! Applying philosophy to everyday problems.* New York, NY: HarperCollins.

Manzoni, A. (1988). *I promessi sposi [Promises spouses]* (E. Raimondi & L. Bottoni. Eds.). Milano: Principato. (Original published 1840)

Moretti, N. (1993) (Producer and Director). *Caro Diario [Dear Diary]* [Motion picture]. ITA: Sacher Film.

Nietzsche, F. (2006). *Thus spoke Zarathustra: A book for all and none* (A. De Caro, & R. B. Pippin, Eds., A. De Caro, Trans.). Cambridge: Cambridge University Press. (Original work published 1883–1885).

Nietzsche, F. (1910). The will of power. An attempted transvaluation of all values (A. M. Ludovicy, Trans.). Books one and two. In O. Levy (Ed.), *The complete works of Friedrich Nietzsche*. Edinburgh & London: T.N. Foulis. (Original work published 1901)[§]

Nordenstrom, J. (2006). *Evidence-based medicine in Sherlock Holmes' footsteps.* New York: Blackwell.

Nathan, P. E., Stuart, S. P., & Dolan, S. L. (2000). Research on psychotherapy efficacy and effectiveness: between Scylla and Charybdis. *Psychological Bulletin, 126,* 964–981.

Odiorne, G. S. (1979). *MBO II. A System of Managerial Leadership for the 80s* [it. Trans.: *MBO*, Milano: Sperling & Kupfer, 1985].

Owens,L. (Ed, 1981). *The complete Hans Christian Andersen fairy tales.* New York, NY: Avenel Books.

Peirce, C. S. (1935–1966). *Collected Papers* (C. Hartshorne, P. Weiss, & A. W. Burks. Eds.), Cambridge, MA: Harvard University Press.

Perry, C. J. G. (1965). Psychiatric selection of candidates for space missions. *Journal of the American Medical Association, 194,* 841–844.

Peterson C., & Seligman, M. E. P. (2004). *Character strengths and virtues: A handbook and classification*, Oxford: Oxford University Press.

Pinn, V. W., Harden J. T., & Blehar M. C. (2002). *Outreach notebook: for the inclusion, recruitment and retention of women and minority subjects in clinical research.* U.S. Department of Health & Human Services, Public Health Service, National Institutes of Health Publication No. 03–7036. Retrieved from http://www4.od.nih.gov/orwh/outreach.pdf.

Racker, H. (1968). *Transference and countertransference*. London: Karnac Books.

Rapaport, D. (1967). *The theoretical implications of diagnostic testing procedures.* In M. M. Gill (Ed.) (1967), *The collected papers of David Rapaport* (334-356). New York: Basic Books. (Original work published 1950)

Ravaglia, G. (2003). Psicoterapia "evidence-based." Retrieved September, 15, 2004, from http://www.risorse-psicoterapia.org/movimento_est.htm.

Rocci, L. (1974). *Vocabolario greco-italiano [Greek-Italian Dictionary]*. Milano—Roma—Napoli—Città di Castello: Società Editrice Dante Alighieri—Società Editrice S. Lapi.

Roncaglia, G. C. (2006). *Il jazz e il suo mondo [Jazz and its world]*. Torino, ITA: Einaudi.

Roudinesco, E. (1999). *Pourquoi la psychanalyse? [Why psychoanalysis]*. Paris: Fayard.

Sanders Thompson, V. L., Bazile, A., & Akbar M. (2004). African Americans' perceptions of psychotherapy and psychotherapists. *Professional Psychology: Research and Practice, 1,* 19–26.

Seligman, M. E. P. (1991). *Learned Optimism*. New York: Simon & Schuster.

Seligman, M. E. P. (2002). *Authentic happiness*. New York: Free Press.

Shelder J., Mayman, M., & Manis, M. (1993). The illusion of mental health. *American Psychologist, 48,* 11, 1117–1131.

Sloan, R. P., Bagiella, E., Van de Creek, L., Hover, M., Casalone, C., Hirsch, T., Hasan, Y., Kreger, R., & Polous, P. (2000). Should physicians prescribe religious activities? *New England Journal of Medicine, 342,* 1913–1916.

Snowdon, D. A. (2001). *Aging with grace*. New York: Bantam.

Soldz, S. (2006). Models and meanings: Therapist effects and the stories we tell. *Psychotherapy Research, 16,* 173–177.

Sorokin, P.A. (1956), *Fads and foibles in modern sociology and related sciences*. Chicago, IL: H. Regnery.

Spielberger, C. D., Gorsuch, R. L., & Lushene. R. E. (1970). Manual for the State-trait anxiety inventory. Palo Alto, CA: Consulting Psychologists Press.

Stampa, P. (1990). "Malpractice." Una nota su alcune condizioni epistemologiche e conseguenze pratiche dell' errore in psicologia clinica ["Malpractice". Consideration on some epistemological conditions and practical consequences of the error in clinical psychology]. In P. Colamonico, G. Montesarchio, C. Saraceni (Eds.), *Psicodiagnostica e psicoterapia: "parliamo di errori"* (pp. 147–159). Roma: SIRP (Società Italiana per la Ricerca Psicodiagnostica).

Stampa, P. (2006). Il Piè-veloce Achille ha sorpassato la tartaruga? Una nota sul silenzio degli psicologi nei processi della c. d. "globalizzazione" [Has The fleet foot Achilles surpass the turtle? Considerations on the silence of the psychologist on the dynamics of the so called "globalisation"]. *Rivista di Psicologia Clinica [On line Journal]. Teoria e metodi dell'intervento,* 2 3. Retrieved from http://www.rivistadipsicologiaclinica.it/italiano/numero2_3/Stampa.htm.

Stone, A. A. (1989), A Response to Dr Klerman, *The Harvard Medical School Mental Health Letter*, July, 4–5.

Vaillant, G. E. (2003). Mental health. *American Journal of Psychiatry, 160,* 1373–1384.

Wade, P., & Berstein, B. L. (1991). Cultural sensitivity training and counselor's race: Effects on Black female clients' perception and attrition. *Journal of Counseling Psychology, 38,* 9–15.

Wakefield, J. C. (1992). Disorder as harmful dysfunction: A conceptual critique of DSM-III-R's definition of mental disorder. *Psychological Review, 99,* 232–247.

Wakefield, J. C. (1997). When is development disordered? Developmental psychopathology and the harmful dysfunction analysis of mental disorder. *Development & Psychopathology, 9,* 269–290.

Wakefield, J. C. (1999). Evolutionary versus prototype analyses of the concept of disorder. *Journal of Abnormal Psychology, 108,* 373–399.

Wakefield, J. C. (2004). Realtà e valori nel concetto di salute mentale: il disturbo come disfunzione dannosa [Fact and value in the concept of mental disorder: Disorder as harmful Dysfunction]. *Psicoterapia e Scienze Umane, 38*(4), 439–464.

Wakefield, J. C. (2005). Il concetto di salute mentale: una critica a Vaillant [A critique of Vaillant's concept of positive mental health]. *Psicoterapia e Scienze Umane, 39*(1), 91–96.

Wampold, B. E., & Bolt, D. M. (2006). Therapist effects: Clever ways to make them (and everything else) disappear. *Psychotherapy Research, 16,* 184–187.

Ward, E. C. (2005). Keeping it real: A grounded theory study of African American clients engaging in counseling at a Community Mental Health Agency. *Journal of Counseling Psychology, 4,* 471–481.

Webster's New World Dictionary (1977), New York, NY: Harper Collins.

Weinberger, J., & McClelland D. C. (1990). Cognitive vs traditional motivational models. In R. Sorrentino, & T. Higgins (Eds.). *Handbook of motivation and cognition* (562–597). New York: Guilford Press.

Westen, D., Morrison, K., & Thompson–Brenner, H. (2004). The empirical status of empirically supported psychotherapies: Assumptions, findings, and reporting in controlled clinical trials. *Psychological Bulletin, 130,* 631–663.

Westen, D. (2006). *Making Clinical Research Empirically Relevant* [Lecture notes]. Rome, ITA: University of Rome "La Sapienza." Electronic version: Gazzillo, F., & Lingiardi, V. (Eds.) (2007) Making clinical research empirically relevant: Drew Western's lecture at the Sapienza (14 June 2006). Rivista di psicologica clinica, 1. Retrieved from http://www.rivistadipsicologiaclinica.it/english/number1_07/Gazzillo_Lingiardi.htm.

Wilson, W. (1967). Correlates of avowed happiness. *Psychological Bulletin, 67,* 294–306.

Wilson, G. (1998). Manual-based treatment and clinical practice. *Clinical Psychology: Science & Practice, 5,* 363–375.

Zittel, C., & Westen, D. (2003). *The countertransference questionnaire.* (unpublished manuscript). Emory University.

[§] Nietzsche was not ready, when he died, for an edition of the work first published in 1901 as Vol. XV of *Grossoktav-Ausgabe* (Naumann, & Leipzig, 1901). A second edition in 1906 was overseen by Peter Gast and Elizabeth Förster-Nietzsche (the philospoher's sister) in Vols. IX–X of *Taschen-Ausgabe,* an enriched and expanded version of the first edition, and the one on which almost all the later editions were based.

ABOUT THE AUTHORS

Kenneth R. Cabell. He studies psychology at Clark University, with a focus on cultural psychology and semiotics. His research involves using the complex views of phenomena in psychoanalysis and applying them in a semiotic-cultural framework. He is an editorial associate of *Culture & Psychology* (Sage). Address: Kenneth R. Cabell, Clark University, Psychology Department, 950 Main Street, Worcester, MA 01610, USA. Email: KCabell@Clarku.edu

Renzo Carli. Full Professor of Clinical Psychology. He teaches at the first Faculty of Psychology, Sapienza University of Rome. In 1982, he founded, with M. Bertini and R. Canestrari, the Rivista di Psicologia Clinica. Since 2006, he is Editor of the same journal in its online and bi-linguistic form (Rivista di Psicologia Clinica/Journal of Clinical Psychology), published at: http://www.rivistadipsicologiaclinica.it. He has published about two hundred scientific papers on Italian and foreign journals and twenty-four volumes. He is psychoanalyst, affiliated to the Italian Psychoanalytical Society and of the International Psychoanalitical Association. He developed the theoretical construct of collusion as an extension of psychoanalytic theory to social interaction based on experimentation in this area. He has proposed instruments in detecting the collusion into cultural processes that characterize the social organisations and cultures: Indicators of Organisational Development and Emotional Analysis of Text. He is the President of the "Studio di Psicosociologia" (SPS) in Rome. He directs the 4-year school of psychoanalytic psychotherapy, organised by Studio di Psicosociologia (SPS) in Rome and recognised by the MIUR (Italian Ministery for University and Research). Email: renzo.carli@uniroma1.it.

Nicolas Favez. Associate Professor at the University of Geneva since Fall 2007, where he teaches family clinical psychology, and he is the head of the Research Unit of the Centre for Family Studies in the Institute for Psychotherapy of Lausanne. He served for 8 years as a research and teaching assistant at the University of Geneva with Professor D. N. Stern (1991–1997). He worked then as an Educational Psychologist, doing home interventions in high-risk families with infants and toddlers (1996–2004). He was Associate Professor at the University of Lausanne (2005–2007). Professional address: FPSE, Uni Mail, 40 Boulevard du Pont-d'Arve, CH-1211 Geneva 4. Email: nicolas.favez@unige.ch.

Maria Francesca Freda. Associated Professor in Clinical Psychology at the Faculty of Philosophy and Literature of Naples' University "Federico II." She is president of the Master Degree Course in Dynamic, Clinical and Community Psychology. She works on the psychosocial intervention in institutions, with particular attention towards educational and health institutions. Many of her studies are on narrative as a methodology for the elaboration of experience's meaning. Her current interests concern the study of narratives as a device of the psychological clinical intervention, area of study in which she published *Narrazione e Intervento in Psicologia Clinica [Narration and Intervention in Clinical Psychology*] (Liguori, Napoli, 2009). Email: mariafrancesca.freda@unina.it.

Fiammetta Giovagnoli. Psychologist, psychotherapist and specialist in clinical psychology. She works as teacher at the first Faculty of Psychology, Sapienza University of Rome and at the four-years school of psychoanalytic psychotherapy organised by "Studio di Psicosociologia" (SPS) in Rome. She is engaged in research and intervention on the cultural processes of organisational contexts. She is a member of the editorial board of the Journal of Clinical Psychology http://www.rivistadipsicologiaclinica.it. Email: fiammetta.giovagnoli@uniroma1.it.

Massimo Grasso. Clinical psychologist and psychotherapist. Full Professor of Clinical Psychology at the Faculty of Psychology, University of Rome "La Sapienza." Training and supervising psychotherapist at many psychoanalytic psychotherapy institutes and at the National Mental Health Service. Co-editor of the on-line journal Rivista di Psicologia Clinica/Journal of Clinical Psychology. His clinical and research interests are mainly directed to the study of methodological and theoretical problems in clinical psychology and psychotherapy. On these issues, he has published over 180 scientific papers and many books. Email: massimo.grasso@uniroma1.it.

Sergio Salvatore. Full Professor of Dynamic Psychology at the University of Salento (Lecce, Italy). His scientific interests are mainly based on the